OSTEOPOROSIS: DIAGNOSIS AND MANAGEMENT

Edited by

PIERRE J MEUNIER, MD
Department of Rheumatology
and Bone Diseases
Pavillon F, Edouard Herriot Hospital,
69437 Lyon Cedex 3, France

MARTIN DUNITZ

© Martin Dunitz Ltd 1998

First published in the UK in 1998 by
Martin Dunitz Ltd
The Livery House
7-9 Pratt Street
London NW1 0AE

A CIP catalogue record for this book is available from the British Library.

ISBN 1–85317–412–2

Composition by Wearset, Boldon, Tyne and Wear
Printed and bound in Great Britain, by
Biddles Ltd, Guildford and King's Lynn

Contents

Contributors

Patrick Ammann MD
Division of Bone Diseases
Department of Internal Medicine
University Hospital
1211 Geneve 14
Switzerland

Nigel Arden MSc MRCP
MRC Environmental Epidemiology Unit
Southampton General Hospital
Tremona Road
Southampton SO16 6YD
UK

Jean-Philippe Bonjour MD
Division of Bone Diseases
Department of Internal Medicine
University Hospital
1211 Geneve 14
Switzerland

Marie-Claire Chapuy PhD
INSERM Unite 403, Pavillon F
Hôpital Edouard Herriot
Place d'Arsonval,
69437 Lyon Cedex 03
France

Cyrus Cooper DM MRCP
MRC Environmental Epidemiology Unit
Southampton General Hospital
Tremona Road
Southampton SO16 6YD
UK

Pierre D Delmas MD PhD
INSERM Unite 403, Pavillon F
Hôpital Edouard Herriot
Place d'Arsonval,
69437 Lyon Cedex 03
France

Richard Eastell MD FRCP
Department of Human Metabolism
and Clinical Biochemistry
The University of Sheffield
Clinical Sciences Centre
Northern General Hospital
Herries Road
Sheffield S5 7AU
UK

Genevieve Fraikin PhD
Unité d'Exploration du Metabolisme Osseux
CHU Brull
45 quai Godefroid Kurth
4020 Liège
Belgium

Harry K Genant MD
Musculoskeletal Radiology
University of California
505 Parnassus Avenue
Suite M392, Box 0628
San Francisco, CA- 94143-0628
USA

Patrick Garnero PhD
INSERM Unite 403, Pavillon F
Hôpital Edouard Herriot
Place d'Arsonval,
69437 Lyon Cedex 03
France

Carlo Gennari MD
Istituto di Patologia Speciale Medica
Universita' degli Studi di Siena
Nuovo Policlinico 'Le Scotte' Viale Bracci
53100 Siena
Italy

Claus C Glüer PhD
Department of Diagnostic Radiology
Medical Physics Research Group
Christian-Albrechts Universität zu Kiel
Kiel
Germany

Christiane Gosset PhD
Department of Public Health and Epidemiology
CHU Sart-Tilman
Bâtiment B23
4000 Liège
Belgium

Didier Hans PhD
Osteoporosis and Arthritis Research Group
University of California
San Francisco
350 Parnassus Avenue
Suite 908
San Francisco, CA-94117
USA

Robert P Heaney MD
Creighton University
2500 California Plaza
Omaha NE 68178
USA

Michael Jergas MD
Department of Radiology
St. Josef-Hospital
Gudrunstr. 56
D-44791 Bochum
Germany

Olof Johnell MD
Department of Orthopaedics
Malmo Hospital
Malmö
Sweden

Paul Lips MD
Afdeling Endocrinologie
Academisch Ziekenhuis Vrije Universiteit
Portbus 7057
The Netherlands

Pierre J Meunier MD
INSERM Unite 403, Pavillon F
Hôpital Edouard Herriot
Place d'Arsonval,
69437 Lyon Cedex 03
France

Gregory R Mundy MD
Division of Endocrinology and Metabolism
The University Of Texas
Health Science Center at San Antonio
7703 Floyd Curl Drive
San Antonio
Texas 78284-7877
USA

Christopher F Njeh PhD
Medical Physics Department
Queen Elizabeth Hospital
Edgbaston
Birmingham B15 2TH
UK

Ranuccio Nuti MD
Cattedra di Medicina Interna
Universita' degli studi di Siena
Nuovo Policlinico 'Le Scotte' Viale Bracci
53100 Siena
Italy

Jean-Yves L Reginster MD
Unité d'Exploration du Metabolisme Osseux
and Department of Public Health and
Epidemiology, University of Leige
4000 Liège
Belgium

Ian R Reid MD
Faculty of Medicine and Health Science
The University of Auckland
Private Bag 92019
Auckland
New Zealand

Johann D Ringe MD
Med Klinik IV Klinikum Leverkusen
Akadem Lehrkrankenhaus
University of Cologne D–51375 Leverkusen
Germany

René Rizzoli MD
Division of Bone Diseases
Department of Internal Medicine
University Hospital
1211 Geneve 14
Switzerland

Ego Seeman MD
Department of Endocrinology
Austin and Repatriation Medical Centre
University of Melbourne,
Melbourne
Australia

Chris P Spencer MRCOG
Wynn Department of Metabolic Medicine
Imperial College School of Medicine
21 Wellington Road
London NW8 9SQ
UK

John C Stevenson MB FRCP
Wynn Department of Metabolic Medicine
Imperial College School of Medicine
21 Wellington Road
London NW8 9SQ
UK

Preface

It is stating the obvious to say that the continuous increase in life expectancy during the last century has made osteoporosis a major health issue worldwide, having significant medical, social and economic consequences. The lifetime cumulative fracture risk for a 50-year-old Caucasian woman without intervention approaches 40 per cent, and the predictions of the epidemiologists, based upon the projected rapid expansion of the elderly population, are pessimistic. These predictions could lead us to consider fragility fractures as an inevitable price to pay for longer life. This pessimism is unjustified because major advances have been made and are still in progress to identify the risk of fracture before the fracture itself occurs – which represents an irreversible event – and to develop, on a large scale, preventative strategies. The aim of this book is not to cover exhaustively all aspects of osteoporosis from basic science to treatment, but to provide the reader with a concise description of some innovative aspects of osteoporosis research, not covered in classical textbooks. Each of the 17 chapters explains the state-of-the-art in a domain where substantial advances have been achieved in recent years.

Thus, the epidemiology chapter by Arden and Cooper is focused on future projections and genetic epidemiology. The chapter on bone remodelling by Mundy emphasizes the cellular events involved in the remodelling sequence, which are the target for pharmacologic tools used in the prevention of bone loss. Jergas and Genant discuss the current definition of osteoporosis and review the studies demonstrating the association between low bone density and fractures. A substantial chapter by Hans, Glüer and Njeh updates the recent major advances in the growing field of ultrasonic evaluation of osteoporosis and describes the

many quantitative ultrasonic systems available. Garnero and Delmas discuss in detail the clinical usefulness of biochemical markers of bone remodelling for prognostic assessment and monitoring of the treatment of osteoporotic patients. Distal forearm and humerus fractures, which clinically reveal osteoporosis in many patients and are predictors of later osteoporotic fractures, are covered for the first time in full by Johnell. Hormonal replacement therapy for the prevention and treatment of osteoporosis, estrogens and the new selective estrogen receptor modulators (SERM) are reviewed by Spencer and Stevenson. In the chapter on bisphosphonates for the treatment of osteoporosis, Reginster, Gosset and Fraikin discuss the recent studies on aminobisphosphonates and cyclical bisphonates. The controversial issue of fluoride salts for the treatment of osteoporosis is approached in the chapter on stimulators of bone formation by Ringe, where other bone-forming agents such as parathyroid hormone, strontium or IGF–1 are also discussed.

The important role of calcium and vitamin D supplements for treatment of osteoporosis is emphasized in the chapter by Gennari and Nuti, who also discuss the past and future of calcitonin and anabolic steroids. Calcium and vitamin D are discussed again in the chapter by Heaney, but are seen from the nutritional angle. He also details the role of exercise among the non-pharmacologic tools of prevention. Eastell describes his personal approach to the practical management of the patient with osteoporotic vertebral fracture, and his pragmatic views will be very helpful for the prescriber. Pathophysiology and prevention of hip fractures in elderly people are covered by Chapuy and myself because of the importance of these fractures as a source of morbidity and mortality in the elderly population. Positive results of calcium–vitamin D supplements for preventing hip fractures in very elderly women suggest that it is never too late to prevent such fractures.

Osteoporosis in men, which is a growing public health problem, has been extensively covered by Seeman, who stresses the current absence of any randomized controlled trial using spine or hip fracture rates as end points in men. The pathogenesis and management of glucocorticoid–induced osteoporosis, which is the most important form of secondary osteoporosis, are thoroughly described by Reid. Quality of life assessment is an important part of the evaluation of new therapies of osteoporosis, and specific indices and questionnaires are now available for epidemiology or clinical trials, as described by Lips. The last chapter by Ammann, Rizzoli and Bonjour details the preclinical evaluation of new therapeutic agents for osteoporosis which have a crucial role in the development of new preventative and curative antiosteoporotic therapies.

All these chapters have been written by international experts in their respective areas, and I am very grateful that they were willing to take time from their heavy commitments to make these contributions. Their kind and effective cooperation also represents a sign of friendship, and I have been touched by their response.

As this book goes to press, I hope it will be successful in both educating and stimulating its readers. Much progress has been made, but there is still a long way to go before we will eradicate all fragility fractures.

Pierre J Meunier

1

Present and future of osteoporosis: epidemiology

N Arden and C Cooper

CONTENTS • **Limitations of WHO criteria** • **The size of the problem** • **Site-specific fracture epidemiology** • **Economic costs** • **Future projections** • **Genetic epidemiology** • **The influence of early environment**

Osteoporosis is defined as a 'disease characterised by low bone mass and microarchitectural deterioration of bone tissue, leading to enhanced bone fragility and a consequent increase in fracture risk'.[1] The term 'osteoporosis' was first coined in the nineteenth century in France and Germany as a histological description of aged human bone, emphasizing its apparent porosity. The diagnosis has evolved through phases of criteria based on histologically measured bone volume, physically measured bone mass and the occurrence of fractures. The main advantage in a fracture-based diagnosis (with the possible exception of vertebral fracture) is that this is a discrete event which can be diagnosed using a simple algorithm. The main disadvantage is that diagnosis is unacceptably delayed in a disease where prevention, at present, is the best form of treatment.

Recent advances in bone densitometry have provided the means to measure bone mineral density (BMD) accurately, reproducibly and with minimal radiation exposure. Prospective studies indicate that the risk of osteoporotic fracture increases continuously as BMD declines with a one and a half- to a three-fold increase risk of fracture for each standard deviation fall in BMD.[2] There does not seem to be a threshold value for BMD above which the fracture risk is stable, and the risk gradient for this relationship is as steep as that between blood pressure and stroke. The main advantage of a density-based diagnosis is that it will allow early diagnosis and therefore early initiation of preventive strategies.

The WHO has recently proposed that both low BMD and fracture be combined in a stratified definition of osteoporosis[3] (Figure 1.1). There are four categories:

1. Normal: BMD not more than 1 standard deviation below the young adult mean.
2. Osteopenic: BMD between 1 and 2.5 standard deviations below the young adult mean.
3. Osteoporosis: BMD more than 2.5 standard deviations below the young adult mean.
4. Established (or severe) osteoporosis: BMD more than 2.5 standard deviations below the young adult mean in the presence of one or more fragility fractures.

Using this 2.5 standard deviation cut-off it is estimated that 30% of postmenopausal Caucasian women have osteoporosis at the hip, spine or forearm,[4] which is similar to the lifetime risk of fracture for a 50-year-old woman at one of these three sites.[5]

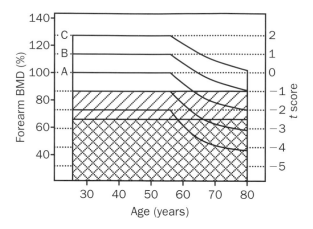

Figure 1.1 Bone mineral content at the distal forearm in women expressed as a percentage of young healthy adults. The solid lines denote the mean values with age (category A) ± 2 s.d. (categories B and C). The hatched area denotes women with osteopenia and the cross-hatched area women with osteoporosis. (Reproduced with permission from Kanis et al.[4])

LIMITATIONS OF WHO CRITERIA

Bone mineral density is a normally distributed variable in the population and there is a significant overlap between BMD in normal and fracture populations, so that, in cases of vertebral fracture, a lumbar spine BMD that is 2 standard deviations below the young adult mean has a sensitivity and specificity for fracture of only around 60%.[6] Furthermore, a woman of 50 with a radial BMD that is equal to the young adult mean has a 15% lifetime risk of hip fracture compared with a 25% lifetime risk for a 50-year-old woman with a radial BMD that is 2.5 standard deviations below the young adult mean.[7] This poor discrimination reflects the multifactorial pathogenesis of osteoporotic fractures, which includes aspects of bone microarchitecture and trauma not measured by simple densitometry. These criteria are therefore useful in population-based measurements but less useful in an individual patient for diagnostic and therapeutic decision-making.

Most of the large population-based databases used to define normal ranges on modern dual energy X-ray absorptiometry (DXA) machines consist of white women. Ideally, separate reference ranges should be developed for men, children before skeletal maturity and different racial groups. For men, whose risk of fracture is lower than that of women, it may be possible to use stricter criteria based on female reference ranges, for example, using 3–4 standard deviations below normal as the criterion for osteoporosis.[4] This works well in most Western societies, but would not be applicable for populations where men have a similar risk of fracture to women, such as the Maoris of New Zealand.[8] Asian women have a much lower BMD than white women and therefore must have a separate reference range; however, despite the lower BMD, they also have a lower rate of hip fracture than white women which also warrants separate differential criteria.[9] The rates of hip and vertebral fractures vary by up to 13-fold between racially similar populations within the same continent[10,11] and therefore, ideally, population-specific reference ranges are needed. More data are required to decide the level (continent, country, region) at which specific reference ranges are appropriate.

Likewise, there are systematic differences in bone density measurements obtained using different equipment, and again it is important to consider this in comparing data from various populations.

THE SIZE OF THE PROBLEM

Using the WHO criteria, it has been estimated that most American women under the age of 50 have normal BMDs and osteoporosis is rare (Figure 1.2). With advancing age, an increasing number of women have osteoporosis, so that by the age of 80 years 27% are osteopenic and 70% are osteoporotic at the hip, lumbar spine or forearm. Sixty per cent of the osteoporotic group will already have experienced one or more osteoporotic fractures. Table 1.1 shows

Table 1.1 Proportion (%) of Rochester, Minnesota, women with BMD more than 2.5 standard deviations below the mean for young normal women

Age group (years)	Lumbar spine (%)	Either hip site (%)	Midradius (%)	Spine, hip or midradius (%)
50–59	7.6	3.9	3.7	14.8
60–69	11.8	8.0	11.8	21.6
70–79	25.0	24.5	23.1	38.5
≥80	32.0	47.5	50.0	70.0
Total	16.5	16.2	17.4	30.3

Reproduced with permission from Melton.[12]

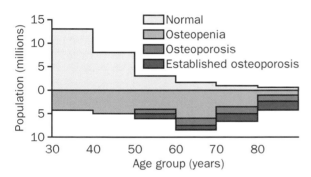

Figure 1.2 Estimated skeletal status of white American women using the WHO criteria. Osteopenia and osteoporosis are defined as WHO criteria at hip, spine or distal forearm. (Reproduced with permission from Melton.[5])

the site specificity of these data. It is estimated that, in the USA, 16.8 million (54%) of post-menopausal white women are osteopenic and a further 9.4 million (30%) are osteoporotic.[12]

Alternatively, we can examine the prevalence and incidence of osteoporotic fractures but unfortunately there are few data available. The prevalence of vertebral fractures varies depend-ing on the definition of fracture used, but is estimated at between 10% and 25% in women aged 50 and over.[10,13] There were an estimated 1.66 million hip fractures occurring worldwide in the over-35s in 1990, with about 50% occur-ring in Europe and North America.[14]

Another approach is to assess the fracture burden. Using Monte Carlo simulations in a Markov model on a hypothetical cohort of 10 000 men and women aged 50 years at base-line, it has been possible to estimate the lifetime risk of fracture, given the known fracture inci-dence rates from the USA. The estimated life-time risk of sustaining an osteoporotic fracture is 39.7% for women and 13.1% for men. The risk for a symptomatic vertebral fracture is 15.6% for women and 5% for men. The risks for hip fracture are 17.5% and 6.0% and, for distal fore-arm fracture, 16.0% and 2.5% for women and men respectively.[5] The comparable figures for British men and women are 15–25% lower.

SITE-SPECIFIC FRACTURE EPIDEMIOLOGY

Appendicular fractures exhibit a bimodal distri-bution with an initial peak at age 10–20 years, which is generally attributed to traumatic frac-tures. The second peak in people aged over 50

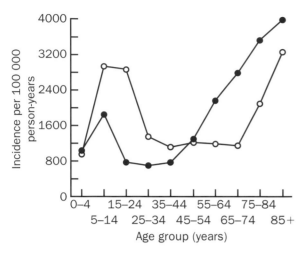

Figure 1.3 Age- and sex-specific incidence of limb fractures: ○, men; ●, women. (Reproduced with permission from Garraway et al.[15])

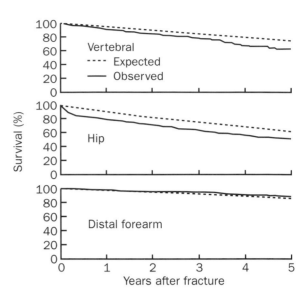

Figure 1.4 Five-year survival after the diagnosis of fracture. (Reproduced with permission from Cooper et al.[16])

years corresponds with osteoporotic fractures associated with only moderate trauma[15] (Figure 1.3).

Hip fracture

Hip fracture is the most serious complication of osteoporosis and is associated with considerable morbidity and mortality (Figure 1.4). The 5-year survival rate after hip fracture is 82% of that expected, with most of the excess deaths occurring in the first 6 months.[16] The incidence of hip fracture increases exponentially with age in both sexes (Figure 1.5) with rates of 2 per 100 000 person-years among women aged less than 35 years to 3032 per 100 000 person-years in women aged 85 years or older; in men the rates are 4 and 1909 respectively.[17] Ninety per cent of fractures occur in those aged over 50 years and 52% in those aged over 80 years.[11,17] The increased incidence results from a combination of declining BMD and an increased incidence of falls with advancing age.[18]

Although 90% of hip fractures are a consequence of falls from standing height or less,[19] only 1% of falls lead to a fracture. Falls that result in a hip fracture tend to occur on a hard surface, with the patient falling straight down or sideways, landing directly on the hip without the fall being broken by protective responses.[20] Fifty per cent of these falls are the result of slipping or tripping, 20% of syncope, 20–30% of loss of balance and the rest of miscellaneous factors.[21]

In most Western populations, the incidence of hip fracture is about twice as high in women as in men. As there are more elderly women than men, however, about 80% of all hip fractures occur in women.[14] There are several populations, including the Maoris in New Zealand[8] and the Bantus in South Africa,[22] in which the incidence in men is equal to or greater than that in women. The explanation for this is unknown but neither population exhibits the dramatic rise in incidence with age seen in the West. There is a marked racial variation in incidence with fracture rates being lower in Black and Asian people.[23] In Blacks, this may result from

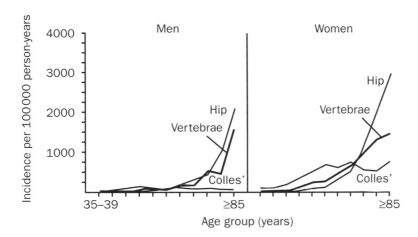

Figure 1.5 Age-specific incidence rates for hip, vertebral and distal forearm fractures in men and women. (Reproduced with permission from Cooper and Melton.[17])

an increased peak BMD, lower rates of bone loss and a lower risk of falls. Asians, however, have lower BMD than Whites, but still have lower fracture rates;[9] this may be explained partly by shorter stature and altered hip geometry.[24]

There is also marked variation in fracture incidence between countries, with higher rates in Scandinavia than in comparable populations in western Europe and Oceania.[23] One study reports a 13-fold difference in age-standardized risk within southern Europe[11] with a north–south gradient, and another with a similar variation within the USA.[26] In the USA, the age-adjusted rate in white women increases with decreasing latitude, socioeconomic deprivation, decreased January sunlight, decreasing water hardness, the proportion of the population drinking fluoridated water and the percentage of land in agricultural use. Regional variations did not correspond with obesity, cigarette smoking, alcohol consumption or Scandinavian heritage[26] (Figure 1.6).

Fractures occur more frequently during the winter months in temperate climates in both the northern and southern hemispheres. As most fractures occur indoors, this cannot be explained entirely by an increase in outdoor falls during icy winter weather conditions. Alternative explanations include decreased neuromuscular coordination and vitamin D deficiency in the winter months.[26]

Vertebral fracture

Compared with hip fractures the epidemiology of vertebral fractures is less well characterized. The predominant reasons for this are the lack of a universally accepted diagnostic criterion and the high proportion of asymptomatic vertebral fractures. Early definitions of fracture relied on subjective assessment of wedge, crush and biconcave deformities, a technique with poor reproducibility. More recently, the development of definitions based on vertebral morphometry with fixed cut-off values, which have increased specificity,[27] have permitted more reliable work in the field. Less than a third of vertebral deformities present to medical practitioners[28] and only 2–8% necessitate hospital admission. The association between pain and morphometric deformity is stronger when using more stringent criteria for diagnosis (a reduction in ratio of 4 standard deviations or s.d.), with 80% of these cases seeking medical attention.[28] Severe vertebral deformities have a predilection for the thoracolumbar junction, T10–L1, whereas mild deformities are more evenly distributed throughout the thoracolum-

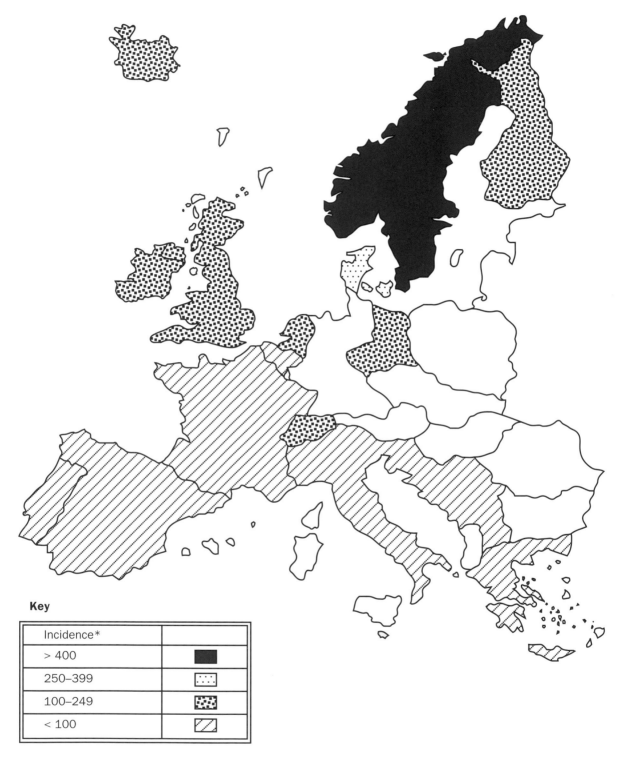

Key

Incidence*	
> 400	■
250–399	▦
100–249	▨
< 100	▧

* Crude rate/100000 of the population aged 50 years or over.

Figure 1.6 European incidence of hip fracture in women.

bar spine. Over 90% of fractures in women occur as the result of mild or moderate trauma; however, this proportion is only 55% in men.[29] Vertebral fractures are associated with a similar increased mortality at 5 years as hip fractures. However, the increase in mortality is gradual over this period, compared with hip fracture.

The incidence of clinical vertebral fractures increases with age in both sexes (see Figure 1.5): men exhibit an exponential increase similar to that seen with the hip, whereas women exhibit a more gradual increase.[28,29] The incidence of radiological fractures in American white women has been estimated at 18 per 1000 person-years, which is almost three times as great as the hip fracture rate.[29] The age-adjusted prevalence of radiological fractures has been estimated at between 8% and 25% in women over 50 years, depending on the definition used.[10,13,29] Prospective studies of clinical fractures suggest a female excess with a ratio of 2 : 1; however, the ratio narrows with age reaching parity over 80 years of age.[30] More recently, a large prevalence study of 15 570 European men and women has suggested an equal sex incidence.[10] In this study there is a geographical variation in prevalence with higher rates in Scandinavia, although there is only a threefold variation between European countries compared with an elevenfold variation in hip fracture rates.

Wrist fracture

Distal forearm fractures, most of which are of the Colles type, display a different pattern of incidence compared with that of hip or vertebral fractures. There is a greater female predominance than in other osteoporotic fractures, with an age-adjusted women : men ratio of 4 : 1, with 85% of fractures occurring in women.[31] The incidence in men is relatively constant between 20 and 80 years of age, in contrast to women where there is a linear increase in incidence up to 60 years of age, after which the incidence plateaus (see Figure 1.5). The reason for the plateau in women may relate to the cessation of the rapid trabecular bone loss that

occurs after the menopause or by the different types of fall with advancing age. A Colles' fracture results from a fall onto the outstretched hand:[20] with advancing years women walk more slowly, and tend to fall sideways or straight down onto the hip, often failing to break the fall with the hand as a result of the loss of the protective reflexes.

There is a geographical variation in the incidence of distal forearm fracture which is of similar magnitude, generally paralleling that of hip fractures. However, as only 20% of cases with distal forearm fractures are hospitalized, this variation may be partially explained by methodological problems of differential case ascertainment.[32] Distal forearm fractures exhibit a greater winter rise in incidence than hip and vertebral fractures (Figure 1.7). A greater proportion of falls leading to distal forearm fracture occur outdoors than for hip fracture,[20] suggesting that a seasonal variation in fall incidence may partially explain this seasonal variation in fracture types. Incidence rates increase during periods of freezing weather;[33] however, other factors are involved because less than 10% of fractures result directly from a fall on snow- or ice-covered surfaces.[15]

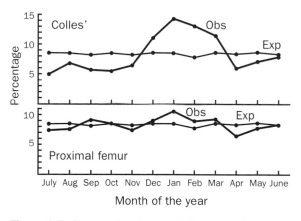

Figure 1.7 Observed and expected seasonal distribution of distal forearm and hip fractures. (Reproduced with permission from Melton LJ III. Epidemiology of fractures. In: *Etiology, Diagnosis and Management*, 2nd edn (Riggs BL, Melton LJ III, eds). Lippincott-Raven.)

Distal forearm fractures are not associated with an increased mortality[16] and were traditionally thought to be free of long-term disability. More recent data suggest that, although less than 1% of patients become dependent as a result of the fractures, only 50% report a good functional outcome at 6 months.[34] This results from long-term complications including algodystrophy, neuropathies and post-traumatic arthritis.

Other fractures

Fractures at several other sites, including the proximal humerus, pelvis and proximal tibia, exhibit the features of osteoporotic fractures. There is an excess of these fractures in women, incidence rates increase with advancing age and most result from only mild or moderate trauma. Furthermore, these fractures are associated with low appendicular bone mass with a similar magnitude to hip and vertebral fractures.[35]

ECONOMIC COSTS

The financial costs of osteoporosis are difficult to estimate accurately, because they include acute hospital care, long-term residential care and more indirect costs, including loss of working days and pharmacological preventive strategies. In England and Wales, the cost of osteoporotic fractures in 1990 was estimated at £742 million p.a.[36] In France an estimated 56 000 hip fractures alone cost about FF3.5 billion p.a. In the USA, the total cost of fractures is estimated at US$20 billion p.a. with over US$8 billion attributed to hip fractures.[30] The vast majority of these costs are accounted for by direct costs, including inpatient and outpatient hospital care and nursing home care (Table 1.2). They include an estimated 3.4 million hospital bed days per year, resulting from 253 000 hospitalizations.[30] In England and Wales, hip fracture patients occupy up to 20% of all orthopaedic beds.

Being elderly, hip fracture patients often have concurrent medical conditions and a high risk of developing complications such as pressure sores and pneumonia. Almost one-third of hip fracture patients become dependent after the fracture[37] with up to 19% requiring long-term nursing home care as a result of their fracture.[39] In the USA over 60 000 nursing home admissions annually are attributed to hip fracture, so that 8% of nursing home beds are occupied by hip fracture patients.[39] Non-institutionalized subjects experience 7 million restricted activity days p.a. which equates to 62.5 days per fracture.[39] Indirect costs such as loss of earnings are not a major component of the total costs of hip fracture, because most patients are retired and hence few working days are lost. Distal forearm fractures, which occur at a younger age, may result in a relatively greater loss of earnings.

Table 1.2 Estimated cost of hip fractures by type of cost; 1988

Type of cost	Cost (US$ million)
Direct costs	
Hospital inpatient services	3077
Hospital outpatient services	778
Physician services	403
Other practitioner services	11
Drugs	5
Nursing home care	1565
Pre-payments and administration	339
Non-health sector goods and services	875
Indirect costs	
Morbidity	1415
Mortality[a]	260
Total	8728

[a] Present value of lifetime earnings discounted at 4%.
Modified with permission from Praemer et al.[30]

FUTURE PROJECTIONS

Estimations of future fracture rates are based on projections of the size, age and sex distribution of the world population, and of the age-adjusted incidence rates for fracture. Most estimates assume a constant age-adjusted fracture rate; however, there is convincing evidence that the age-adjusted rates have increased in both sexes in most societies over the last 50 years. More recently, however, the increase appears to have reached a plateau or even partially reversed in some countries. In England and Wales, the age-adjusted incidence rose by 61% between 1968 and 1978, but then stabilized between 1979 and 1985.[40] Similarly the age-adjusted rates in women in Sweden doubled between 1950 and 1987, before declining over the next 4 years.[41] Studies in the USA and Canada have demonstrated increasing age-adjusted rates in men and women over 50 years of age up to 1984.[42] In Rochester, Minnesota, the age-adjusted rates in women increased by more than threefold between 1930 and 1950, but then slowly declined for the next 40 years.[43] The age-adjusted rates in men rose steadily from 1930 to 1980 before starting to decline.

The reason for the initial increase in incidence rates was variously attributed to changes in risk factors for osteoporosis and falling or to the increased rates of oophorectomy.[43] The most likely risk factor to account for these changes is the decline in levels of physical activity associated with increasing urbanization and mechanization with time. A second possible explanation is that the elderly population is becoming increasingly frail; this hypothesis is supported by data showing that the increased incidence in Rochester was mainly accounted for by the oldest age groups (Figure 1.8).[43] The explanation for the reversal of this trend is less clear because no specific population-based strategies have been employed; however, the increasing availability of medical care may be important. Alternatively, the initial increase in incidence may have resulted from a cohort effect adversely influencing bone mass or the risk of falling.

Assuming a constant age-specific rate of fractures, the total number of fractures and hence the cost to society will increase over the next 50 years as a result of an increase in the elderly population. In the USA, the number of people aged 65 and over is predicted to rise from 32 million to 69 million between 1990 and 2050,

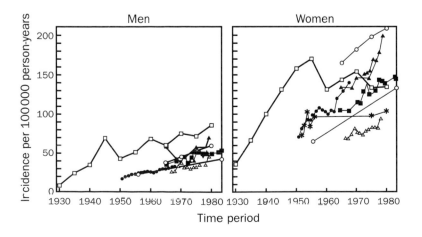

Figure 1.8 Incidence of hip fractures over time as reported from various studies. □, Rochester, MN; ■, USA; ◇, Oxford; ◆, Frenen county, Denmark; △, the Netherlands; ▲, Göteborg, Sweden; ○, Uppsala, Sweden; ●, New Zealand; *, Dundee. (Reproduced with permission from Melton et al.[43])

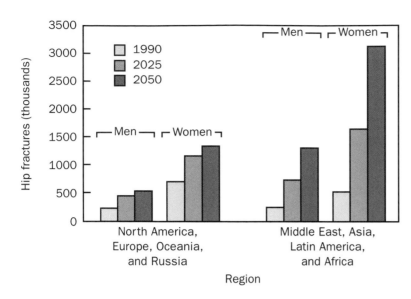

Figure 1.9 Estimated number of hip fractures (in thousands) for men and women in different regions of the world in 1990, 2025 and 2050. (Modified from Cooper et al.[14])

and the over 85s from 3 to 15 million.[14] This could lead to a threefold increase in the number of hip fractures in the USA by 2040. In the UK, hip fractures are projected to increase from 46 000 in 1985 to 60 000 in 2016[44] and from 10 150 to 18 550 from 1986 to 2011 in Australia.[45] At present about 50% of all hip fractures in the elderly population occur in Europe and North America[14] where the populations of over 65s are set to double in the next 50 years. The number of over 65s worldwide is, however, predicted to increase almost fivefold from 323 million to 1555 million by 2050 (Figure 1.9). This is explained by the projected rapid expansion of the elderly populations of Latin America and Asia, which could increase the estimated number of hip fractures worldwide from 1.66 million in 1990 to 6.26 million in 2050, with only 25% occurring in Europe and North America.

GENETIC EPIDEMIOLOGY

One of the first references to a possible genetic component to osteoporosis came from the Greek philosopher Herodotus in 430 BC. On walking through the battlefield of Pelusium some 40 years after the battle, he noted that 'if you strike the Persian skulls, even with a pebble, they are so weak that you break them; but the Egyptian skulls are so strong that you may smite them with a stone and you will scarcely break them in'.[46] Additional support for a genetic component is provided by studies demonstrating that a family history of a fracture is an independent predictor of fracture at that site with relative risks of 1.5–3.[47]

Over the last three decades, numerous family and twin studies have been performed to quantify the heritability or genetic component of a trait. Heritability is defined as the proportion of population variance of a trait explained by genetic factors. Most family studies have examined the parent–offspring and sibling–sibling correlations in BMD, giving correlation coefficients of 0.28–0.59.[48,49] This suggests, but does not quantify, a major genetic component. Several authors have proceeded to produce a heritability estimate from family studies with estimates of 0.51–0.58 at the radius and 0.70 for

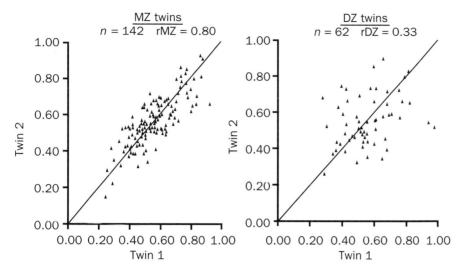

Figure 1.10 Scatterplot of lumbar spine bone mineral density in monozygotic and dizygotic postmenopausal twins, rMZ and rDZ are the intraclass correlation coefficients for monozygotic and dizygotic twins.

the femoral neck.[48–50] Unfortunately, family studies cannot separate familial co-variance resulting from genetic factors from that caused by shared environment, which may over-estimate the extent of heritability.

Twin studies

The classic twin study, which compares the co-variance of monozygotic (MZ) and dizygotic (DZ) twins, tends to reduce the bias introduced by shared environment between family members. Numerous twin studies have now been performed which have consistently demonstrated a major genetic component to peak bone mass at all sites measured, in both women and men, with heritability estimates of up to 0.92[51,52] (Figure 1.10). Anatomical sites with a high trabecular bone content consistently appear to have a greater genetic component than those sites composed predominantly of cortical bone. Postmenopausal BMD also appears to be under strong genetic control with heritabilities of up to 0.87.[53,54] There are no published data on the genetic component of postmenopausal bone loss; however, bone loss at the midradius in

men is almost entirely environmentally determined (heritability 0.02),[55] and change in BMD in a small study of predominantly pre-menopausal women demonstrated a heritability of 0.76 for lumbar spine and 0.20 for femoral neck.[56] Although requiring larger studies, this would suggest a greater genetic component to bone loss in trabecular bone compared with cortical bone.

Twin studies have also demonstrated a genetic component to biochemical markers of bone turnover in postmenopausal women, with heritability estimates of 0.38–0.98 for markers of bone formation and 0.36–0.86 for markers of bone resorption.[57] Hip axis length and quantitative ultrasonography of the calcaneus, both independent predictors of hip fracture, have a major genetic component with heritability estimates of 0.53–0.62.[54]

The vitamin D receptor gene

Interest has recently focused on the vitamin D receptor gene since the publication of a twin study suggesting that polymorphisms at this locus explained 75% of the genetic variance of

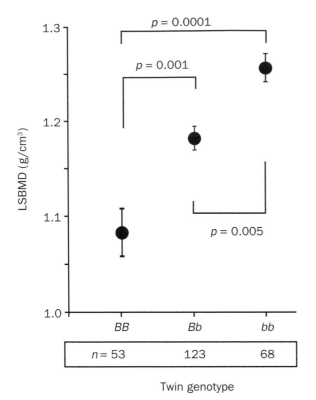

Figure 1.11 Lumbar spine BMD in dizygous twins according to vitamin D receptor genotype. (Reproduced with permission from Morrison et al.[58])

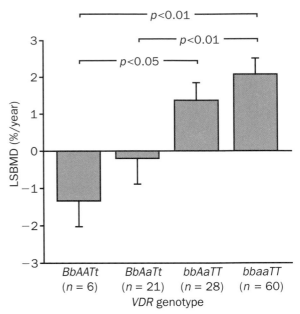

Figure 1.12 Rate of change of lumbar spine BMD (LSBMD) during 1α-hydroxyvitamin D therapy according to vitamin D receptor genotype. (Modified from Tokita et al.[65])

BMD[58] (Figure 1.11). There have now been numerous studies examining the association of the vitamin D receptor gene and BMD with conflicting results. Several twin and population-based studies have confirmed an association, but these explain considerably less than 75% of the genetic variance previously reported.[59,60] Other studies have failed to find any association[61,62] and, more interestingly, two studies have found a statistically significant association between vitamin D receptor gene (VDR) polymorphisms and BMD in the opposite direction to the original studies.[63]

There are several potential explanations for these discrepancies. First, many of the negative studies were small and underpowered. Second, there may be important environmental–genetic interactions obscuring the association in some of the negative studies. The VDR polymorphisms can modify the therapeutic response to both calcium[64] and vitamin D[65] (Figure 1.12). As the policies of dietary supplementation of calcium and vitamin vary around the world, this may explain some of the discrepant results. Finally, the polymorphisms of the VDR gene, to which no functional significance has yet been attached, may be in linkage disequilibrium with a novel osteoporosis susceptibility locus mapping nearby on chromosome 12. As recombination between the VDR gene and the putative osteoporosis gene may occur at each meioisis, linkage disequilibrium may vary between populations.

Other genes

Several other candidate genes are under investigation at present, some of which look promising from early data but all of which need confirmation in larger studies. Polymorphisms at the Sp1 binding motif of the gene for α1 chain of type I collagen are over-represented in patients with osteoporotic fracture and are associated with a low BMD at the lumbar spine.[66] Polymorphisms of the oestrogen receptor gene are associated with lumbar spine and total body BMD in a population of postmenopausal Japanese women;[67] however, provisional reports in British women demonstrate no association.

THE INFLUENCE OF EARLY ENVIRONMENT

Although the genotype possessed by any individual is an established determinant of the peak bone mass attained during growth, and may also contribute to determining the subsequent loss of bone, environmental factors clearly interact with the genome. The conventional means of studying such gene–environment interactions rests upon investigation of current lifestyle (for example, diet, exercise, cigarette smoking and alcohol consumption) among individuals whose genotype and BMD have been measured. However, the growth trajectory of the skeleton appears to be established during the first 2–3 years of life,[68] and it might be that environmental influences have a more profound influence on gene expression during critical periods of early life than several decades later.

Recent retrospective cohort studies have suggested that weight in infancy is a significant predictor of skeletal size and mineral content in the lumbar spine and femoral neck of women during adulthood.[69,70] These relationships are most pronounced during young adulthood (say, around the age of 21 years), but are also observed in late adulthood (during the seventh decade of life). The mechanism underlying these associations is believed to be the programming of a range of metabolic and endocrine systems. 'Programming' is the term used for persisting changes in structure and function caused by environmental stimuli during critical periods of early development.[71] One of the best examples of this phenomenon is the life-long effect of early exposure to sex hormones on sexual physiology. A female rat injected with testosterone propionate on the fifth day after birth develops normally until puberty, but fails to ovulate or show normal patterns of female sexual behaviour thereafter.[72] Pituitary and ovarian function are normal, but the release of gonadotrophin by the hypothalamus has been irreversibly altered from the cyclical female pattern of release to the tonic male pattern. If the same injection is given at 20 days of age, it has no effect. Thus, there is a critical time at which the animal's sexual physiology is sensitive and can be permanently changed. Other animal experiments have shown that, when the protein or energy intake of the mother during pregnancy and lactation is lowered, the offspring are smaller than they would otherwise have been.[73]

In general, the earlier in life that undernutrition occurs, the more likely it is to have permanent effects on body weight and length. The precise timing and mechanism of skeletal programming are unknown. Symmetrical, but slow, postnatal growth is a characteristic of fetal adversity during the third trimester. There are several means whereby such adversity could compromise the skeleton. These include interaction with gene expression of various endocrine systems (for example, the growth hormone/insulin-like growth factor I (IGF-1) axis, the hypothalamic/pituitary/gonadal axis or the parathyroid/vitamin D axis). In the epidemiological studies, a stronger relationship between weight in infancy and adult height is observed among men than among women, although the findings with regard to bone mineral content are more marked among women than men. This discrepancy might be explained by the differential effects of gonadal steroids and the growth hormone/IGF-I axis on skeletal growth. Further evidence for the programming of gonadal function in women comes from the observation that birthweight is a significant predictor of menarchal age after accounting for the effects of childhood body build.[74]

Further exploration of the genetic and early environmental programming of skeletal growth and metabolism may shed light on novel means whereby bone health might be improved.

REFERENCES

1. Consensus Development Conference. Prophylaxis and treatment of osteoporosis. *Am J Med* 1991; **90:** 107–10.
2. Cummings SR, Black DM, Nevitt MC et al, for the Study of Osteoporotic Fractures Research Group. Bone density at various sites for prediction of hip fractures. *Lancet* 1993; **341:** 72–5.
3. World Health Organization. Assessment of Fracture Risk and its Application to Screening for Postmenopausal Osteoporosis. *WHO Technical Report Series.* Geneva: WHO, 1994.
4. Kanis JA, Melton LJ, Christianson C, Johnston CC, Khaltaev N. The diagnosis of osteoporosis. *J Bone Miner Res* 1994; **9:** 1137–41.
5. Melton LJ III, Chrischilles EA, Cooper C, Lane AW, Riggs BL. How many women have osteoporosis? *J Bone Miner Res* 1992; **7:** 1005–10.
6. Overgaard K, Hansen MA, Riis BJ, Christiansen C. Discriminatory ability of bone mass measurements (SPA and DEXA) for fractures in elderly postmenopausal women. *Calcif Tissue Int* 1992; **50:** 30–5.
7. Suman V, Atkinson EJ, O'Fallon WM, Black DM, Melton LJ III. A nomogram for predicting lifetime hip fracture risk from radius bone mineral density and age. *Bone* 1993; **14:** 834–46.
8. Stott S, Gray DH. The incidence of femoral neck fracture in New Zealand. *NZ Med J* 1980; **91:** 6–9.
9. Ross PD, Norimatsu H, Davis JW et al. A comparison of hip fracture incidence among native Japanese, Japanese Americans, and American Caucasians. *Am J Epidemiol* 1991; **133:** 801–9.
10. O'Neill TW, Felsenberg D, Varlow J et al. The prevalence of vertebral deformity in European men and women: The European vertebral osteoporosis study. *J Bone Miner Res* 1996; **11:** 1010–18.
11. Ellfors I, Allander E, Kanis JA et al. The variable incidence of hip fracture in Southern Europe: The MEDOS study. *Osteoporosis Int* 1994; **4:** 253–63.
12. Melton LJ III. How many women have osteoporosis now? *J Bone Miner Res* 1995; **10:** 175–7.
13. Spector TD, McCloskey EV, Doyle DV, Kanis JA. Prevalence of vertebral fracture in women and the relationship with bone density and symptoms: The Chingford study. *J Bone Miner Res* 1993; **7:** 817–22.
14. Cooper C, Campion G, Melton LJ III. Hip fractures in the elderly: A worldwide projection. *Osteoporosis Int* 1992; **2:** 285–9.
15. Garraway WM, Stauffer RN, Kurland LT, O'Fallon WM. Limb fractures in a defined population. I. Frequency and distribution. *Mayo Clin Proc* 1979; **54:** 701–7.
16. Cooper C, Atkinson EJ, Jacobsen SJ, O'Fallon WM, Melton LJ III. Population-based study of survival following osteoporotic fractures. *Am J Epidemiol* 1993; **137:** 1001–5.
17. Cooper C, Melton LJ III. Epidemiology of osteoporosis. *Trends Endocrinol Metab* 1992; **314:** 224–9.
18. Winner SJ, Morgan CA, Evans JG. Perimenopausal risk of falling and incidence of distal forearm fracture. *BMJ* 1989; **289:** 1486–8.
19. Gallagher JC, Melton LJ, Riggs BL, Bergstralh E. Epidemiology of fractures of the proximal femur in Rochester, Minnesota. *Clin Orthop* 1980; **150:** 163–71.
20. Nevitt MC, Cummings SR, and the Study of Osteoporotic Fractures Research Group. Type of fall and risk of hip and wrist fractures: The study of osteoporotic fractures. *J Am Geriatr Soc* 1993; **41:** 1226–34.
21. Clark ANG. Factors in fracture of the female femur: A clinical study of the environment, physical, medical and preventative aspects of this injury. *Geront Clin* 1968; **10:** 257–70.
22. Solomon L. Osteoporosis and fracture of the femoral neck in the South African Bantu. *J Bone Joint Surg [Br]* 1968; **50-B:** 2–13.
23. Melton LJ III. Differing patterns of osteoporosis across the world. In: *New Dimensions in Osteoporosis in the 1990s* (Chesnut CH III, ed.). Asia Pacific Conference Series No. 125. Hong Kong: Excerpta Medica, 1991: 13–18.
24. Nakamura T, Turner CH, Yoshikawa T et al. Do variations in hip geometry explain differences in hip fracture risk between Japanese and white Americans. *J Bone Miner Res* 1994; **9:** 1071–6.

25. Jacobsen SJ, Goldberg J, Miles TP, Brody JA, Stiers W, Rimm AA. Regional variation in the incidence of hip fracture: US white women aged 65 years and older. *JAMA* 1990; **264**: 500–2.

26. Melton LJ III. Epidemiology of age related fractures. In: *The Osteoporotic Syndrome: Detection, Prevention and Treatment* (Avioli LV, ed.). New York: Wiley-Liss, 1993: 17–18.

27. McCloskey EV, Spector TD, Eyres KS et al. The assessment of vertebral deformity. A method for use in population studies and clinical trials. *Osteoporosis Int* 1993; **3**: 138–47.

28. Cooper C, Atkinson EJ, O'Fallon WM, Melton LJ III. The incidence of clinically diagnosed vertebral fractures: A population-based study in Rochester, Minnesota, 1985–1989. *J Bone Miner Res* 1992; **7**: 221–7.

29. Melton LJ III, Lane AW, Cooper C, Eastell R, O'Fallon WM, Riggs BL. Prevalence and incidence of vertebral deformities. *Osteoporosis Int* 1993; **3**: 113–19.

30. Praemer A, Furner S, Rice DP. *Musculoskeletal Conditions in the United States.* Rosemont, IL: American Academy of Orthopaedic Surgeons, 1992, 145–70.

31. Owen RA, Melton LJ III, Johnson KA, Ilstrup DM, Riggs BL. Incidence of Colles' fracture in a North American community. *Am J Public Health* 1982; **72**: 605–7.

32. Garraway WM, Stauffer RN, Kurland LT, O'Fallon WM. Limb fractures in a defined population. II. Orthopedic treatment and utilisation of health care. *Mayo Clin Proc* 1979; **54**: 708–13.

33. Miller SWM, Evans JG. Fractures of the distal forearm in Newcastle: an epidemiological survey. *Age Ageing* 1985; **14**: 155–8.

34. Kaukonen JP, Karaharju EO, Porras M, Lüthje P, Jakobsson A. Functional recovery after fractures of the distal forearm. *Ann Chir Gynaecol* 1988; **77**: 27–31.

35. Seeley DG, Browner WS, Nevitt MC, Genant HK, Scott JC, Cummings SR, for the Study of Osteoporotic Fractures Research Group. Which fractures are associated with low appendicular bone mass in elderly women? *Ann Intern Med* 1991; **115**: 837–42.

36. Department of Health, Advisory Group on Osteoporosis. Department of Health, 1994.

37. Jensen JS, Bagger J. Long-term social prognosis after hip fractures. *Acta Orthop Scand* 1982; **53**: 97–101.

38. Chrischilles EA, Butler CD, Davis CS, Wallace RB. A model of lifetime osteoporosis impact.

Arch Intern Med 1991; **151**: 2026–32.

39. Holbrook TL, Grazier K, Kelsey JL, Stauffer RN. *The Frequency of Occurrence, Impact and Cost of Selected Musculoskeletal Conditions in the United States; RB.* Chicago: American Academy of Orthopedic Surgeons, 1984.

40. Spector TD, Cooper C, Lewis AF. Trends in admissions for hip fracture in England and Wales, 1968–85. *BMJ* 1990; **300**: 1173–4.

41. Gullberg B, Duppe H, Nilsson B et al. Incidence of hip fractures in Malmo, Sweden (1950–1991). *Bone* 1993; **14**: S23–9.

42. Rodrigues JG, Sattin RW, Waxweiler RJ. Incidence of hip fractures, United States, 1970–83. *Am J Prev Med* 1989; **5**: 175–81.

43. Melton LJ III, O'Fallon WM, Riggs BL. Secular trends in the incidence of hip fractures. *Calcif Tissue Int* 1987; **41**: 57–64.

44. Hoffenberg R, James OFW, Brocklehurst JC et al. Fractured neck of femur: Prevention and management. Summary and recommendations of a report of the Royal College of Physicians. *J R Coll Physicians Lond* 1989; **23**: 8–12.

45. Lord SR, Sinnett PF. Femoral neck fractures: Admissions, bed use, outcome and projections. *Med J Aust* 1986; **145**: 493–6.

46. Herodotus, 430 BC. *The Persian Wars.* Book III, Chapter 12.

47. Fox KM, Cummings SR, Threets K. Family history and risk of osteoporotic fracture. *J Bone Miner Res* 1994; **9**(suppl 1): S153

48. Krall EA, Dawson-Hughes B. Heritable and lifestyle determinants of bone mineral density. *J Bone Miner Res* 1993; **8**: 1–9.

49. Tylavski FA, Bortz AD, Hancock RL, Anderson JJB. Familial resemblance of radial bone mass between premenopausal mothers and their college age daughters. *Calcif Tissue Int* 1989; **45**: 265–72.

50. Lutz J. Bone mineral, serum calcium and dietary intakes of mother/daughter pairs. *Am J Clin Nutr* 1986; **44**: 99–106.

51. Pocock N, Eisman J, Hopper JL, Yeates M, Sambrook P, Eberl S. Genetic determinants of bone mass in adults. *J Clin Invest* 1987; **80**: 706–10.

52. Slemenda CW, Christian JC, Williams CJ, Norton JA, Johnston CC Jr. Genetic determination of bone mass in adult women: a re-evaluation of the twin model and the potential importance of gene interaction on heritability estimates. *J Bone Miner Res* 1991; **6**: 561–7.

53. Flicker L, Hopper JL, Rodgers L, Kaymakci B, Green R, Wark JD. Bone density determinants in

elderly women: a twin study. *J Bone Miner Res* 1995; **10:** 1607–13.

54. Arden NK, Baker J, Hogg C, Baan K, Spector TD. The heritability of bone mineral density, ultrasound of the calcaneus and hip axis length: a study of postmenopausal twins. *J Bone Miner Res* 1996; **11:** 530–4.

55. Slemenda CW, Christian JC, Redd T, Reister TK, Williams CJ, Johnston CC Jr. Long term bone loss in men: effects of genetic and environmental factors. *Ann Intern Med* 1992; **117:** 286–91.

56. Kelly PJ, Nguyen T, Hopper J, Pocock N, Sambrook P, Eisman J. Changes in axial bone density with age: A twin study. *J Bone Miner Res* 1993; **8:** 11–17.

57. Garnero P, Arden NK, Griffiths G, Delmas PD, Spector TD. Genetic influence on post-menopausal bone turnover: a twin study. *J Clin Endocrinol Metab* 1996; **81:** 140–6.

58. Morrison NA, Qi JI, Tokita A et al. Prediction of bone density from vitamin D receptor alleles. *Nature* 1994; **367:** 284–7.

59. Spector TD, Keen RW, Arden NK et al. Influence of vitamin D receptor genotype on bone mineral density in postmenopausal women: A twin study in Britain. *BMJ* 1995; **310:** 1357–60.

60. Yagamata Z, Miyamura T, Tijima S et al. Vitamin D receptor gene polymorphism and bone mineral density in healthy Japanese women. *Lancet* 1994; **344:** 1027.

61 Hustmyer FG, Peacock M, Hui S, Johnson CC, Christian JC. Bone mineral density in relation to polymorphisms at the vitamin D receptor locus. *J Clin Invest* 1994; **94:** 2130–4.

62. Garnero P, Borel O, Sornay-Rendu E, Delmas PD. Vitamin D receptor polymorphisms do not predict bone turnover and bone mass in healthy premenopausal women. *J Bone Miner Res* 1995; **10:** 1283–8.

63. Uitterlingen AG, Pols HAP, Burger H et al. A large-scale population-based study of the association of vitamin D receptor gene polymorphisms with bone mineral density. *J Bone Miner Res* 1996; **11:** 1241–8.

64. Krall EA, Parry P, Lichter JB, Dawson-Hughes B. Vitamin D receptor alleles and rates of bone loss: influences of years since menopause and calcium intake. *J Bone Miner Res* 1995; **10:** 978–84.

65. Tokita A, Watanabe T, Miura Y et al. Vitamin D receptor gene RFLP and bone mineral density in Japanese. *Lancet* 1995; **345:** 1238–9.

66. Grant SF, Reid OM, Blake G, Herd R, Fogelman I, Ralston SW. Reduced bone density and osteoporosis associated with a polymorphic Sp1 binding site in the colagen type I alpha 1 gene. *Nature Genet* 1996; **14:** 203–5.

67. Kobayashi S, Satoshi I, Hosoi T et al. Association of bone mineral density with polymorphisms of the estrogen receptor gene. *J Bone Miner Res* 1996; **11:** 306–11.

68. Johnston FE. Somatic growth of the infant and pre-school child. In: *Human Growth: A Comprehensive Treatise*, Vol 2 (Faulkner F, Tanner JM, eds). New York: Plenum Press, 1986: 3–24.

69. Cooper C, Cawley M, Bhalla A et al. Childhood growth, physical activity and peak bone mass in women. *J Bone Miner Res* 1995; **10:** 940–7.

70. Cooper C, Fall C, Egger P, Hobbs R, Eastell R, Barker D. Growth in infancy and bone mass in later life. *Ann Rheum Dis* 1997; **56:** 17–21.

71. Barker DJP. Programming the baby. In: *Mothers, Babies and Disease in Later Life* (Barker DJP, ed.). London: BMJ Publishing Group, 1994: 14–36.

72. Barraclough CA. Production of anovulatory, sterile rats by single injections of testosterone propionate. *Endocrinology* 1961; **68:** 62–7.

73. Widdowson EM, McCance RA. The effect of finite periods of undernutrition at different ages on the composition and subsequent development of the rat. *Proc R Soc Lond [Biol]* 1963; **158:** 329–42.

74. Cooper C, Kuh D, Egger P, Wadsworth M, Barker D. Childhood growth and age at menarche. *Br J Obstet Gynaecol* 1996; **103:** 814–17.

2

Bone remodeling and mechanisms of bone loss in osteoporosis

GR Mundy

Disorders of bone remodeling are among the most common public health problems in the Western World. The most common of the bone diseases is osteoporosis, which affects 25% of the aging female population and 5–10% of the male population. Although we are still ignorant of many of the important cellular and molecular events involved in normal bone remodeling, advances in cell and molecular biology in the last decade have clarified some of the mechanisms responsible for normal physiological bone resorption and bone formation, as well as some of the means by which bone remodeling can become dysfunctional and result in bone loss. In this chapter, a review will be presented of current concepts of bone remodeling in health and in the osteoporotic population.

NATURAL HISTORY OF THE SKELETON

The changes in total body bone mass with age are shown diagrammatically in Figure 2.1. Bone mass reaches a maximum about 10 years after linear growth stops, probably begins to decrease during the fourth decade, and declines to half its maximum value by the age of 80. Peak bone mineral density (bone mass), which is reached in the 30s, is less in women than it is

in men, and less in white people than in black. Women of all ethnic groups show an additional accelerated phase of bone loss, which occurs for about 10 years after the cessation of ovarian function. It has been estimated that a woman can expect to lose 35% of her cortical bone and 50% of her cancellous bone as she ages, and a man can expect to lose about two-thirds of these amounts.[1-3] It has been estimated that about a half the loss in cancellous bone results from the menopause, and about a half from the aging process. It remains controversial precisely

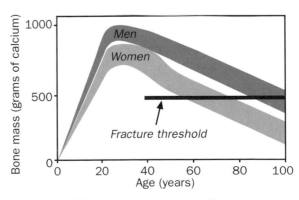

Figure 2.1 Changes in bone mass with age.

when bone mass starts to decline, and whether there is a similar accelerated phase of bone loss in both cancellous and cortical bone after the menopause. Different measuring techniques have given slightly different answers.

The bones of the adult skeleton consist of either cortical (or compact) bone or cancellous (or trabecular) bone. Current evidence indicates that cortical bone and cancellous bone do not change with age in exactly the same way, and for this reason should be considered as two separate functional entities. The differences are most likely to reside in the different environments of the bone cells in cortical or cancellous bone. Bone remodeling cells on cancellous bone surfaces are in intimate contact with the cells of the marrow cavity, which produce a variety of potent osteotropic cytokines. It is possible that the cells in cortical bone, which are more distant from the influences of these cytokines, are influenced more by the systemic osteotropic hormones such as parathyroid hormone and 1,25-dihydroxyvitamin D. Osteoclasts and osteoblasts in cancellous bone may be controlled primarily by factors produced by adjacent bone marrow cells. The proportions of cortical and cancellous bone vary at the different sites in the skeleton where osteoporotic fractures frequently occur. Cancellous bone is relatively prominent in the vertebral column, the most common site of fracture associated with osteoporosis. In the lumbar spine, cancellous bone comprises more than 66% of the total, whereas in the intertrochanteric area of the femur bone is composed of 50% cortical and 50% cancellous. In the neck of the femur, the bone is 75% cortical and 25% cancellous, but in the midradius more than 95% of the bone is cortical.

REMODELING OF CORTICAL AND CANCELLOUS BONE

Cortical bone

Cortical bone is dense or compact bone. It makes up 85% of the total bone in the body, and is relatively most abundant in the long

bone shafts of the appendicular skeleton. The volume of cortical bone is regulated by the formation of periosteal bone, remodeling within haversian systems and endosteal bone resorption. Cortical bone is removed primarily by endosteal resorption and resorption within the haversian canals. The latter leads to increased porosity of cortical bone. However, periosteal bone formation continues to increase the diameter of cortical bone throughout life. Cortical bone loss probably begins during the fifth decade (according to most studies) and there is an acceleration of cortical bone loss that occurs for 5–10 years after the menopause. This accelerated phase of cortical bone loss continues for 15 years and then gradually slows. There is irrefutable evidence that estrogen replacement therapy after the menopause helps preserve cortical bone. In later life, women with osteoporosis lose cortical bone at similar rates to those of premenopausal women. Loss of cortical bone is the major predisposing factor for fractures that occur in the hip and around the wrist. Cortical bone is particularly prone to increased resorption in patients with primary hyperparathyroidism.

Cancellous bone

Although cancellous bone makes up only 15% of the skeleton, the changes that occur in this type of bone after the age of 30 determine whether the most important clinical features of osteoporosis will occur. Depending on the technique used, decline in cancellous bone mass begins in mid-adult life, occurring earlier than the decline in cortical bone mass.[4] However, other studies have disagreed with these findings, and suggested that the decline in cancellous bone mass begins later, after ovarian function ceases.[5] Riggs and Melton[6] suggest that acceleration in cancellous bone loss occurring at the time of the menopause is not as prominent as the accelerated loss of cortical bone mass that occurs at this time. The loss of cancellous bone, which occurs with aging, is not the result simply of a generalized thinning of the bone plates, but rather is the result of complete perforation and fragmentation of some trabeculae.[7,8] As cancellous bone has a broad surface area, resorption may be modulated by focal osteoclastic resorption, in turn regulated by local hormonal factors produced by cells in the bone marrow microenvironment, including marrow cells as well as other types of bone cells.

THE REMODELING OF BONE

All of the diseases of bone occur as a consequence of the effects of the disease process on the cellular events in the normal bone remodeling cycle. Thus, understanding of the control mechanisms responsible for these cellular events is the key to understanding the pathophysiology of age-related bone loss and osteoporosis. The adult skeleton is in a dynamic state, being continually broken down and reformed by the coordinated actions of osteoclasts and osteoblasts on trabecular surfaces and in haversian systems. Current concepts of bone remodeling or turnover are based on the morphologic observations of Frost and colleagues,[9] who observed that bone formation in human adults occurred almost exclusively at sites that had recently undergone osteoclastic resorption. This turnover or remodeling of bone occurs in focal and discrete packets throughout the skeleton. It is now recognized that the remodeling of each packet takes a finite period of time (estimated to be about 3–4 months). The remodeling which occurs in each packet (called a bone remodeling unit by Frost[10]) is geographically and chronologically separated from other packets of remodeling. This suggests that activation of the sequence of cellular events responsible for remodeling is locally controlled, possibly by an autoregulatory mechanism, perhaps by autocrine or paracrine factors generated in the bone microenvironment. The sequence is always the same – osteoclastic bone resorption followed by osteoblastic bone formation to repair the defect. The new bone that is formed is called a bone structural unit (BSU).[10]

Osteoclast activation is the initial step in the remodeling sequence. Osteoclasts are activated in specific focal sites by mechanisms that are still not understood. Osteoclast activation may occur as a result of interactions that take place between integral membrane proteins (integrins) on osteoclast cell membranes and proteins in bone matrix containing RGD (arginine–glycine–asparagine) amino acid sequences (for example, osteopontin). Miyauchi et al[11] have demonstrated such a phenomenon in vitro. Osteoclast activation may also be caused by stimulatory signals produced by local cells in the osteoclast microenvironment such as immune cells, but this does not explain what the trigger for activation of immune cells might be. The resorptive phase of the remodeling process has been estimated to last 10 days. This period is followed by repair of the resorption defect by a team of osteoblasts, which are attracted to the site of the resorption defect and then proceed to make new bone. This part of the process takes about 3 months. The initial events in the formation phase are possibly unidirectional migration (chemotaxis) of osteoblast precursors to the site of the defect, followed by enhanced cell proliferation. The complete sequence of the cellular events that occur at the bone surface during the remodeling process has been described in detail by Baron et al[12] from studies on the alveolar bone of the rat, and by Boyce et al[13] from studies of the calvarial bone of the mouse. The technique of Boyce et al, in particular, lends itself readily to use as a model to study the effects of drugs or factors on the normal bone remodeling sequence. The cellular events that occur in these models are similar to those in adult human bone.

All of the diseases of bone are superimposed on this normal cellular remodeling sequence. In diseases such as primary hyperparathyroidism, hyperthyroidism and Paget's disease, in which osteoclasts are activated, there is a compensatory and (approximately) balanced increase in the formation of new bone. However, there are also a number of well-described conditions in which osteoblast activity does not completely repair the defect left by previous resorption and replace all of the bone removed. The most obvious example is myeloma, usually characterized by punched-out lytic bone lesions with little new bone formation.[14] In myeloma, there appears to be a specific defect in osteoblast maturation.[15] There are probably increased numbers of osteoblasts around the edges of the lytic lesions, but the osteoblasts fail (in the great majority of patients) to synthesize more than thin osteoid seams. In solid tumors associated with malignancy, there is also a failure of bone formation to repair resorptive defects in patients dying from their malignancy.[16] In elderly patients with osteoporosis, there is a decrease in mean wall thickness, presumably reflecting the inability of osteoblasts to repair adequately the resorptive defects made during normal osteoclastic resorption.[17] It should also be stressed that progressive bone loss, beginning at about 35 years of age (depending on the bone), occurs in all humans and is indicative of a 'physiological' imbalance between resorption and formation.

Although bone formation usually occurs on sites of previous osteoclastic resorption in normal adult humans, there are several special situations in which osteoblasts may lay down new bone on surfaces not previously resorbed. Two examples are osteoblastic metastases associated with tumors such as carcinoma of the prostate and breast, and during prolonged exposure to pharmacological doses of fluoride therapy. However, in most physiological and pathological circumstances, the coupling of bone formation to previous bone resorption occurs faithfully. The cellular and humoral mechanisms that are responsible for mediating the coupling process (or disrupting it, as in the diseases described above) are still not clear. Several theories have been proposed to account for coupling. Almost 20 years ago, Rasmussen and Bordier[18] suggested that the osteoclast, once it finishes the resorptive phase of the remodeling sequence, undergoes fission to form mononuclear cells which are the precursors of osteoblasts. It is now widely accepted that osteoclasts and osteoblasts have different origins. Osteoclasts arise from hemopoietic stem cells, or at least stem cells in the marrow environment that have the capacity to circulate. Osteoblasts, in contrast, arise from stromal mesenchymal cells. Many workers have favored the notion that coupling is humorally mediated – an

osteoblast-stimulating factor (such as insulin growth factors I and II, IGF-I IGF-II, or transforming growth factor β, TGFβ) is released during the process of osteoclastic bone resorption and the stimulation of osteoblast activity leads to new bone formation.[19] A variation on this humoral concept is that the factor that stimulates resorption also acts directly (but slowly) on osteoblasts to cause their activation and subsequent new bone formation. Another hypothesis to explain coupling, distinct from those mentioned above, is that, as osteoblasts normally line bone surfaces, once the phase of osteoclastic resorption is over osteoblasts merely reline the bone surface and repair the resorptive defect without the necessity for involvement of a humoral mediator that is specifically generated as a consequence of resorption.

Obviously, understanding this sequence of cellular events may lead to clarification of the mechanism of decreased osteoblast activity that occurs in age-related bone loss, and possibly the pathophysiology of osteoporosis, as well as the specific defects in osteoblast function which occur in malignancies such as myeloma, breast cancer and prostate cancer. Based on observations, made possible in recent years, of the effects of stimulatory factors such as TGFβ on bone in vivo,[20] a hypothesis for how coupling may be mediated is proposed, based on interpretation of the data available. Before this model is described, the events that are likely to be important in both the resorption and formation phases of the remodeling sequence will be reviewed, together with the local osteotropic factors that may be responsible for mediating these events.

Cellular events involved in the resorption phase of the remodeling sequence

Osteoclast activation
The osteoclast is the major and possibly the sole bone-resorbing cell. Other cells that have been thought capable of resorbing bone include osteocytes, monocytes, tumor cells and osteoblasts. However, there is no conclusive evidence that any of these cause significant

bone resorption in vivo. Thus, in considering the bone resorption that occurs during normal bone remodeling, attention is focused on the events that are happening in the osteoclast and its precursors. Osteoclast activity and the capacity of osteoclasts to resorb bone are, however, modulated by other cells in its microenvironment, including other types of bone cells, mesenchymal stromal cells and immune cells such as monocytes and lymphocytes.

The precursors of osteoclasts are hemopoietic mononuclear cells which are resident in the bone marrow.[21] Osteoclast precursors that are mononuclear circulate in the peripheral blood. These cells do not differentiate into osteoclasts unless they are in the bone microenvironment, lying adjacent to endosteal bone surfaces. Identifiable osteoclasts cannot be seen at sites distant from the bone surface. The stem cell for the osteoclast, which is resident in the bone marrow, is a pluripotent stem cell that has the capacity, in response to appropriate stimuli, to differentiate along other lineages including those of the formed elements of the blood. The colony-forming unit for the granulocyte--macrophage series (GM-CFU) lies in the osteoclast lineage. As for other types of cells, the life cycle of the osteoclast involves proliferation and differentiation of pluripotent or uncommitted precursors, but then undergoes a specific series of steps that are unique for this cell. These steps include: fusion to form the multinucleated cell; attachment to bone surfaces which is mediated by integrins on the osteoclast cell membrane; polarization which leads to realignment of intracellular organelles; and the formation of a specialized area of the cell membrane known as the ruffled border, associated with expression of a specific set of genes. This set of genes is required for the resorption process including (1) the vacuolar ATPase proton pump and (2) the *src* proto-oncogene, as well as the expression of proteolytic enzymes required for bone destruction in the resorption pocket under the ruffled border. The final step is apoptosis of the osteoclast and cessation of bone resorption. A myriad of cytokines generated in the bone microenvironment has been identified; these modulate osteoclast formation and action. Some of these

cytokines are important and some essential, such as the monocyte–macrophage colony-stimulating factor (M-CSF). These cytokines include stimulators of osteoclastic bone resorption as well as inhibitors, namely interferon-γ, interleukin-1 (IL-1) receptor antagonists, TGFβ and IL-4. Among these local factors the arachidonic acid metabolites should be considered; the most notable of these are the leukotrienes, which activate osteoclasts to resorb bone, and the prostaglandins of the E series, which transiently inhibit osteoclast activity but ultimately lead to increased osteoclastic resorption.

Fusion

During the process of osteoclast formation, mononuclear progenitor cells fuse to form mature multinucleated osteoclasts. This process is clearly important in osteoclastic bone resorption and, the more nuclei an osteoclast has, the more effective it is during bone resorption. It has been clearly demonstrated that this process occurs by fusion rather than by nuclear division. It has also been previously shown that the process is enhanced by 1,25-dihydroxyvitamin D. However, this hormone is not essential for the process, because osteoclast multinucleation occurs in conditions of 1,25-dihydroxyvitamin D lack such as chronic renal failure.

The molecular mechanisms by which osteoclasts may fuse have recently been clarified. It is possible that osteoclast precursors utilize a similar mechanism to that used by trophoblastic cells in the placenta. These trophoblastic cells of the placenta use (E)-cadherin, a hemophilic calcium-dependent cell attachment molecule, to fuse and become multinucleated cells. In studies performed to determine if a similar mechanism was used by osteoclasts, Mbalaviele et al[22] showed, both in vitro and in vivo, using immunohistochemistry and immunocytochemistry, that osteoclasts and their precursors express (E)-cadherin. To show that expression of (E)-cadherin was a functional phenomenon, both neutralizing antibodies and synthetic peptide antagonists to (E)-cadherin were utilized in studies in vitro of murine marrow cultures where osteoclasts are formed.[23] These two different types of inhibitors of (E)-cadherin function interfered with osteoclast formation, suggesting that expression of functional (E)-cadherin is important in osteoclast formation and subsequent bone resorption. It was also possible that other members of the cadherin family may be important in this process, not just in the formation of osteoclasts, but also in cell–cell contact which occurs between osteoclasts and other cells in the bone microenvironment.[24]

Tyrosine kinases in bone resorption
A number of tyrosine kinases are clearly important in both osteoclast formation and osteoclastic bone resorption. The receptor tyrosine kinase *c-fms* is probably required for normal osteoclast formation. This is the receptor that mediates the effects of M-CSF; absence of M-CSF leads to impaired osteoclast formation and a form of osteoporosis.[25,26] However, there are also non-receptor tyrosine kinases which are involved in osteoclastic bone resorption. Mice that are deficient in expression of the proto-oncogene *c-src* by targeted disruption of the gene also develop osteoporosis, but a different form of osteoporosis from that found in M-CSF deficiency. In this form of osteoporosis, osteoclasts are present but do not become polarized and form ruffled borders. As the *src* non-receptor tyrosine kinase is regulated by other tyrosine kinases, and may have downstream tyorsine kinases as substrates, it appears likely that there is a hierarchy of tyrosine kinases that are involved in the process of osteoclastic bone resorption as well as osteoclast formation. These tyrosine kinases and their substrates provide important potential targets for the development of new inhibitors of osteoclastic bone resorption.

Osteoclast apoptosis
Morphologic evidence of apoptosis occurs in the osteoclast at the conclusion of the normal phase of osteoclastic bone resorption during bone remodeling. Osteoclast apoptosis is apparent from characteristic morphologic changes in the osteoclast, including condensation of nuclear chromatin, and by separation of osteoclasts from the bone surface. Studies, both in vitro and in vivo, show that this process may be regulated by the same hormones that are responsible for osteoclast formation, but in an inverse manner. In other words, hormones such as parathyroid hormone, 1,25-dihydroxyvitamin D and IL-1, which stimulate osteoclast formation, inhibit osteoclast apoptosis. In contrast, TGFβ is an inhibitor of osteoclast formation, although it promotes osteoclast apoptosis (programmed cell death). Moreover, drugs that are inhibitors of bone resorption, such as the bisphosphonates and estrogen, are powerful inducers of osteoclast apoptosis. Osteoclast apoptosis is a relevantly recently observed phenomenon, and its importance in osteoclastic bone resorption relative to the events involved in osteoclast formation is not yet clear. However, it is possible that the effects of important agents in osteoporosis, such as estrogen and the bisphosphonates, has as a final common pathway the inducement of osteoclast apoptosis. Osteoclast apoptosis may be particularly important for the effects of estrogen on bone. Parfitt[27] has suggested that, during estrogen deficiency, osteoclasts are particularly active and this could be explained by their having a prolonged life as a result of the absence of this apoptotic stimulus. This may be the reason why extreme perforation of trabecular bone plates occurs and for labeling the osteoclasts 'killer' osteoclasts.[28]

Cellular events involved in the formation phase of the remodeling sequence

The specific cellular events involved in osteoblastic bone formation are chemotaxis, proliferation and differentiation of osteoblasts, followed by formation of mineralized bone and cessation of osteoblast activity. The initial event must be the chemotactic attraction of osteoblasts or their precursors to the sites of the resorption defect. This is probably mediated by local factors produced during the resorption process. Resorbing bone has been shown to produce chemotactic factors for cells with osteoblast characteristics in vitro.[29,30] One mediator that may be responsible for this effect is TGFβ, because active TGFβ is released by resorbing bone cultures. Structural proteins such as collagen or the bone Gla protein could also be involved, because type I collagen and bone Gla protein and their fragments had the same effect.[29,30] More recently, it has been shown that TGFβ, which is enriched in the bone matrix and released as a consequence of bone resorption, is also chemotactic for bone cells.[31] However, TGFβ is not the only potential chemoattractant. Platelet-derived growth factor (PDGF) is chemotactic for some mesenchymal cells, monocytes, neutrophils and smooth muscle cells.[32–35] Perhaps a combination of chemotactic factors is responsible for attraction of osteoblast precursors to resorption sites.

The second event involved in the formation phase of the coupling phenomenon is proliferation of osteoblast precursors. This is probably mediated by local osteoblast growth factors released during the resorption process. There are several leading candidates for these factors, which represent autocrine and paracrine factors, including members of the TGFβ superfamily (TGFβ1 and -2). In addition, PDGF causes proliferation of cells with osteoblast characteristics. IGF-1 and -2 and the heparin-binding fibroblast growth factors (HB-FGFs) also cause osteoblast proliferation.

The third event of the formation phase is the differentiation of the osteoblast precursor into the mature cell. Several of the bone-derived growth factors can cause the appearance of markers of the differentiated osteoblast phenotype, including expression of alkaline phosphatase activity, type I collagen and osteocalcin synthesis. Most prominent of these are IGF-1 and BMP-2. Active TGF inhibits osteoblast differentiation in vitro, which suggests that its role may be to 'trigger' the process, after which it is removed or becomes inactivated, and the increased pool of precursors then undergoes differentiation.

The final phase of the formation process must be cessation of osteoblast activity. The resorption lacunae are usually repaired either completely or almost completely. It is not known how this is achieved. One possibility is that factors produced during this process decrease osteoblast activity. Under the appropriate circumstances, one such factor could, again, be TGFβ. Active TGFβ decreases differentiated function in osteoblasts and, as noted above, is expressed by osteoblasts as they differentiate.[36]

The coupling of bone resorption to bone formation

Osteotropic factors that could be involved in the coupling phenomenon are TGFβ, bone morphogenetic proteins (BMPs), IGF-1 and -2, PDGF and HB-FGFs. This area has also been recently reviewed by Canalis et al.[37,38] These factors are likely to be released locally from bone as it resorbs, or by bone cells activated as a consequence of the resorption process. They may then act in a sequential manner to regulate all the cellular events required for the formation of bone.

The TGFβ superfamily may be particularly important in the coupling that links bone formation to prior bone resorption. Prolonged primary cultures of fetal rat calvarial osteoblasts show that the BMPs are expressed as these cells differentiate to form new bone, in parallel with other differentiation markers such as osteocalcin and alkaline phosphatase. Transient exposure of these cells to TGFβ stimulates proliferation of the osteoblasts (continued exposure inhibits the formation of mineralized bone expression of differentiation markers). BMP-2 and BMP-4 lead to increased numbers of mineralized nodules. The following events probably occur during normal bone remodeling, based on in vitro observations. Bone resorption leads to the release of active TGFβ, as has been shown previously. Exposure of osteoblast precursors to active TGFβ causes increased proliferation. However, this exposure is transient and, as a consequence, the proliferating cells undergo differentiation and express bone morphogenetic proteins. This is associated with expression of differentiation markers such as alkaline phosphatase, osteocalcin and type I collagen. Mineralized bone nodules form, so the bone resorption process results in a cascade of growth factors that are responsible for the subsequent events. Initially, the most abundant growth factor in the bone matrix, namely TGFβ, is released in an active form as a consequence of resorption. TGFβ then stimulates proliferation of osteoblast precursors and attracts osteoblast precursors to the site of the resorption defect.[39,40] The proliferating osteoblasts then begin to differentiate to form more mature osteoblasts and express differentiation markers such as osteocalcin and alkaline phosphatase, and also the bone morphogenetic proteins. These bone morphogenetic proteins are then responsible for an autostimulatory effect on the osteoblasts and the formation of mineralized bone nodules. Of course, it is unlikely that the TGFβ superfamily members are acting alone. Other growth factors, such as the IGFs, HBFGFs, and PDGFs, are also likely to have an effect on osteoblast proliferation and differentiation. These factors are all bone growth stimulants. Recently, it has been shown that FGFs have comparable osteoblast stimulating effects on bone to those of TGFβ.[41]

Role of growth factors in bone formation
Although the HBFGFs have always been thought to be potent proliferative agents for bone cells, it is only recently that their importance in bone growth and development has been fully appreciated. This arose as a result of observations that a number of disorders of impaired skeletal development are caused by point mutations in the FGF receptor family. Thus, achondroplasia results from a point mutation in FGF receptor 3, Crouzon's syndrome from a point mutation in FGF receptor 2 and Jackson–Weiss syndrome also from a point mutation in receptor 2.[42,43] Not only are these growth peptides important in skeletal development in endochondral bone, they are also likely to play an important role in normal adult bone formation. Certainly, when administered exogenously, they have very powerful effects on stimulating bone formation in vivo in rodents. This occurs when administered either locally or systemically to aged rats that have been ovariectomized.[44] Similar effects are seen with both FGF-1 and FGF-2.

TGFβ and its binding proteins
TGFβ has a complex relationship with several different types of binding proteins, which may modulate its activity in the bone microenvironment. The major binding protein is a bone matrix protein related to the fibrillin family; unfortunately this is called the latent TGFβ-binding protein (LTBP). It appears likely that this LTBP is stored covalently bound to TGFβ in the bone matrix, and that the release of TGFβ from the bone matrix requires proteolytic cleavage of TGFβ from this LTBP. This proteolytic cleavage step may be a critical event involved in normal bone remodeling. However, this is not all that is required for the release of active TGFβ. The binding of TGFβ to LTBP in the bone matrix is via its precursor, and there must be subsequent release of the active TGFβ moiety from the precursor molecule. This could involve not only proteolytic mechanisms, but also an acidic microenvironment, which of course is present under the ruffled border of the osteoclast. Cleavage of TGFβ precursor from LTBP may be mediated by plasmin.[45] Cells of the osteoblast phenotype express plasminogen activator when incubated with osteotropic hormones such as parathyroid hormone.[46]

TGFβ and receptors
TGFβ is one of the most abundant proteins in the bone matrix, and probably plays an important role in normal bone turnover. Recent observations have indicated the potential importance of this role.[47] These workers have shown that, when TGFβ expression is targeted to osteoblasts with the use of an osteocalcin promoter, osteoblast-specific over-expression of TGFβ-2 from the osteocalcin promoter causes profound changes in bone remodeling, including progressive bone loss with increases in both bone resorption and bone formation.

The most convincing evidence that IGF-1 may play a role as a coupling factor has been provided by the work of Canalis et al[37,38] in cultures of embryonic rat calvariae. They found that parathyroid hormone stimulated expression of IGF-1 by calvarial cultures upon transient exposure, and suggested that this production of IGF-1 is responsible for subsequent bone formation. However, this is unlikely to be the only mechanism involved.

Hence, as with hemapoiesis and differentiation of multipotent hemapoietic stem cells, bone formation may represent a complex multi-hierarchical organization of the cells in the osteoblast lineage. It is possible that the actions of the bone-derived growth factors could be coordinated in a similar way to the one suggested for the hemopoietic growth factors. These factors may work as a cascade, as suggested for TGFβ and the BMPs, or they may act in concert. Walker et al[48] have suggested that the distinct CSFs for macrophages and granulocytes act on hemopoietic progenitor cells by causing direct effects on target cells; indirect effects are also caused by altering the expression of receptors for other factors and therefore altering the cells responsive to these other factors. They have proposed that the capacity of each CSF to down-modulate other CSF receptors parallels its biological effects. Such a hierarchical modulation of receptors and the potential for alteration, by one growth factor, of the target cell's responses to other growth factors are also applicable to the osteoblast cell lineage. There is much evidence to suggest that there are synergistic as well as inhibitory interactions between the growth factors acting on osteoblasts; for example, TGFβ, PDGF, IGF-1 and -2, and BMPs may all influence osteoblasts directly, but also modulate the response of osteoblasts to these other growth regulatory factors.[49-54] The potential interactions between these factors are extraordinarily complex, probably as complex as the interactions of the CSFs in hemopoiesis, but it is essential to unravel them to understand local control of bone formation. It is probable that the complicated interactions between those factors released locally in active form, as a consequence of the resorption process, are responsible for the carefully coordinated formation of new bone, which occurs at these sites.

PATHOPHYSIOLOGY OF AGE-RELATED BONE LOSS AND OSTEOPOROSIS

The pathogenesis of osteoporosis must be considered in the light of the natural history of the skeleton and the characteristics of age-related bone loss. These changes are of two types: the changes in bone mass that occur with advancing age, and the specific changes in cancellous bone microarchitecture that occur in the vertebral bodies and the necks of femora of osteoporotic individuals. Both are important for the increased bone fragility that occurs at these sites.

The natural history of the skeleton and the changes in bone mass that occur with age have been discussed above. The changes in bone mass with age are illustrated in Figure 2.1. Bone mass reaches a maximum after linear growth stops, starts to fall at about 30 years and declines to half its maximum value by 80 or 90 years. Women have less bone mass at their peak than men and show an accelerated phase of bone loss for 10 years after the menopause. This loss involves endosteal and haversian resorption and loss of cancellous bone, particularly in the vertebrae, without replacement by new bone.

The low bone mass that is common with advancing age results from a combination of suboptimal peak bone mass attained in early adult life, and from increased rates of bone loss which occur after middle age. Osteoporotic bones are prone to fracture because of low bone mass, architectural abnormalities at both the micro- and macro-levels, and acute trauma. The relative importance of each of these in the causation of osteoporotic fracture depends on the fracture site.

Attainment of peak bone mass

Peak bone mass, which is attained in early adult life, is dependent primarily on genetic factors; it is also, however, influenced considerably by dietary calcium intake during adolescence and by physical activity. Genetic factors have been obvious because there are differences in peak bone mass in various ethnic groups. For example, Blacks have greater peak bone mass than Caucasians who, in turn, have greater peak bone mass than oriental people, particularly Japanese. There is no question that genetic factors have a powerful influence on the attainment of peak bone mass. This has been apparent from twin studies for more than 20 years, because it was known that monozygotic twins have much closer concordance of bone mineral density than dizygotic twins.[55] The issue is which genes are the most important. In recent years, most attention has been focused on the vitamin D receptor gene. Morrison et al[56] reported that polymorphisms in this gene were closely associated with peak bone mass in monozygotic twins, and that these polymorphisms accounted for most of the genetic effect. Another group reported no association,[57] and there have been many conflicting reports (cited in Garnero et al[58]). More recently, the Sydney group has indicated that further study of Australian twin pairs does not confirm their original findings. This does not mean that there is no effect of the vitamin D receptor gene polymorphisms, but rather that it is not as prominent as first thought. Since then, roles for other gene polymorphisms, including those for collagen type I, estrogen receptor, IL-6 and TGFβ have been suggested. Other influences that are clearly important during adolescence, in the attainment of peak bone mass, are physical activity, dietary calcium intake and factors influencing the progression of puberty.[59] In fact, evidence is probably even stronger for dietary calcium intake than it is for physical activity. Delayed puberty has deleterious consequences on attainment of peak bone mass in women, and probably also in men.

Rates of bone loss with advancing age

The factors that affect peak bone mass (genetic and environmental factors) and the factors that cause progressive loss of bone mass after midlife (aging, menopause and environmental factors) are shown in Figure 2.2.

Bone loss occurs in all individuals after middle life, the mechanisms of which are multifactorial. They are caused by complicated changes in bone cell activity during bone remodeling, and these cellular changes depend on the major factor that is operative at any point in time. The major factors causing bone loss after middle life

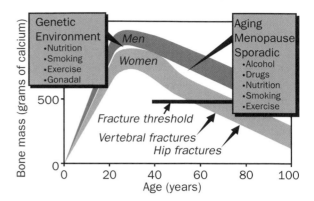

Figure 2.2 Important factors that influence attainment of peak bone mass, and influence rates of bone loss in later adult life.

include sex hormone deficiency, disuse, and calcium and vitamin D deficiency. The rates of bone loss after abrupt hormonal withdrawal are exponential, whereas the rates of loss as a result of disuse or calcium and vitamin deficiency are more gradual.[60] As sex hormone withdrawal is usually abrupt in women, this may be the reason that women have such a rapid phase of accelerated bone loss after the menopause, whereas men lose bone slowly in keeping with a more gradual decline in sex hormone production. The loss of bone associated with the menopause is probably relatively greater in cancellous bone than in cortical bone. It has been estimated that about two-thirds of the bone loss in old women can be ascribed to the menopause, and about one-third to aging.[2] Although not all workers might agree with these estimates, there is no disagreement on the major role that estrogen deficiency plays in bone loss in women. The importance of other factors such as disuse and dietary calcium and viatamin D deficiency are considered below.

Pathophysiology of osteoporotic fracture

Osteoporotic fractures occur most commonly in the hip and the vertebral bodies, although they also occur at the wrist. The fractures occur because of low bone mass, architectural abnormalities in the skeleton and acute trauma. The factors responsible for peak bone mass and the rate of bone loss after middle life have been considered earlier. Here, disturbances in bone architecture and falls are considered.

Bone microarchitecture

Bone loss associated with advanced age and estrogen deficiency in women is accompanied by a disturbance of bone microarchitecture.[7,61,62] There is focal perforation of cancellous bone plates caused by osteoclastic resorption, leading to loss of connectivity of these horizontal plates (or 'struts') and the presence of 'unconnected' vertical rods and bars dispersed throughout the marrow cavity. This has two important consequences. First, it places the remaining cancellous bone at a major structural disadvantage and increases the chances of compression or crush fractures in those bones that are rich in cancellous bone, such as the vertebral bodies. Unconnected vertical rods are liable to buckling and fracture, particularly if further thinned by states of high bone turnover. The mean thickness of cancellous bone plates is approximately 100–150 µm, whereas osteoclasts cause resorption defects of 50–100 µm during normal remodeling. Parfitt has suggested that focal perforations in cancellous bone plates could result from increased osteoclast activity (caused by so-called 'killer' osteoclasts), or to normal osteoclastic resorption defects occurring in relatively thin plates, an event that would be increased in frequency when activation of remodeling sites is increased (for example, by estrogen deficiency after the menopause)[27] or osteoclast lifespan is enhanced by inhibition of apoptosis.[28] Second, it may create a situation where there is no bone structure on which new bone formation can occur, even if osteoblasts can be stimulated to make new bone. The vertebral fracture rate presumably can be inhibited either by reducing rates of bone remodeling, which reduces erosion of the vertical rods, or by factors that stimulate bone formation leading to thickening of the rods. It is still debatable whether these changes in connectivity of horizontal struts, which occur in older women, can be corrected by formation-stimulating agents, although recent data suggest that it may be possible with some agents.[44]

Femoral neck geometry

There is some evidence to suggest that the geometry of the femoral neck may be an important predictor of future fracture, and that patients with particularly long femoral necks are more likely to have a fracture of the hip. One study showed that the length of the hip axis increased by 1 standard deviation between 1950 and 1990 in New Zealand, corresponding to the author's increase in fracture incidence.[63,64]

FACTORS THAT INFLUENCE SKELETAL INTEGRITY DURING AGING

Non-hormonal

Bone cell senescence

Although there is no direct evidence, it appears likely that age-related bone loss results partly from decreased functional capacity of bone cells associated with the aging process, which leads to impaired bone formation relative to bone resorption. Several histomorphometric studies have shown that, in elderly individuals, the cavities formed by resorbing osteoclasts are incompletely filled by osteoblasts after completion of a remodeling cycle. This abnormality is known as decreased mean wall thickness.[18] It could result theoretically either from decreased capacity of osteoblasts to form new bone, caused by an inherent cellular defect or from decreased production of local growth regulatory factors (coupling factors) which are required to stimulate normal new bone formation. It is likely that both are important. However, the fact that fractures heal in elderly people does show that osteoblasts can function normally in old people, albeit often more slowly than in young people.

Diet

There is very convincing evidence to link dietary calcium deficiency with osteoporosis.

Calcium deficiency in animals such as cats, rodents and dogs causes osteoporosis.[65] Calcium balance studies in osteoporotic patients have consistently revealed that these patients are in negative calcium balance, with dietary calcium intake insufficient to account for calcium losses in feces, urine and sweat.[65] Calcium absorption from the gut declines in all individuals with aging for many reasons, including changes in the gut epithelium and decreased synthesis and/or responsivitiy to vitamin D.[66] Normal young individuals can adapt by increasing the fractional absorption of calcium by the gut, but this capacity is reduced in elderly people.[65,67] As early data come mainly from cross-sectional rather than longitudinal studies, it is not surprising that there have been some disagreements on how much dietary calcium is required to prevent negative calcium balance. Nordin et al[68] believe that it is 500 mg/day, whereas Heaney et al[69] estimate that postmenopausal women require 1500 mg/day. More recently, several studies have shown that children receiving modest calcium supplements during the pre-teen years achieve higher peak bone mass than those with unsupplemented diets.[59] After middle age, increasing calcium intake has modest effects on the changes that are occurring in bone mass in the first 5 years after the menopause, but much greater effects thereafter (see below).

Dietary calcium deficiency has also been implicated as a pathogenic factor from other data. Dietary calcium intake is less in females than in males at all ages, and particularly in adolescent females, in whom calcium intake is not sufficient to maintain normal calcium balance. Moreover, epidemiologic studies in Hungary have revealed that populations with low dietary calcium intakes have increased incidence of hip fracture and decreased cortical bone mineral density, as measured by cortical metacarpal thickness.[70] Just how dietary calcium deficiency could cause bone loss is unclear. It is possible that it could lead to secondary hyperparathyroidism, which, in turn, could cause cortical bone loss. This has been reinforced by studies showing that calcium and vitamin D supplements decrease hip fracture rates in elderly people and suppress plasma parathryoid hormone concentrations.[71] Alternatively, as evidence exists that estrogen may stimulate, 1,25-dihydroxyvitamin D production, increased calcium requirements after the menopause could result from estrogen deficiency, leading to decreased production of 1,25-dihydroxyvitamin D, which would cause decreased gut absorption of calcium.[2]

Protein malnutrition is occasionally present in patients with osteoporosis. It is usually associated with alcoholism, malabsorption or nephrotic syndrome in most Western societies. Excess alcohol intake may be an independent factor impairing bone remodeling, and particularly osteoblast function (see below). High protein diets can cause a negative calcium balance, probably because of renal calcium losses associated with impaired renal tubular calcium reabsorption.[65] There is a high prevalence of osteoporosis in patients with lactase deficiency,[72] which is possibly related to decreased tolerance to dairy foods and subsequent dietary calcium lack.

Ethnic Influences

There are quite marked differences in the prevalence of osteoporosis in different ethnic groups. Osteoporosis is much less common in African–Americans[73] and in Mexican Americans[74] than in white or Asian people. The reasons for these differences are not clear. However, as bone mineral density shows a higher concordance between monozygotic twins than between dizygotic twins, genetic factors are likely to be important.[55] In African–Americans, it appears likely that peak bone mass is greater.[75] Bone mass and osteoporotic hip fracture are poorly correlated in Japanese individuals, possibly because cultural differences lead to stronger musculature of the pelvic girdle in traditional Japanese people, and subsequent decreased propensity to fall.

The studies of Eisman and colleagues[76,77] may shed light on genetic influences on peak bone mass, and possibly also on rates of bone loss. This group has suggested that there is a positive correlation between patterns of expression of the vitamin D receptor gene and bone mass, as well as with markers of bone turnover such as serum osteocalcin. It is possible that changes in vitamin D receptor function may be one of the determinants in the genetic component of peak bone mass, although there are also likely to be many others.

Environmental Influences

Epidemiologic evidence suggests that tobacco intake, alcoholism and inadequate sunlight are associated with increased propensity to osteoporosis.[78,79] Moreover, increased coffee ingestion, and particularly caffeine intake, has been linked to osteoporosis.[78] Inadequate sunlight exposure causes decreased formation of vitamin D, which in turn causes decreased calcium absorption from the gut. The importance of marginal vitamin D deficiency in the pathogenesis of osteopenia associated with aging is probably greater in Europe than it is in the USA, where sunlight and fortified foods make vitamin D deficiency very rare.

Physiologic stresses and illnesses

Pregnancy and lactation may have a protective effect on the skeleton, because patients who have had multiple pregnancies seem to be less prone to osteoporosis. There is, however, a small subset of patients who have a severe and reversible form of osteoporosis during pregnancy. Obesity is also protective. Immobilization, and even lack of physical exercise, predispose people to bone loss; bone mass is directly related to lean muscle mass.[75] As muscle mass declines, so too does bone mass.[80] The importance of physical exercise and maintenance of muscle mass is supported by many studies showing that regular physical exercise is good for muscle mass.[81–83]

Hormonal

Gonadal hormones

Osteoporosis has been associated with the postmenopausal state since Fuller Albright noted, over 40 years ago, that 40 of his 42 patients with osteoporosis were postmenopausal women. In recent years, it has clearly been shown that there is accelerated loss of bone, occurring immediately after the menopause, which lasts for about 10 years, but which is relatively much greater in the first 2–3 years.[84,85] This rapid phase of bone loss is reversed by estrogen therapy during these years. The precise mechanism by which estrogen deficiency increases bone resorption is still controversial.

Estrogen lack leads to an increase in activation frequency on bone surfaces, which in turn leads to an increase in osteoclastic bone resorption. Bone formation increases in parallel, but not to the same extent, and the overall result is a loss of bone mass. The mechanisms by which estrogen lack leads to these abnormalities in bone remodeling is unknown, but is the subject of intense investigation and is very controversial.

Possibly, most of the discrepancies between different reports could be explained by the use of different in vitro systems and the problems in extrapolating from different rodent systems to humans. These points notwithstanding, there is evidence at present to suggest that estrogen may mediate its effects indirectly through cytokines and growth factors, including IL-1α, IL-1 receptor antagonist, tumor necrosis factor (TNF), IL-6 and TGFβ; in addition, it also has direct effects on osteoclasts as shown by Oursler et al.[86]

The points about which there is no argument are the morphologic and functional effects of estrogen withdrawal. Estrogen withdrawal either in ovariectomized female rodents or in women is associated with markedly increased osteoclastic bone resorption, with an increase in the numbers of cells at each detectable stage in the osteoclast lineage,[87] including GM-CFU, committed marrow precursors and mature multinucleated osteoclasts. Parfitt[28] has suggested that the osteoclasts are hyperactive and resorb bone more efficiently – he has labeled these cells 'killer' osteoclasts which perforate trabecular bone plates and possibly have an increased lifespan. These effects are reversed by replacement with physiologic doses of estrogen and, under these circumstances, osteoclast apoptosis is enhanced.[88]

How does estrogen mediate these effects?

The arguments in favor of IL-1 being a major mediator of the estrogen effects on bone are that IL-1 production by peripheral blood monocytes is enhanced in women after estrogen withdrawal, and this increased production is reduced by treatment with estrogen.[89,90] Moreover, the effects on bone loss can be reversed by treatment with a specific IL-1 receptor antagonist, which inhibits the effects of IL-1 on bone.[91] The argument that IL-6 is the major mediator comes from the studies of Jilka and Manolagas,[87,92,93] who show that estrogen can inhibit IL-6 production by bone cells and bone marrow stromal cells and that, in ovariectomized mice, neutralizing antibodies to IL-6 block the effects of estrogen withdrawal causing bone loss. The argument for TGFβ is based on in vitro studies in which TGFβ production by bone cells, as well as by osteoclasts, may be regulated by estrogen.[94,95] Also to be mentioned are prostaglandins of the E series, whose production in vivo is also enhanced by estrogen withdrawal.

None of these mechanisms addresses the specific problem with bone formation. After estrogen withdrawal, there is an increase in rates of bone formation, but these do not match those of bone resorption and the result is progressive bone loss. This failure of perfect coupling of formation and resorption is a fundamental part of the mechanism for bone loss, but it is not yet understood.

The molecular mechanisms by which estrogen exerts its effects on bone cells are an area of intense interest, because the design of effective modulators of estrogen action, which mediate the beneficial effects of estrogen without the side effects, is a major aim of many pharmaceutical companies. The role of the newly discovered estrogen receptor in this process is unclear.

Parathyroid hormone

Parathyroid hormone (PTH) secretion is probably normal in many patients with osteoporosis. In a subset of patients, plasma PTH is increased.[96,97] These patients often have so-called type II osteoporosis,[2] characterized by older age and propensity to osteoporotic hip fracture. The senile secondary hyperparathyroidism and risk of hip fracture can be reduced by increasing oral calcium and vitamin D intake.[71]

Harms et al[98] have suggested that PTH is secreted in a pulsatile manner in normal individuals, with bursts of about 6–8 pulses per hour. This has been verified by several other groups.[99,100] Harms et al[98] examined three men with idiopathic osteoporosis and suggested that these pulses of PTH secretion were lost in these individuals. This raises the possibility that non-pulsatile PTH secretion may be related to the bone loss associated with idiopathic osteoporosis. As PTH causes different effects on bone cells when administered in a continuous manner, compared with when it is administered in an intermittent manner, this is not an unreasonable hypothesis. However, Samuels et al[101] were unable to confirm that pulses of PTH secretion are lost in patients with osteoporosis.

The vitamin D endocrine system

Most (but not all) studies have reported that circulating levels of 1,25-dihydroxyvitamin D are decreased in elderly patients, including osteoporotic individuals, by about 30%.[102,103] The reason for decreased 1,25-dihydroxyvitamin D production is not entirely clear, although it is likely that vitamin D metabolism in the kidney is less efficient in elderly people.[104] It is also possible that substrate availability is decreased because of dietary deficiency and decreased exposure to sunlight. Several studies have suggested that there is decreased 1,25-dihydroxyvitamin D production in response to stimuli such as PTH in elderly people,[2,67] although there is no convincing evidence that there is a difference between elderly patients with and those without osteoporosis.

As noted above, recent studies show that hip fractures can be reduced by increasing oral calcium and vitamin D intake in institutionalized elderly people.[71] The serum 25-hydroxyvitamin D concentration should be greater than 80 nmol/l, particularly in the elderly population. Hip fracture risk is increased dramatically if serum 25-hydroxyvitamin D is less than 10 nmol/l.[105]

Calcitonin

Circulating calcitonin concentrations are less in elderly than in young people and less in women than in men at any age.[106,107] Improvements in assay techniques (particularly plasma extraction) have cast some doubt on the age differences,[108] although all workers agree that circulating concentrations of calcitonin in women are less than in men at any given age.

Local regulatory hormones or factors

Bone loss that occurs after midlife is characterized by an imbalance between bone resorption and bone formation, so that there is a relative increase in bone resorption over bone formation. This imbalance means that there is a disturbance in the coupling phenomenon that links resorption and formation, but the precise mechanism is entirely unknown. As coupling probably involves local growth regulatory factors produced in the microenvironment of the remodeling unit, the secret to remodeling imbalance probably lies with abnormal local production of these factors, or abnormal responsivity of bone cells to them. These factors were discussed in more detail earlier, and include the growth regulatory factors that are stored within the bone matrix such as TGFβ, the BMPs, the IGFs and the FGFs.

CONCLUSION

Great advances have been made in the past 10 years in our understanding of the cellular events involved in normal bone remodeling. This has led to new ideas about the mechanisms responsible for the dysfunctions in bone remodeling that are responsible for osteoporosis. Most attention has been focused on the factors responsible for controlling bone cell activity, and how the conditions that predispose to osteoporosis, such as estrogen deficiency, aging and many others, influence these factors. In the next decade, there will almost certainly be more attention given to the cells themselves, and in particular how those conditions such as estrogen deficiency and aging influence expression in osteoclasts and osteoblasts.

ACKNOWLEDGEMENTS

Some of the work described here was supported in part by NIH grants CA40035, AR39529, AR28149, RR1346 and AR07464.

REFERENCES

1. Mazess RB. On aging bone loss. *Clin Orthop* 1982; **165:** 239–52.
2. Riggs BL, Wahner HW, Dunn WL et al. Differential changes in bone mineral density of the appendicular and axial skeleton with aging: Relationship to spinal osteoporosis. *J Clin Invest* 1981; **67:** 328–35.
3. Smith DM, Khairi MRA, Johnston CC Jr. The loss of bone mineral with aging and its relationship to risk of fracture. *J Clin Invest* 1975; **56:** 311–18.
4. Riggs BL, Wahner HW, Melton LJ III et al. Rates of bone loss in the axial and appendicular skeletons of women: Evidence of substantial vertebral bone loss prior to menopause. *J Clin Invest* 1986; **77:** 1487–91.
5. Genant HK, Cann CE, Ettinger B et al. Quantitative computed tomography of vertebral spongiosa: A sensitive method for detecting early bone loss after oophorectomy. *Ann Intern Med* 1982; **97:** 699–705.
6. Riggs BL, Melton LJ III. Involutional osteoporosis. *N Engl J Med* 1986; **314:** 1676–86.
7. Parfitt AM, Matthews CHE, Villaneuva AR et al. Relationship between surface, volume, and thickness of iliac trabecular bone on aging and in osteoporosis: implications for the microanatomic and cellular mechanism of bone loss. *J Clin Invest* 1983; **72:** 1396–409.
8. Kleerekoper M, Villanueva AR, Stanciu J et al. The role of three dimensional trabecular microstructure in the pathogenesis of vertebral

compression fractures. *Calcif Tissue Int* 1985; **37:** 594–7.

9. Hattner R, Etker BN, Frost HM. Suggested sequential mode of control of changes in cell behaviour in adult bone remodelling. *Nature* 1995; **206:** 489–90.

10. Frost HM. Dynamics of bone remodeling. In: *Bone Biodynamics.* Boston: Little & Brown, 1964: 315.

11. Miyauchi A, Alvarez J, Greenfield EM et al. Recognition of osteopontin and related peptides by an $\alpha v \beta 3$ integrin stimulates immediate cell signals in osteoclasts. *J Biol Chem* 1991; **266:** 20369–74.

12. Baron R, Vignery A, Horowitz M. Lymphocytes, macrophages and the regulation of bone remodeling. In: *Bone and Mineral Research* (Peck WA, ed.). Amsterdam: Elsevier, 1984: 175–243.

13. Boyce BF, Yates AJP, Mundy GR. Bolus injections of recombinant human interleukin-1 cause transient hypocalcemia in normal mice. *Endocrinology* 1989; **125:** 2780–3.

14. Snapper I, Kahn A. *Myelomatosis.* Basel: Karger, 1971.

15. Valentin-Opran A, Charhon SA, Meunier PJ et al. Quantitative histology of myeloma induced bone changes. *Br J Haematol* 1982; **52:** 601–10.

16. Stewart AF, Vignery A, Silvergate A et al. Quantitative bone histomorphometry in humoral hypercalcemia of malignancy – uncoupling of bone cell activity. *J Clin Endocrinol Metab* 1982; **55:** 219–27.

17. Darby AJ, Meunier PJ. Mean wall thickness and formation periods of trabecular bone packets in idiopathic osteoporosis. *Calcif Tissue Int* 1981; **33:** 199–204.

18. Rasmussen H, Bordier P. *The Physiological and Cellular Basis of Metabolic Bone Disease.* Baltimore: Williams & Wilkins, 1974.

19. Howard GA, Bottemiller BL, Turner RT et al. Parathyroid hormone stimulates bone formation and resorption in organ culture: evidence for a coupling mechanism. *Proc Natl Acad Sci USA* 1981; **78:** 3204–8.

20. Marcelli C, Yates AJP, Mundy GR. *In vivo* effects of human recombinant transforming growth factor beta on bone turnover in normal mice. *J Bone Miner Res* 1990; **5:** 1087–96.

21. Roodman GD, Ibbotson KJ, MacDonald BR et al. $1,25\text{-}(OH)_2$ vitamin D3 causes formation of multinucleated cells with osteoclast characteristics in cultures of primate marrow. *Proc Natl Acad Sci USA* 1985; **82:** 8213–17.

22. Mbalaviele G, Chen H, Boyce BF et al. The role of cadherin in the generation of multinucleated osteoclasts from mononuclear precursors in murine marrow. *J Clin Invest* 1995; **95:** 2757–65.

23. Mbalaviele G, Nishimura R, Feng J et al. Molecular cloning of a novel cadherin in human osteoclasts (abstract). *J Bone Miner Res* 1995; **10**(suppl 1): 10.

24. Mbalaviele G, Nishimura R, Reddy R et al. Characterization of the molecular mechanisms of heterotypic osteoclast–osteoblast interactions during bone resorption – role of a novel cadherin-6 isoform. *J Bone Miner Res* 1997; **11**(suppl): in press.

25. Felix R, Cecchini MG, Fleisch H. Macrophage colony stimulating factor restores in vivo bone resorption in the OP/OP osteopetrotic mouse. *Endocrinology* 1990; **127:** 2592–4.

26. Wiktor-Jedrzejczak W, Urbanowska E, Aukerman SL et al. Correction by CSF-1 of defects in the osteopetrotic op/op mouse suggests local, developmental, and humoral requirements for this growth factor. *Exp Hematol* 1991; **19:** 1049–54.

27. Parfitt AM. Bone remodeling in the pathogenesis of osteoporosis. *Med Times* 1981; **109:** 80–92.

28. Parfitt AM, Mundy GR, Roodman GD et al. A new model for regulation of bone resorption, with particular reference to the effects of bisphosphonates. *J Bone Miner Res* 1996; **11:** 150–9.

29. Mundy GR, Rodan SB, Majeska RJ et al. Unidirectional migration of osteosarcoma cells with osteoblast characteristics in response to products of bone resorption. *Calcif Tissue Int* 1982; **34:** 542–6.

30. Mundy GR, Poser JW. Chemotactic activity of the gamma-carboxyglutamic acid containing protein in bone. *Calcif Tiss Int* 1983; **35:** 164–8.

31. Pfeilschifter J, Wolf O, Naumann A et al. Chemotactic response of osteoblast-like cells to transforming growth factor β. *J Bone Miner Res* 1990; **5:** 825–30.

32. Deuel TF, Senior RM, Huang JS et al. Chemotaxis of monocytes and neutrophils to platelet-derived growth factor. *J Clin Invest* 1982; **69:** 1046–9.

33. Grotendorst GR, Seppa HEJ, Kleinman HK et al. Attachment of smooth muscle cells to collagen and their migration toward platelet-derived growth factor. *Proc Natl Acad Sci USA* 1981; **78:** 3669–72.

34. Seppa H, Grotendorst G, Seppa S et al. Platelet-derived growth factor is chemotactic for fibrob-

lasts. *J Cell Biol* 1982; **92:** 584–8.

35. Senior RM, Griffin GL, Huang JS et al. Chemotactic activity of platelet alpha granule proteins for fibroblasts. *J Cell Biol* 1983; **96:** 382–5.

36. Dallas S, Snyder SP, Miyazono K et al. Autoinduction of forms of latent transforming growth factor β (L-TGFβ) in bone cells. *J Bone Miner Res* 1992; **7**(suppl).

37. Canalis E, McCarthy T, Centrella M. Growth factors and the regulation of bone remodeling. *J Clin Invest* 1989; **81:** 277–81.

38. Canalis E, Centrella M, Burch W et al. Insulin-like growth factor I mediates selective anabolic effects of parathyroid hormone in bone cultures. *J Clin Invest* 1989; **83:** 60–5.

39. Pfeilschifter J, Bonewald L, Mundy GR. Characterization of the latent transforming growth factor β complex in bone. *J Bone Miner Res* 1990; **5:** 49–58.

40. Gehron-Robey PG, Young MF, Flanders KC et al. Osteoblasts synthesize and respond to transforming growth factor type beta (TGFβ) in vitro. *J Cell Biol* 1987; **105:** 457–63.

41. Dunstan C, Boyce B, Izbicka E et al. Acidic and basic fibroblast growth factors promote bone growth in vivo comparable to that of TGFβ (abstract). *J Bone Miner Res* 1993; **8**(suppl 1): 8.

42. Rousseau F, Bonaventure J, Legeal-Mallet L et al. Mutations in the gene encoding fibroblast growth factor receptor 3 in achondroplasia. *Nature* 1994; **371:** 252–4.

43. Reardon W, Winter RM, Rutland P et al. Mutations in the fibroblast growth factor receptor 2 gene cause Crouzon syndrome. *Nature Genet* 1994; **8:** 98–103.

44. Dunstan CR, Garrett IR, Adams R et al. Systemic fibroblast growth factor (FGF-1) prevents bone loss, increases new bone formation, and restores trabecular microarchitecture in ovariectomized rats. *J Bone Miner Res* 1995; **10**(suppl 1): 279.

45. Bonewald LF, Mundy GR. Role of transforming growth factor beta in bone remodeling. *Clin Orthop Rel Res* 1990; **250:** 261–76.

46. Hamilton JA, Lingelbach S, Partridge NC et al. Regulation of plasminogen activator production by bone-resorbing hormones in normal and malignant osteoblasts. *Endocrinology* 1985; **116:** 2186–91.

47. Erlebacher A, Derynck R. Increased expression of TGFβ-2 in osteoblasts results in an osteoporosis-like phenotype. *J Cell Biol* 1996; **132:** 195–210.

48. Walker F, Nicola NA, Metcalf D et al. Hierarchical down modulation of hemopoietic growth factor receptors. *Cell* 1985; **43:** 269–76.

49. Assoian RK, Grotendorst GR, Miller DM et al. Cellular transformation by coordinated action of three peptide growth factors from human platelets. *Nature* 1984; **309:** 804–6.

50. Massague J. Transforming growth factor β modulates the high affinity receptors of epidermal growth factor and transforming growth factor α. *J Cell Biol* 1985; **100:** 1508–14.

51. Bowen-Pope DF, Dicorletto PE, Ross R. Interactions between the receptors for platelet-derived growth factor and epidermal growth factor. *J Cell Biol* 1983; **96:** 679–83.

52. Seyedin SM, Thomas TC, Thompson AY et al. Purification and characterization of two cartilage-inducing factors from bovins demineralized bone. *Proc Natl Acad Sci USA* 1985; **82:** 2267–71.

53. Roberts AB, Anzano MA, Wakefield LM et al. Type β transforming growth factor: a bifunctional regulator of cellular growth. *Proc Natl Acad Sci USA* 1985; **82:** 119–23.

54. Tucker RF, Shipley GD, Moses HL et al. Growth inhibitor from BSC-1 cells closely related to platelet type B transforming growth factor. *Science* 1984; **226:** 705–7.

55. Smith DM, Nance WE, Kang KW et al. Genetic factors in determining bone mass. *J Clin Invest* 1973; **52:** 2800–8.

56. Morrison NA, Qi JC, Tokita A et al. Prediction of bone density from vitamin D receptor alleles. *Nature* 1994; **367:** 284–7.

57. Hustmyer FG, Peacock M, Hui S et al. Bone mineral density in relation to polymorphism at the vitamin D receptor gene locus. *J Clin Invest* 1994; **94:** 2130–4.

58. Garnero P, Borel O, Sornay-Rendu E, Arlot ME, Delmas PD. Vitamin D receptor gene polymorphisms are not related to bone turnover, rate of bone loss, and bone mass in postmenopausal women: The OFELY study. *J Bone Miner Res* 1996; **11:** 827–34.

59. Johnston CC, Miller JZ, Slemenda CW et al. Calcium supplementation and increases in bone mineral density in children. *N Engl J Med* 1992; **327:** 82–7.

60. Heaney RP. Why does bone mass decrease with age and menopause? In: *Proceedings of the 4th International Symposium on Osteoporosis and Consensus Development Conference* (Christiansen C, ed.). Hong Kong, 1993; 15.

61. Parfitt AM. Age-related structural changes in trabecular and cortical bone: cellular mechanism and biomechanical consequences. a) Difference between rapid and slow bone loss. b) Localized bone gain. *Calcif Tissue Int* 1984; **36:** S123–8.

62. Parfitt AM. Trabecular bone architecture in the pathogenesis and prevention of fracture. *Am J Med* 1987; **82**(suppl 1B): 68–72.

63. Reid IR, Chin K, Evans MC et al. Relation between increase in length of hip axis in older women between 1950s and 1990s and increase in age specific rates of hip fracture. *BMJ* 1994; **309:** 508–9.

64. Faulkner KG, Cummings SR, Black D et al. Simple measurement of femoral geometry predicts hip fracture: the study of osteoporotic fractures. *J Bone Miner Res* 1993; **8:** 1211–17.

65. Heaney RP, Gallagher JC, Johnston CC et al. Calcium nutrition and bone health in the elderly. *Am J Clin Nutr* 1982; **36:** 986–1013.

66. Gennari C. Intestinal calcium transport and aging. In: *Proceedings of the 4th International Symposium on Osteoporosis and Consensus Development Conference* (Christiansen C, ed.). Hong Kong, 1993: 21.

67. Slovik DM, Adams JS, Neer RM et al. Deficient production of 1,25-dihydroxyvitamin D in elderly osteoporotic patients. *N Engl J Med* 1981; **305:** 372–4.

68. Nordin BEC, Horsman A, Marshall DH et al. Calcium requirement and calcium therapy. *Clin Orthop* 1979; **140:** 216–39.

69. Heaney RP, Recker RR, Saville PD. Menopausal changes in bone remodeling. *J Lab Clin Med* 1978; **92:** 964–70.

70. Matkovic V, Kostial K, Simonovic I et al. Bone status and fracture rates in two regions of Yugoslavia. *Am J Clin Nutr* 1979; **32:** 540–9.

71. Chapuy MC, Arlot ME, Duboeuf F et al. Vitamin D3 and calcium to prevent hip fractures in the elderly women. *N Engl J Med* 1992; **327:** 1637–42.

72. Newcomer AD, Hodgson SF, McGill DB et al. Lactase deficiency. Prevalence in osteoporosis. *Ann Intern Med* 1978; **89:** 218–20.

73. Trotter MI, Broman GE, Peterson RR. Densities of bones of white and negro skeletons. *J Bone Joint Surg [Am]* 1960; **42:** 50–8.

74. Bauer RL. Ethnic differences in hip fracture incidence in Bexar County. *Clin Res* 1986; **34:** 358A.

75. Cohn SH, Abesamis C, Yasumura S et al. Comparative skeletal mass and radial bone mineral content in black and white women. *Metabolism* 1977; **26:** 171–8.

76. Kelly PJ, Hopper JL, Macaskill GT et al. Genetic factors in bone turnover. *J Clin Endocrinol Metab* 1991; **72:** 808–13.

77. Morrison NA, Yeoman R, Kelly PJ et al. Contribution of transacting factor alleles to normal physiological variability: vitamin D receptor polymorphism and circulating osteocalcin. *Proc Natl Acad Sci USA* 1992; **89:** 6665–9.

78. Daniell HW. Osteoporosis of the slender smoker: Vertebral compression fractures and loss of metacarpal cortex in relation to postmenopausal cigarette smoking and lack of obesity. *Arch Intern Med* 1976; **136:** 298–304.

79. Seeman E, Melton LJ, O'Fallon WM et al. Risk factors for spinal osteoporosis in men. *Am J Med* 1983; **75:** 977–83.

80. Thompson K, Goltfredsen A, Christiansen C. Is postmenopausal bone loss an age-related phenomenon? *Calcif Tissue Int* 1986; **39:** 123–7.

81. Smith EL, Reddan W, Smith PE. Physical activity and calcium modalities for bone mineral increase in aged women. *Med Sci Sports Exerc* 1981; **13:** 60–4.

82. Aloia JF, Cohn SH, Ostuni JA et al. Prevention of involutional bone loss by exercise. *Ann Intern Med* 1978; **89:** 356–8.

83. Krolner B, Taft B, Nielsen PS et al. Physical exercise as prophylaxis against involutional vertebral bone loss: A controlled trial. *Clin Sci* 1983; **64:** 541–6.

84. Lindsay R, Hart DM, Aitken JM et al. Long-term prevention of postmenopausal osteoporosis by oestrogen: Evidence for an increased bone mass after delayed onset of oestrogen treatment. *Lancet* 1976; **i:** 1038–104.

85. Lindsay R, Hart DM, Forrest C et al. Prevention of spinal osteoporosis in oophorectomised women. *Lancet* 1980; **ii:** 1151–3.

86. Oursler MJ, Osdoby P, Pyfferoen J et al. Avian osteoclasts as estrogen target cells. *Proc Natl Acad Sci USA* 1991; **88:** 6613–17.

87. Jilka RL, Hangoc G, Girasole G et al. Increased osteoclast development after estrogen loss – mediation by interleukin-6. *Science* 1992; **257:** 88–91.

88. Hughes DE, Jilka R, Manolagas S et al. Sex steroids promote osteoclast apoptosis in vitro and in vivo. *J Bone Miner Res* 1995; **10**(suppl).

89. Pacifici R, Rifas L, Teitelbaum S et al. Spontaneous release of interleukin-1 from

human blood monocytes reflects bone formation in idiopathic osteoporosis. *Proc Natl Acad Sci USA* 1987; **84:** 4616–20.

90. Pacifici R, Rifas L, McCracken R et al. Ovarian steroid treatment blocks a postmenopausal increase in blood monocyte interleukin-1 release. *Proc Natl Acad Sci USA* 1989; **86:** 2398–402.

91. Pacifici R, Vannice JL, Rifas L et al. Monocytic secretion of interleukin-1 receptor antagonist in normal and osteoporotic women – effects of menopause and estrogen/progesterone therapy. *J Clin Endocrinol Metab* 1993; **77:** 1135–41.

92. Girasole G, Jilka RL, Passeri G et al. 17 beta-estradiol inhibits interleukin-6 production by bone marrow-derived stromal cells and osteoblasts in vitro – A potential mechanism for the anti-osteoporotic effect of estrogens. *J Clin Invest* 1992; **89:** 883–91.

93. Manolagas SC, Jilka RL. Mechanisms of disease: Bone marrow, cytokines, and bone remodeling – emerging insights into the pathophysiology of osteoporosis. *N Engl J Med* 1995; **332:** 305–11.

94. Oursler MJ. Osteoclast synthesis and secretion and activation of latent transforming growth factor β. *J Bone Miner Res* 1994; **9:** 443–52.

95. Spelsberg TC, Harris SA, Riggs BL. Immortalized osteoblast cell systems (new human fetal osteoblast systems). *Calcif Tissue Int* 1995; **56:** S18–21.

96. Riggs BL, Jowsey J, Kelly PJ et al. Studies on pathogenesis and treatment in postmenopausal and senile osteoporosis. *Clin Endocrinol Metab* 1973; **2:** 317–22.

97. Gallagher JC, Riggs BL, Jerpback CM et al. The effect of age on serum immunoreactive parathyroid hormone in normal and osteoporotic women. *J Lab Clin Med* 1980; **95:** 373–85.

98. Harms HM, Kaptaina U, Kulpmann WR et al. Pulse amplitude and frequency modulation of parathyroid hormone in plasma. *J Clin Endocrinol Metab* 1989; **69:** 843–51.

99. Kitamura N, Shigeno C, Shiomi K et al. Episodic fluctuation in serum intact parathyroid hormone concentration in men. *J Clin Endocrinol Metab* 1990; **70:** 252–63.

100. Samuels MH, Veldhuis J, Cawley C et al. Pulsatile secretion of parathyroid hormone in normal young subjects: Assessment by deconvolution analysis. *J Clin Endocrinol Metab* 1993; **77:** 399–403.

101. Samuels MH, Veldhuis J, Cawley C et al. Pulsatile secretion of parathyroid hormone in normal young subjects: Assessment by deconvolution analysis. *J Clin Endocrinol Metab* 1997: in press.

102. Gallagher JC, Riggs BL, Eisman J et al. Intestinal calcium absorption and serum vitamin D metabolites in normal subjects and osteoporotic patients: Effect of age and dietary calcium. *J Clin Invest* 1979; **64:** 729–36.

103. Tsai K-S, Heath H III, Kumar R et al. Impaired vitamin D metabolism with aging in women: Possible role in pathogenesis of senile osteoporosis. *J Clin Invest* 1984; **73:** 1668–72.

104. Armbrecht HJ, Zenser TV, Davis BB. Effect of age on the conversion of 25-hydroxyvitamin D₃ to 1,25-dihydroxyvitamin D₃ by kidney of rat. *J Clin Invest* 1980; **66:** 1118–23.

105. Cummings SR, Black DM, Nevitt MC et al. Bone density at various sites for prediction of hip fractures. *Lancet* 1993; **341:** 72–5.

106. Heath H III, Sizemore GW. Plasma calcitonin in normal man: Differences between men and women. *J Clin Invest* 1977; **60:** 1135–40.

107. Deftos IJ, Weisman MH, Williams GW et al. Influence of age and sex on plasma calcitonin in human beings. *N Engl J Med* 1980; **302:** 1351–3.

108. Body JJ, Health H III. Estimates of circulating monomeric calcitonin: Physiological studies in normal and thyroidectomized man. *J Clin Endocrinol Metab* 1983; **57:** 897–903.

3

Contributions of bone mass measurements by densitometry in the definition and diagnosis of osteoporosis

M Jergas and HK Genant

CONTENTS • Defining osteoporosis • Which fractures are osteoporotic? • Association between low bone density and fractures • Diagnosing osteoporosis with quantitative ultrasonography • Other predictors of fracture • Diagnosing osteoporosis • Summary and conclusion

DEFINING OSTEOPOROSIS

The term 'osteoporosis' is derived from the Greek language: *osteon* means bone, and *poros* is a small hole. Thus, the term 'osteoporosis' is quite descriptive of the changes in bone tissue that can be observed in this generalized skeletal disease. Nevertheless, the definition of osteoporosis has changed through the years, mostly based on new evidence or new techniques that have become available for its diagnosis. Today, there is a tendency to define osteoporosis by means of quantitative determination of bone mineral density, or bone densitometry. Bone densitometry has played a major role as a means of objective measurement of what radiologists describe subjectively as changes in the radiolucency of the skeleton on conventional radiographs. The current importance of bone densitometry in the clinical diagnosis of osteoporosis is reflected in the definition of osteoporosis given by the Consensus Development Conference 1993, sponsored by the European Foundation for Osteoporosis and Bone Disease, the National Osteoporosis Foundation and the National Institute of Arthritis and Musculoskeletal and Skin Disease:[1]

Osteoporosis is a systemic skeletal disease characterized by low bone mass and microarchitectural deterioration of bone tissue, with a consequent increase in bone fragility and susceptibility to fracture.

The availability of a technique, i.e. bone densitometry in its various applications, clearly finds its expression in many definitions of osteoporosis that are based entirely on bone density; for example, Melton and Wahner[2] proposed a definition of osteoporosis based on it. These authors defined *clinical* osteoporosis as the presence of fractures resulting from minor trauma and simultaneous low bone density below a 'fracture threshold'. The clinical consequences of such a finding would be to start treatment for osteoporosis. The state of low bone density that goes along with a doubling or tripling of the risk for a fracture is defined as osteopenia, and represents an indication for starting prophylactic treatment. The World Health Organization Working Group carried out this approach in its definition of the osteoporosis, which was published in 1994.[3–5] In women osteoporosis can be diagnosed if the

Table 3.1 Diagnostic categories for osteoporosis based on bone density measurements as proposed by Kanis et al[6]

Category	Definition by bone density
Normal	A value for bone mineral density or bone mineral content that is not more than 1 s.d. below the young adult mean value
Low bone mass (or osteopenia)	A value for bone mineral density or bone mineral content that lies between 1 and 2.5 s.d. below the young adult mean value
Osteoporosis	A value for bone mineral density or bone mineral content that is more than 2.5 s.d. below the young adult mean value
Severe osteoporosis (or established osteoporosis)	A value for bone mineral density or bone mineral content more than 2.5 s.d. below the young adult mean value in the presence of one or more fragility fractures

value for bone mineral density (BMD) or bone mineral content (BMC) is 2.5 or more standard deviations below the mean value of a young reference population (*t*-score ≤ -2.5 standard deviations). Kanis and co-workers commented on this definition and gave diagnostic categories that may be applied to white women (Table 3.1).[6]

Thus, today's diagnosis of osteoporosis relies mainly on bone mass measurements. The essential task of bone densitometry in a clinical setting is to identify patients at risk for osteoporotic fractures. Therefore, the association between bone mass and future fractures must be established, and various researchers have studied this association in a prospective fashion.

WHICH FRACTURES ARE OSTEOPOROTIC?

Fractures are the hallmark of osteoporosis, and they often have a substantial impact on a patient's life. There is unanimous agreement that most fractures of the hip, wrist and vertebral body, with no occurrence of trauma, may be attributed to osteoporosis.[7] However, there are a number of other fractures occurring in the

elderly person which may be related to osteoporosis (Figure 3.1).[8] Not all fractures in elderly people are, however, associated with low bone density. In the setting of a large prospective study on the various aspects of osteoporosis in the ageing female population, the 'Study of osteoporotic fractures', Seeley et al[9] studied the relationship between bone mass and a variety of fractures. The authors found that risks for fractures of the wrist, foot, humerus, hip, rib, toe, leg, pelvis, hand and clavicle were significantly related to reduced bone mass at the distal and proximal radius as well as the calcaneus (Figure 3.2).[9] On the other hand, fractures of the ankle, elbow, finger and face were not associated with bone density at any measurement site. Thus, low bone density is associated with most types of fractures in elderly people. Few other studies offer such a detailed review of various fracture sites.

ASSOCIATION BETWEEN LOW BONE DENSITY AND FRACTURES

The first prospective studies to evaluate the association between bone density and fractures were published as early as 1975. Smith and

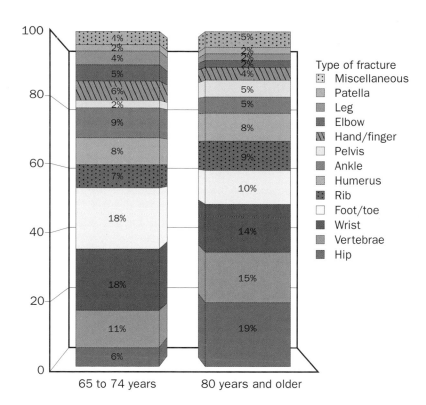

Figure 3.1 Frequency (as percentages) of fracture by type in white women aged 65–74 years, and aged 80 years and older from the 'Study of osteoporotic fractures' 1986–92. Data from Nevitt.[8]

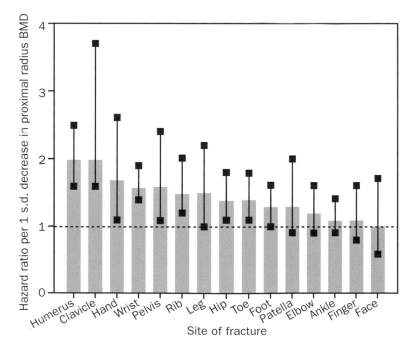

Figure 3.2 Age-adjusted hazard ratios (and 95% confidence interval) of various fractures for a 1 standard deviation decrease in proximal radius bone density. Data from Seeley et al.[9]

co-workers followed 278 women out of an initial study population of 571 white women aged 50 or above who had bone density measurements made of the radius at baseline.[10] After a mean follow-up time of 1.7 years, 31 women had fractures. For both distal and proximal sites at the radius, bone mass was inversely related to fracture incidence. A second study from the same group also used Singh's index of femoral trabecular pattern in addition to radius bone mass for fracture prediction in 106 white women, aged 70–95 years who were residents of a nursing home.[11] Fractures occurred in 29 women after a mean follow-up period of 2.5 years. The authors again noted an association between bone mass at the radius and incident fractures whereas they did not find any correlation between Singh's index and subsequent fracture. The latter observation for Singh's index is probably the result of the difficult assessment of this index.

After these first prospective studies on fracture risk, a number of researchers studied the association between bone density and fracture risk. The aforementioned 'Study of osteoporotic fractures' is probably the largest and most ambitious of a number of epidemiological studies, involving more than 9000 non-black women in four different regions of the USA. What makes it difficult to compare the results from the different epidemiological studies is the way the data were acquired and analysed. Often, Cox's proportional hazards model, or logistic regression analyses with a variety of predictors included in the models, are employed. There are also considerable differences in the populations studied as well as the length of the follow-up period. Table 3.2 lists some characteristics and results of prospective studies for prediction of osteoporotic fractures using bone densitometry. The risk ratios and odds ratios were taken directly from the respective publications.

Single photon (and X-ray) absorptiometry (SPA, SXA) as well as dual photon (and X-ray) absorptiometry (DPA, DXA) have been the most commonly used techniques for assessing bone mass in the context of epidemiological studies. Almost all measures derived from these techniques – bone mineral content (BMC), bone mineral density (BMD) and bone mineral apparent density (BMAD) – have been found to be associated with most types of fractures, especially in women (Table 3.2).[12,13,15–30] In a meta-analysis of prospective studies involving bone densitometry, Marshall and co-workers[31] demonstrated that bone density measurements at the specific site of fracture tend to be slightly superior in predicting fractures at the respective site to bone density measurements at other sites (Figure 3.3), for example, a hip fracture is best predicted by hip bone density. However, what seems to hold true for the hip fracture does not seem to hold true for other sites and appendicular fractures, and Black et al[22] found that measurements of the radius, calcaneus, hip and lumbar spine all provided similar predictive capability of a woman's subsequent risk of wrist fracture.[22] Overall, the different techniques and sites of measurement do not differ considerably in their ability to predict future fracture, and the question of whether one technique is significantly better than others remains controversial.

There are few prospective data for quantitative computed tomography (QCT), even though this method has been applied widely in clinical practice since the early 1980s.[32] Ross and colleagues examined the vertebral fracture incidence in 380 women participating in a pharmaceutical trial, of whom 294 had an axial QCT measurement at baseline as well as DPA measurements of the spine and the femur.[18] Over an average 2.9 years' follow-up time, 47 women experienced new vertebral fractures and 28 women had 'repeat' fractures in previously fractured vertebrae. For women with repeat fractures, rate ratios were higher for QCT measurements than for spinal or femoral DPA, whereas spinal and femoral DPA predicted new (incident) vertebral fractures somewhat better. There was also a strong association of incident vertebral fractures with prevalent fractures. The authors also found that the simultaneous use of two predictors (either two bone density measurements or bone density and prevalent fracture) improved fracture prediction. The latter study is the only published prospective study including QCT measure-

Table 3.2 Summary details from selected prospective studies of bone density and fracture risk

Study	Study population	Time of follow-up (years)	Site/type of fracture (number of patients)	Site/type of measurement	Model/adjustment	Odds/risk ratio
Melton et al[12]	304 women aged 30–94 years	7.8	Spine (mild to moderate trauma; $n < 48$)	BMD spine BMD femoral neck BMD trochanter BMD distal radius BMD midradius	Age adjusted	2.2 (1.4–3.4) 2.0 (1.3–3.1) 1.7 (1.1–2.6) 1.6 (1.0–2.5) 2.5 (1.5–4.2)
			Proximal femur (mild to moderate trauma; $n < 10$)	BMD spine BMD femoral neck BMD trochanter BMD distal radius BMD midradius	Age adjusted	2.3 (1.0–5.4) 2.8 (1.4–5.8) 2.4 (1.1–5.2) 3.1 (1.2–7.8) 1.5 (0.6–3.6)
			Distal forearm (mild to moderate trauma; $n < 15$)	BMD spine BMD femoral neck BMD trochanter BMD distal radius BMD midradius	Age adjusted	1.4 (0.8–2.7) 1.5 (0.8–2.8) 1.6 (0.9–2.8) 2.3 (1.1–4.6) 1.5 (0.7–3.2)
			All sites (mild to moderate trauma; $n < 125$)	BMD spine BMD femoral neck BMD trochanter BMD distal radius BMD midradius	Age adjusted	1.5 (1.1–2.0) 1.6 (1.2–2.2) 1.5 (1.1–1.9) 1.4 (1.0–1.9) 1.5 (1.1–2.1)
Stegman et al[13]	131 Roman Catholic nuns	24	All sites ($n < 31$)	BMC radius	Adjusted for age and effective time postmenopausal	1.7 (1.1–2.6)[a] 1.9 (1.1–3.3)[b]
Hui et al[14]	386 free living white women	6.7	Forearm ($n = 7$) All sites ($n = 35$)	BMC radius	Age adjusted	3.6 (1.9–6.8) 2.6 (2.0–3.4)
	135 white women living in retirement home	5.5	Forearm ($n = 10$) Hip ($n = 30$) All sites ($n = 54$)			1.2 (0.7–2.2) 1.9 (1.4–2.7) 1.5 (1.2–2.0)
Hui et al[15]	386 free living white women	6.7	All sites ($n = 35$)	BMC radius BMD radius BMAD radius	Unadjusted	3.1 3.2 3.4
	135 white women living in retirement home	5.5	All sites ($n = 54$)	BMC radius BMD radius BMAD radius		1.7 1.7 1.6
Wasnich et al[16]	699 Japanese American women aged 43–80 years	3.6	Spine ($n = 39$)	BMD calcaneus BMD distal radius BMD spine	Age adjusted; risks calculated for 2 s.d. difference	6.9 (4.3–10.6) 5.7 (3.6–8.7) 3.9 (2.4–6.2)
Ross et al[17]	897 postmenopausal women	>4	Spine ($n = 61$)	BMD distal radius BMD proximal radius BMD calcaneus BMD spine	Age adjusted; risks calculated for 2 s.d. difference	3.6 (2.2–6.8) 4.0 (2.3–7.3) 5.8 (3.2–10.5) 5.0 (2.8–9.1)
Ross et al[18]	380 women in clinical trial (294 with baseline QCT measurements)	2.9	All spine fractures (repeat and new; ($n = 57$)	QCT spine BMD (DPA) spine BMD femoral neck BMD Ward's area BMD trochanter	Age adjusted; risks calculated for 2 s.d. difference	5.1 (2.8–9.1) 3.6 (2.0–6.6) 2.8 (1.4–5.6) 3.9 (2.0–7.3) 4.8 (2.6–8.8)
			New spine fracture ($n = 47$)	QCT spine BMD (DPA) spine BMD femoral neck BMD Ward's area BMD trochanter		4.8 (2.5–9.1) 5.8 (2.9–11.6) 5.2 (2.2–12.4) 3.8 (1.9–7.5) 5.3 (2.7–10.3)
Gärdsell et al[19]	1076 women	13	Distal radius ($n = 66$)	BMD distal radius BMD midradius	Age adjusted	1.5 1.7
			Proximal humerus ($n = 35$)	BMD distal radius BMD midradius		1.9 1.7
			Hip, cervical ($n = 28$)	BMD distal radius BMD midradius		1.9 2.5

Table 3.2 Continued

Study	Study population	Time of follow-up (years)	Site/type of fracture (number of patients)	Site/type of measurement	Model/adjustment	Odds/risk ratio
			Hip, trochanter (*n* = 17)	BMD distal radius		2.7
				BMD midradius		3.4
			All hip (*n* = 43)	BMD distal radius		2.5
				BMD midradius		3.2
			Spine (*n* = 70)	BMD distal radius		1.7
				BMD midradius		2.6
Gärdsell et al[20]	654 men from various studies	11 (*n* = 61)	Fragility fracture	BMD radius	Unadjusted; risk ratio for lowest vs highest quintile	13
Cummings et al[21]	8134 non-black women aged 65 and above	1.8	Hip (*n* = 65)	BMD total femur	Age adjusted	2.7 (2.0–3.6)
				BMD femoral neck		2.6 (1.9–3.6)
				BMD intertrochanteric		2.5 (1.9–3.3)
				BMD trochanter		2.7 (2.0–3.6)
				BMD Ward's area		2.8 (2.1–3.6)
				BMD spine		1.6 (1.2–2.1)
				BMD distal radius		1.6 (1.2–2.1)
				BMD proximal radius		1.5 (1.2–1.9)
				BMD calcaneus		2.0 (1.5–2.7)
Black et al[22]	8134 non-black women aged 65 and above	0.1–1.9 (0.7)	All sites (*n* = 191)	BMD total femur	Age adjusted	1.4 (1.2–1.6)
				BMD femoral neck		1.4 (1.2–1.7)
				BMD intertrochanteric		1.4 (1.2–1.7)
				BMD trochanter		1.4 (1.2–1.6)
				BMD Ward's area		1.4 (1.2–1.6)
				BMD spine		1.4 (1.2–1.6)
				BMD distal radius		1.5 (1.3–1.8)
				BMD proximal radius		1.4 (1.2–1.7)
				BMD calcaneus		1.3 (1.1–1.5)
			Wrist (*n* = 37)	BMD total femur	Age adjusted	1.5 (1.1–2.1)
				BMD femoral neck		1.7 (1.1–2.4)
				BMD intertrochanteric		1.3 (0.9–1.9)
				BMD trochanter		1.5 (1.1–2.1)
				BMD Ward's area		1.4 (1.0–2.0)
				BMD spine		1.6 (1.1–2.3)
				BMD distal radius		1.8 (1.3–2.6)
				BMD proximal radius		1.6 (1.1–2.4)
				BMD calcaneus		1.8 (1.3–2.6)
Black et al[23]	Random sample of 501 women from the 'Study of osteoporotic fractures'	3.7	Spine (*n* = 22)	BMD distal radius	Age adjusted	1.8 (1.1–3.1)
				BMD proximal radius		1.6 (1.0–2.6)
				BMD calcaneus		2.7 (1.5–4.7)
Seeley et al[24]	9704 non-black women aged 65 and above	5.9	Ankle (*n* = 191)	BMD distal radius	Age adjusted	1.1 (1.0–1.3)
					multivariable	1.2 (1.0–1.4)
			Foot (*n* = 204)		Age-adjusted	1.3 (1.1–1.5)
					multivariable	1.3 (1.1–1.5)
Nguyen et al[25]	1080 women aged 60 and above	3.2	All atraumatic fractures (*n* = 192)	BMD femoral neck	Adjusted for quadriceps strength and body sway	2.4 (1.9–3.0)
	709 men aged 60 and above	3.2	All atraumatic fractures (*n* = 89)	BMD femoral neck	Adjusted for quadriceps strength and body sway	2.0 (1.5–2.6)

Table 3.2 Continued

Study	Study population	Time of follow-up (years)	Site/type of fracture (number of patients)	Site/type of measurement	Model/adjustment	Odds/risk ratio
Cheng et al[26]	188 women aged 75 years 133 women aged 80 years 103 men aged 75 years 57 men aged 80 years	29–34 months	Non-spine fractures in seventeen 75 year olds, ten 80 year olds Non-spine fractures in three 75 year olds, six 80 year olds	BMD calcaneus BMD calcaneus	75 year olds 80 year olds 75 and 80 year olds	3.4 (1.4–8.1) 1.3 (0.2–5.9) 3.6 (1.2–14.9)
Torgerson et al[27]	1857 women aged 47–51 years	2	Self-reported non-spine and non-hip fractures (n = 44)	BMD spine BMD femoral neck BMD Ward's area BMD trochanter BMD spine	Unadjusted Multivariate analysis	1.9 (1.3–2.6) 1.1 (1.0–2.8) 1.4 (1.0–1.9) 1.1 (0.8–1.5) 1.6 (1.2–2.3)

[a] Odds ratio for prospective study design. [b] Odds ratio for retrospective study design.
Odds or risk ratios were taken directly from the articles.
Abbreviations: BMC, bone mineral content; BMD, bone mineral density; BMAD, bone mineral apparent density.
For the study by Stegman et al[13] odds ratios are given for a prospective and a retrospective study design.

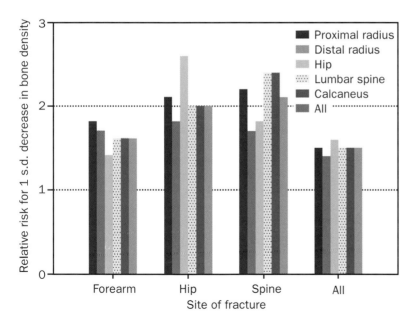

Figure 3.3 Relative risk of fracture for a 1 standard deviation decrease in bone density below the age-adjusted mean from the summary of a meta-analysis of prospective studies.[31] The results are given for various fracture sites as well as various sites of bone density measurements.

ments at baseline. However, there are many cross-sectional studies investigating the association between bone density and vertebral fracture either only for QCT, or for QCT in comparison to other modalities. Most of these studies show a superior diagnostic capability of QCT with respect to discriminating patients with fractures from those without.[33–39] A recent cross-sectional study by Ito and colleagues,[40] however, showed that QCT trabecular bone

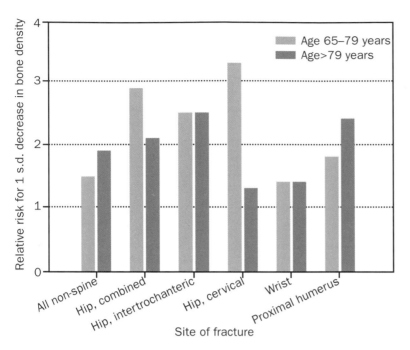

Figure 3.4 Relative risk of various fractures for a 1 standard deviation decrease in femoral neck bone densities in women aged 65–79 years, and 80 years and over. Data are derived from a prospective study involving 8699 women who were followed for an average of 4.9 years.[41]

density was not superior to projectional bone density measurements of the calcaneus and the ultradistal forearm in the oldest study participants, aged 70–79 years, whereas in younger study participants QCT provided the best discrimination between women with and without fractures.[40] This observation has to be confirmed in further studies.

As a vast number of retrospective, or cross-sectional, studies on bone density measurements exist, an important question is whether cross-sectional study designs are valid for the evaluation of bone densitometry techniques and for the assessment of fracture risk. Stegman et al[13] compared prospective and retrospective study designs for assessing fracture risk within a 24-year cohort study. They found that the estimates of relative risk of low-trauma fracture determined from a cohort study, and the odds ratio determined from a nested case-control study within the cohort, did not differ substantially. For each one decrement of Z-scores of forearm BMC, the adjusted relative risk ratio

for the prospective study design was 1.67, whereas the odds ratio determined from the most recent BMC Z-score measurements was 1.87. Thus, these two measures from prospective and retrospective study designs are similar, and the experience from several prospective and retrospective studies indicates that the results from these two types of studies may be comparable if carefully designed.[31] Nevertheless, prospective studies will probably be required, especially when new techniques are evaluated and risk factors other than, and in addition to, bone density are assessed.

Based on results from some prospective studies, the value of bone densitometry for fracture prediction in very old patients has been questioned. In a prospective study by Gärdsell and co-workers,[19] the authors found that BMC measured at the radius was associated with subsequent fractures in women aged 50–79 years, but fractures of the radius and the humerus as well as femoral neck fractures did not show the same strong association with BMD as women aged 80 years or older as in the younger study population. In the same study vertebral fractures showed a clear association with bone density at all ages. Similar results were reported by Hui et al[14] who studied elderly residents at a retirement home and a group of free living women (Table 3.2). Nevitt and colleagues[41] studied the predictive value of bone mass in a larger group of women from the 'Study of osteoporotic fractures', and some results are shown in Figure 3.4. The authors found that, for non-spine fractures, and wrist and humerus fractures, a strong association with bone density existed. Fractures of the proximal femur were associated with bone density in all women. However, only trochanteric but not femoral neck fractures were associated with bone density in the oldest women. These results indicate that femoral neck fractures may be associated with factors other than bone density in elderly women and that efforts to maintain bone mass after the age of 80 may reduce the risk of trochanteric, but not of femoral neck, fractures. Another important result from this study was that the excess risk of fracture of women with below-median bone density was greater in women aged 80 years and over compared with younger women. The study of Nevitt et al clearly demonstrates that bone density continues to be strongly associated with overall fracture risk in women aged 80 and over. Nevertheless, one must be aware that some limitations may exist for bone densitometry in the prediction of certain types of fracture in elderly patients.

Looking at the average follow-up period of the various studies on bone densitometry, bone mass is significantly associated with incident fracture even in the studies with the longest follow-up period of 24 years.[13] The fact that bone density is a predictor of fractures over such a long period of time may be an argument for the importance of peak bone mass for future fracture. Hansen et al[42] found, in a 12-year prospective study, that radial bone density was associated with future Colles' fractures, but it failed to predict vertebral fractures. They found that an increased rate of bone loss existed in patients who later had vertebral fractures. From these results it was concluded that a baseline scan, combined with a single estimation of bone loss, may identify women at risk for developing osteoporotic fracture. Both peak bone mass and bone loss resulting in a low bone mass may be important predictors of future fractures. However, the current evidence from other studies also suggests that the influence of initial bone mass on current bone mass and fracture risk is greater than that of bone loss in women up to the age of 70 years.[14,19,30,43] It is estimated that, 12 years after the menopause, about 30% of the variance in density measurements may be explained on the basis of differential bone loss rates. There is, however, evidence that knowledge about bone loss will improve the estimate of ultimate bone density.

DIAGNOSING OSTEOPOROSIS WITH QUANTITATIVE ULTRASONOGRAPHY

Quantitative ultrasonography (QUS) is one of the latest additions to the diagnostic toolbox of osteoporosis. This method, applied in the form of speed of sound (SOS) measurements, as well as broadband ultrasound attenuation (BUA) measurements, has been used in industrial materials testing for a long time. The evolution in microelectronics made the easy application of QUS to the diagnosis of osteoporosis possible. Quantitative ultrasonography is a radiation-free method and, thus, researchers as well as clinicians have embraced this technology enthusiastically, as indicated by the large number of studies published recently. It is also not a simple measure of bone density, but rather a measure of other qualitative properties of the bone. Clinical studies show that QUS measures often correlate poorly with bone density measures at various sites. Several researchers have studied the association between QUS measures and osteoporotic fractures, and some ongoing epidemiological studies on osteoporosis have included this method in their protocols. Most results that exist on this association are still derived from cross-sectional studies. Table 3.3 lists published prospective studies focusing on QUS measurements. The earliest prospective

Table 3.3 Summary details of prospective studies of quantitative ultrasonography and fracture risk

Study	Study population	Time of follow-up (years)	Site/type of fracture (number of patients)	Site/type of measurement	Model/adjustment	Odds/risk ratio
Porter et al[44]	1414 women aged 70 and above	2	Hip (n = 73)	BUA calcaneus	Combinations with cognisance and mobility	Not given
Heaney et al[45]	130 postmenopausal women, no vertebral fracture	2	Spine (n = 19)	SOS patella	None	2.4 (1.3–4.3)
					Age adjusted	2.1 (1.1–3.9)
Hans et al[46]	5662 women aged 75 or above	2	Hip (n = 115)	BUA calcaneus	Unadjusted	2.1 (1.7–2.6)
				SOS calcaneus		1.9 (1.5–2.3)
				BMD femoral neck		2.1 (1.7–2.5)
				BUA calcaneus	Adjusted for age, weight and centre	2.0 (1.6–2.4)
				SOS calcaneus		1.7 (1.4–2.1)
				BMD femoral neck		1.9 (1.6–2.4)
				BUA calcaneus	Adjusted for age, weight and centre and including all BUA, SOS and femoral neck BMD in the model	1.7 (1.3–2.2)
				SOS calcaneus		1.1 (0.6–1.4)
				BMD femur		1.8 (1.5–2.3)

Abbreviations: BUA, broadband ultrasound attenuation; SOS, speed of sound; BMD, bone mineral density.

study on QUS was published in 1990 by Porter and colleagues.[44] They measured BUA in 1414 women aged 70 or above, who were living in private or local authority homes for elderly people or in geriatric hospitals. Seventy-three women subsequently fractured a hip during the follow-up period of 2 years. Women with a low BUA score and poor cognisance had a higher incidence of fracture than those with a high BUA score and good cognisance who were less mobile. These factors were partly independent. Heaney and colleagues[45] reported on ultrasonic transmission velocity measurements at the patella in 130 postmenopausal women who were free of vertebral fracture at baseline and followed over 2 years. Of these women, 19 developed fractures, and age-adjusted relative risk for the ultrasonic measurement was 2.1. Neither study considered bone density measurements. Hans and co-workers[46] studied prospectively the association of QUS, both BUA and ultrasonic transmission velocity at the heel, and hip fracture in 5662 women from the French EPIDOS study. During the average follow-up period of 2 years, 115 new hip fractures occurred in the study population. The relative risks of hip fracture were 2.0 and 1.7 per 1 standard deviation reduction in BUA and ultrasonic transmission velocity, respectively, as compared with a relative risk of 1.9 per 1 standard deviation reduction in femoral neck bone density. After inclusion of femoral neck density into a multivariate model, the ultrasonic variables remained predictive of hip fracture.

There are a number of retrospective studies worth mentioning because they represent further evidence of the diagnostic capability of QUS (Table 3.4). Bauer and co-workers[50] studied BUA as well as bone density measurements of the hip, spine and the whole body in 442 women enrolling in a clinical trial. After adjusting for age, weight and clinic, the relative risk for vertebral fracture was 1.8 (95% confidence interval or CI = 1.4–2.3) for each standard deviation reduction in BUA; for each standard deviation reduction in bone density, the relative risk was 1.7 at the femoral neck and 2.2 at the spine. Adjustment for spine, hip or whole body BMD did not significantly alter the association

between BUA and vertebral fracture. Glüer and co-workers[51] recently published a cross-sectional study on 4698 women from the 'Study of osteoporotic fractures' population who had received BUA measurements at the heel as well as BMD measurements at the spine, hip and calcaneus. In a multivariate logistic regression analysis, age, BUA and BMD of the calcaneus were independently associated with hip fractures, vertebral fractures at study baseline and recent vertebral fractures. The combination of femoral neck density and BUA showed only marginal improvement in the receiver operating characteristics (ROC) area. Further results from a number of retrospective studies are given in Table 3.4.[47–49,51–53]

OTHER PREDICTORS OF FRACTURE

The association between geometric properties of bone and biomechanical properties, such as that between the cross-sectional area and the fracture load in vertebrae or that of the minimum of the moment of inertia, the cross-sectional area and forearm fracture force, is known from in vitro studies. An early technique for assessing skeletal status, the measurement of the cortical thickness, represents a measurement of a geometric property of bone. Cortical thickness has been found to be related to age and bone density.[55–57] Several cross-sectional studies show an association between cortical thickness measures and prevalent fractures. A prospective, nested, case-control study for the prediction of hip fracture using metacarpal thickness was presented by Jergas and co-workers[58] for the 'Study of osteoporotic fracture' research group. The combined cortical thickness and the cortical index provided a predictive capability (odds ratios between 1.7 and 2.2 per standard deviation decrease) similar to that of bone density measurements at the calcaneus and the radius (odds ratios between 1.8 and 2.0).

Even though cortical thickness may be regarded as an architectural property of bone, it certainly reflects bone density and, thus, one may not necessarily expect cortical thickness to

Table 3.4 Summary details of selected retrospective (cross-sectional) studies of quantitative ultrasonography and fracture risk

Study	Study population	Site/type of fracture (number of patients)	Site/type of measurement	Model/adjustment	Odds/risk ratio
Stegman et al[47]	809 women aged 50 and above	Low trauma fracture after age 40 ($n = 204$)	SOS patella BMD radius BMD ulna	Age adjusted	1.5 (1.2–1.9) 1.6 (1.3–2.0) 1.8 (1.5–2.3)
		All fractures after age 40 ($n = 314$)	SOS patella BMD radius BMD ulna	Age adjusted	1.2 (1.0–1.5) 1.5 (1.2–1.8) 1.6 (1.3–1.9)
	498 men aged 50 and above	Low trauma fracture after age 40 ($n = 44$)	SOS patella BMD radius BMD ulna	Age adjusted	1.6 (1.1–2.3) 1.7 (1.2–2.4) 1.9 (1.3–2.7)
		All fractures after age 40 ($n = 163$)	SOS patella BMD radius BMD ulna	Age adjusted	1.7 (1.3–2.1) 1.5 (1.2–1.9) 1.5 (1.2–1.9)
Stegman et al[48]	874 women aged 50 and above	Spine ($n = 201$)	SOS patella	Age adjusted	1.2 (1.0–1.5)
	522 men aged 50 or above	Spine ($n = 182$)	SOS patella	Age and bone mass not significant in logistic regression model	1.3 (1.1–1.5)
Stewart et al[49]	50 women with recent hip fracture, 50 age-matched controls	Hip ($n = 50$)	BUA calcaneus	Authors performed ROC analyses	No results given for logistic regression analyses
Bauer et al[50]	442 women aged 55–80 enrolled in a	Spine ($n = 131$) BUA calcaneus	BUA calcaneus	Unadjusted Adjusted for age, weight and clinic	1.6 (1.3–2.1) 1.8 (1.4–2.3)
			BUA calcaneus	Adjusted for age, weight, clinic and femoral neck BMD	1.6 (1.2–2.1)
			BUA calcaneus	Adjusted for age, weight, clinic and spine BMD	1.5 (1.1–2.0)
			BUA calcaneus	Adjusted for age, weight, clinic and whole body BMD	1.6 (1.2–2.1)
			BMD femoral neck	Adjusted for age, weight and clinic	1.7 (1.3–2.1)
			BMD femoral neck	Adjusted for age, weight, clinic and BUA	1.5 (1.2–1.9)
			BMD spine	Adjusted for age, weight and clinic	2.2 (1.7–2.9)
			BMD spine	Adjusted for age, weight, clinic and BUA	2.0 (1.5–2.6)
			BMD whole body	Adjusted for age, weight and clinic	1.9 (1.5–2.3)
			BMD whole body	Adjusted for age, weight, clinic and BUA	1.5 (1.1–2.1)
Turner et al[51]	Baseline measurements in 336 women aged 60 or older enrolled in a clinical trial	Spine at baseline ($n = 22$) History of hip fracture after age 58 ($n = 22$)	BUA calcaneus SOS calcaneus BMD spine	Authors performed ROC analyses	No results given for logistic regression analyses
Schott et al[52]	43 women with recent hip fracture and 86 age-matched controls	Hip ($n = 43$)	BUA calcaneus SOS calcaneus BMD femoral neck	Adjusted for height and weight	3.7 (2.0–6.6) 2.7 (1.7–4.5) 2.3 (1.4–3.7)

Table 3.4 Continued

Study	Study population	Site/type of fracture (number of patients)	Site/type of measurement	Model/adjustment	Odds/risk ratio
Gonnelli et al[53]	304 white women	Spine (*n* = 225)	BUA calcaneus	Unadjusted	3.1
				Adjusted for BMD	2.0
			SOS calcaneus	Unadjusted	4.6
				Adjusted for BMD	2.3
			BMD spine	Unadjusted	6.5
Glüer et al[54]	4798 women aged 65 and older from the 'Study of osteoporotic fractures'	Spine at baseline (*n* = 812)	BUA calcaneus	Adjusted for age, centre and equipment	1.5 (1.4–1.6)
			BMD spine		1.5 (1.4–1.6)
			BMD calcaneus		1.5 (1.4–1.6)
			BMD femoral neck		1.7 (1.5–1.8)
		Recent vertebral fractures (*n* = 168)	BUA calcaneus		1.7 (1.4–2.1)
			BMD spine		1.9 (1.6–2.3)
			BMD calcaneus		1.8 (1.5–2.1)
			BMD femoral neck		2.0 (1.6–2.4)
		Hip (*n* = 106)	BUA calcaneus		1.9 (1.5–2.4)
			BMD spine		1.5 (1.2–1.9)
			BMD calcaneus		1.9 (1.5–2.4)
			BMD femoral neck		2.6 (2.0–3.4)
		All fractures (*n* = 1550)	BUA calcaneus		1.5 (1.4–1.6)
			BMD spine		1.4 (1.3–1.5)
			BMD calcaneus		1.5 (1.4–1.6)
			BMD femoral neck		1.6 (1.5–1.7)
	Subgroup of 1571 women	Vertebral fracture at study baseline (*n* = 259)	BUA calcaneus	Adjusted for age, centre and equipment	1.5 (1.3–1.7)
			SOS calcaneus		1.6 (1.3–1.9)
		Recent vertebral fractures (*n* = 43)	BUA calcaneus		2.3 (1.6–3.5)
			SOS calcaneus		2.3 (1.5–3.5)
		Hip (*n* = 34)	BUA calcaneus		1.4 (1.0–2.1)
			SOS calcaneus		1.6 (1.0–2.4)
		All fractures (*n* = 477)	BUA calcaneus		1.4 (1.2–1.6)
			SOS calcaneus		1.4 (1.2–1.6)

Abbreviations: BUA, broadband ultrasound attenuation; SOS, speed of sound; BMD, bone mineral density.

be predictive of a particular type of fracture. However, there are architectural bone properties specific for a type of fracture. Hip axis length is probably the geometric measure that has received the most attention as indicated by a number of recent cross-sectional and prospective studies. It can be measured on radiographs and on DXA images – on the latter using a highly reproducible automated procedure.[59] Hip axis length is associated with hip fracture risk independent of age, height, weight and femoral bone density. In a prospective, nested, case-control study of 64 women with hip fracture and a random sample of 134 women from the 'Study of osteoporotic fractures', Faulkner and colleagues[60] found that each standard deviation increase in hip axis length nearly doubled the risk of hip fracture (odds ratio = 1.8; CI = 1.3–2.5). It is not associated with age and not predictive of fractures other than hip fractures.[61,62] Measuring a number of different geometric parameters from hip radiographs, Glüer et al[63] found that four measurements independently predicted hip fracture: reduced thickness of the femoral shaft cortex and of the femoral neck cortex, reduction in an index of tensile trabeculae, and a wider trochanteric region. Two analyses by Nakamura et al[64] and Cummings et al[65] indicate that differences in geometric measures, including hip axis length, may explain differences in the rates of hip fracture of white, Asian and black women. Based on hip axis length, Cummings and colleagues[65] estimated that Asian women would have a 47% lower risk and black women a 32% lower risk of hip fracture than white women because of their shorter hip axis.

Ross and colleagues[66] measured vertebral depth from conventional radiographs in 804 women, of whom 100 developed new vertebral fractures on serial radiographs with the mean length of observation between radiographs of 8 years. Vertebral depth was a consistent predictor of incident vertebral fracture with an age-adjusted odds ratio of 1.23, even improving when certain measures of bone density were included (odds ratio up to 1.45).

In a number of patients fractures are not only an expression of a traumatic event but also of impaired skeletal status. Thus, one may expect patients with fractures to be at a higher risk for subsequent fractures, and several authors have studied this association, for example, prevalent vertebral deformities are associated with subsequent vertebral deformities and also with non-spine fractures, and vice versa.[17,18,20,23,67–70] The increased risk for subsequent fracture in patients with pre-existing fractures, in part independent of bone density, may be accounted for by systemic effects of osteoporosis or shared risk factors of certain fractures. In a retrospective case control study, Karlsson et al[71] found that even patients with non-osteoporotic fractures early in life may be at an increased risk for fragility fractures later in life.

There is a long list of risk factors associated with osteoporotic fractures idependent of bone density. In a large number of studies, age is significantly associated with prevalent and incident fracture.[72] This association is independent of bone mass and most other measures. Thus, it must be concluded that additional factors which are reflected by age must play an important role in osteoporotic fracture. These factors may be related to bone quality but also to other risk factors not yet accounted for. An extensive review of risk factors for hip fracture derived from the prospective 'Study of osteoporotic fractures' was published by Cummings and colleagues.[73] Aside from having low calcaneal bone density, women at an increased risk were those who had maternal history of hip fracture or previous fractures of any type after the age of 50; who were taller at age 25; who rated their own health as fair to poor; who had previous hyperthyroidism; who had been treated with long-acting benzodiazepines or anticonvulsant drugs; who ingested greater amounts of caffeine; or who spent 4 hours a day or less on their feet. Further findings associated with an increased risk of hip fracture were the inability to rise from a chair without using the arms, poor depth perception, poor contrast sensitivity and tachycardia at rest. Thus, fracture risk in osteoporosis is multifactorial, and knowledge of these risk factors must be taken into consideration for effective treatment of osteoporosis and prevention of its consequences.

DIAGNOSING OSTEOPOROSIS

The variety of risk factors for osteoporotic fracture may leave some doubt about the extent to which it is possible to diagnose osteoporosis. There is indeed some need for clarification about the role of bone density. What seems to be a relatively simple concept for diagnosing osteoporosis, the use of a threshold as proposed by the Working Group of the WHO, needs some further thought. The use of this threshold is derived from the concept of a so-called 'fracture threshold'. From epidemiological studies, it is known that the rate of prevalent fractures increases substantially below a certain value. For clinical use, the 'fracture threshold' is set mostly at a relatively arbitrary level of 2 standard deviations below the mean for a young normal population. From a clinical perspective, this concept offers significant guidance for therapeutic and diagnostic procedures. On the other hand, the term 'fracture threshold' in its literal sense may be misleading because of the substantial overlap between fracture and non-fracture patients. Speaking in terms of bone mass, an absolute discrimination between these groups is not possible. Furthermore, this discrimination is not the point of bone mass measurements. Rather they should be used for an estimate of the risk of future fractures, and risk must be understood as the possibility of an untoward event (the fracture), not as absolute prediction. Osteoporosis should be understood as the lower part of a continuum of bone density, with the greatest risk among those subjects with lowest absolute BMD values ('gradient of risk').[72,74]

Apart from these very basic limitations of a fracture threshold, there are some quite practical considerations which make use of a fracture threshold based on a t-score, as proposed by the Working Group of the WHO; these are quite controversial.[75] Probably the most important issue is the use of an appropriate reference database. Recent studies have shown that there may be limited agreement between a manufacturer's reference database and data derived from a study population. For example, mean values for the femoral neck data from the National Health and Nutrition Examination Survey population were about 3–5% lower than the manufacturer's reference values, and the standard deviations were 26–30% higher.[76] When comparing German normative data with a manufacturer's reference database, Lehmann et al[77] found good agreement for the female normative data. However, the data for their male reference population (30–39 years) were 7% lower than the manufacturer's reference values. There are various reasons for such discrepancies, and the most obvious ones lie in the different sampling procedures of the various studies. Furthermore, across manufacturers, comparable BMD values (using the recently proposed conversion standard[78]) yield slightly different t-scores.[75]

The t-score cut-off points between different

sites of BMD measurement, even within the same region, e.g. total hip, femoral neck or trochanter, will identify different proportions of patients and will create different risk groups (Figure 3.5).[75,79] This is even more so when looking at multiple anatomical sites, such as spine and hip: densitometric results from different sites disagree in a large number of patients. In a population-based study from Rochester, MN (USA), the proportion of women aged 80 years and older with a bone density more than 2 standard deviations below the mean of young normal women is 48% when measured at the lumbar spine, 67% for either hip site, 68% for the midradius, and rises to 84% for the combination of all measurements.[80]

Currently, there are very few data to show whether a combination of multiple sites may improve the diagnostic capability or fracture prediction as compared with measuring BMD at only one site. A prospective study of multiple-site BMC measurements was presented by Wasnich and co-workers[16] who reported that a combination of two sites strengthened the relationship to incident spinal fracture. Black et al,[81] on the other hand, found that a combination of femoral neck and lumbar spine BMD for identifying elderly women at high risk for hip fracture was no better than using femoral neck BMD alone and adjusting the respective thresholds. Similarly, Genant and co-workers[79] presented results for combinations of hip BMD and spinal, calcaneal or radius BMD for the prediction of hip fractures in 5568 women from the 'Study of osteoporotic fractures'.[79] The authors found that, when hip BMD was available, no additional information was gained from secondary measurements at the other sites. However, if BMD was low at the hip, low bone density at the calcaneus or the distal radius increased the risk of hip fracture. This result is in accordance with a cross-sectional study by Jergas et al[82] who found that a combination of spinal and femoral BMD did not improve the prediction of prevalent vertebral fracture. It must be said, however, that, even though adjusting thresholds for a single site measurement may identify a similar number of women at risk for fracture compared with multiple site

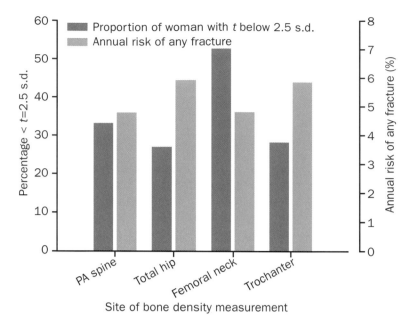

Figure 3.5 Using a *t*-score of 2.5 standard deviations (s.d.) as diagnostic threshold, different proportions of patients are identified as being osteoporotic depending on the site or subregion measured. The use of such a threshold also creates different risk groups as indicated by the site-specific annual risk for any fracture. Data from Black et al.[75]

measurements, it is of concern that different women may be identified as at risk. Therefore, although there may not be a compelling reason for routine bone densitometry of both spine and hip in one patient, any evidence of artefacts, which make BMD results of one site unreliable, e.g. anatomical variations and severe degenerative changes or fractures, make it useful to measure a second site for the assessment of a person's bone mineral status. For general clinical practice, the interpretation and value of multiple site measurements are uncertain.

There is no question that, in times of tight financial constraints, the relative merits and imperfections of bone density measurements for the diagnosis of osteoporosis and the estimate of future fracture risk must spark a controversial discussion.[83–86] Nevertheless, taking into account all risk factors associated with fracture risk, bone densitometry still represents the most consistent predictive tool that is currently available. The predictive capability of bone density is comparable in its magnitude to that of blood pressure for stroke and better than that

of serum cholesterol for coronary artery disease;[87,88] still there is a wide overlap between those patients who will develop a fracture and those who will not. Therefore, rather than being considered a screening tool, the application of bone densitometry should remain confined to certain groups at risk for osteoporosis and to those people receiving drug therapy for osteoporosis.[89–92] The cost-effectiveness of therapeutic intervention, based on densitometric results, has been estimated as comparable with the treatment of mild hypertension to prevent stroke.[93] Further studies on the cost-effectiveness of therapy are necessary in the light of new emerging therapeutic concepts in osteoporosis, as well as the increased costs created by osteoporotic fractures. However, even though cost-effectiveness is an important issue, which has become increasingly relevant, it should not drive the provision of health care.

Several authors have developed models for estimating a woman's lifetime risk of having a hip fracture based on bone density and age.[94–96] The concept of lifetime risk appears to be very appealing for clinical use because it offers some advantages over the existing concept that relies solely on bone density. Applying a nomogram directly to estimate a woman's hip fracture risk, as proposed by Suman,[96] may facilitate the practical application of such a concept. So far, this approach has been proposed only for prediction of hip fracture, and models for prediction of fractures at other sites still need to be developed. It also has to be remembered that low bone density does not entirely account for an increased risk of fracture. Other factors, such as an increased risk of falling and bone properties other than density, are also of great importance. Concepts using current knowledge to determine a patient's risk for osteoporosis more exactly may finally relieve the relatively simplistic approach of a *t*-score of its duty. In any case, the treatment of a patient for osteoporosis does not depend only on bone density but in addition on a number of clinical findings.[97]

SUMMARY AND CONCLUSION

Bone densitometry is an established tool for the diagnosis of osteoporosis, and bone mineral density is significantly associated with the risk of future fracture as shown in many prospective studies. This association is partly independent of age and other significant predictors of fracture such as falls, cognisance and mobility. The differences between the various densitometric techniques in predicting future osteoporotic fracture of any type are marginal. However, it seems that bone density measurements at the site of fracture do perform better than measurements at other sites. In general, retrospective, or cross-sectional, and prospective study designs seem to deliver comparable results. There is currently no evidence that measuring a second site improves the diagnostic capability of bone densitometry. However, measuring a second site may identify a number of different patients at risk for osteoporosis.

From long-term prospective studies, it can be concluded that peak bone density and bone loss are important predictors of subsequent fracture, and that fracture can be predicted over a longer period of time. Bone density predicts fracture even in very elderly people. However, some fractures, such as the femoral neck fracture, may be more strongly influenced by other risk fractures at this higher age.

Quantitative ultrasonography has a predictive capability similar to bone densitometry without showing a close correlation to the quantitative measures of bone density. Considering the results from the first prospective studies, quantitative ultrasonography may soon be an alternative to bone density measurements in clinical practice. From the perspective that bone densitometry and quantitative ultrasonography independently predict fractures, these measures actually seem complementary rather than competitive.

Simple geometric measures of the bones, such as hip axis length and vertebral depth, may also be derived from images of bone densitometry scans and are also predictive of hip fracture or vertebral fracture independent of bone density. In addition, prevalent fractures are strong predictors of future fracture and must be considered when therapeutic intervention is planned. Overall, there are various risk factors that contribute to the fragility of bone and the occurrence of osteoporotic fracture. The concept of using a threshold for bone density based on a comparison with young normal people to define osteoporosis is a concept that does not do justice to the complexity of the disease, even though bone density must currently be regarded as the most important contributor to osteoporotic fractures. Future concepts for determining a person's lifetime risk for fractures and to draw therapeutic decisions must be based on a risk profile for that person, the profile consisting of bone mineral density, bone geometry, bone structure and a number of additional clinical risk factors.

REFERENCES

1. Consensus Development Conference. Diagnosis, prophylaxis, and treatment of osteoporosis. *Am J Med* 1993; **94:** 646–50.

2. Melton LJ III, Wahner HW. Defining osteoporosis. *Calcif Tissue Int* 1989; **45:** 263–4.

3. World Health Organization. *Assessment of fracture risk and its application to screening for postmenopausal osteoporosis. WHO technical report series.* Geneva: WHO, 1994.

4. Kanis JA, WHO Study Group. Assessment of fracture risk and its application to screening for postmenopausal osteoporosis: synopsis of a WHO report. *Osteoporosis Int* 1994; **4:** 368–81.

5. Kanis JA, Devogelaer J-P, Gennari C. Practical guide for the use of bone mineral measurements in the assessment of treatment of osteoporosis: a position paper of the European foundation for osteoporosis and bone disease. *Osteoporosis Int* 1996; **6:** 256–61.

6. Kanis JA, Melton LJ III, Christiansen C, Johnston CC, Khaltaev N. The diagnosis of osteoporosis. *J Bone Miner Res* 1994; **9:** 1137–41.

7. Melton LJ III, Thamer M, Ray NF et al. Fractures attributable to osteoporosis: report from the National Osteoporosis Foundation. *J Bone Miner Res* 1997; **12:** 16–23.

8. Nevitt MC. Epidemiology of osteoporosis. *Rheum Dis Clin North Am* 1994; **20:** 535–59.

9. Seeley DG, Browner WS, Nevitt MC, Genant HK, Scott JC, Cummings SR. Which fractures are associated with low appendicular bone mass in elderly women? *Ann Intern Med* 1991; **115:** 837–42.

10. Smith DM, Khairi MRA, Johnston CC Jr. The loss of bone mineral with aging and its relationship to risk of fracture. *J Clin Invest* 1975; **56:** 311–18.

11. Khairi MRA, Cronin JH, Robb JA et al. Femoral trabecular-pattern index and bone mineral content measurement by photon absorption in senile osteoporosis. *J Bone Joint Surg [Am]* 1976; **58A:** 221–6.

12. Melton LJ III, Atkinson EJ, O'Fallon WM, Wahner HW, Riggs BL. Long-term fracture prediction by bone mineral assessed at different skeletal sites. *J Bone Miner Res* 1993; **8:** 1227–33.

13. Stegman MR, Recker RR, Davies KM, Ryan RA, Heaney RP. Fracture risk as determined by prospective and retrospective study designs. *Osteoporosis Int* 1992; **2:** 290–7.

14. Hui SL, Slemenda CW, Johnston CC. Baseline measurement of bone mass predicts fracture in white women. *Ann Intern Med* 1989; **111:** 355–61.

15. Hui SL, Slemenda CW, Carey MA, Johnston CC Jr. Choosing between predictors of fractures. *J Bone Miner Res* 1995; **10:** 1816–22.

16. Wasnich RD, Ross PD, Davis JW, Vogel JM. A comparison of single and multi-site BMC measurements for assessment of spine fracture probability. *J Nucl Med* 1989; **30:** 1166–71.

17. Ross PD, Davis JW, Epstein RS, Wasnich RD. Pre-existing fractures and bone mass predict vertebral fracture incidence in women. *Ann Intern Med* 1991; **114:** 919–23.

18. Ross PD, Genant HK, Davis JW, Miller PD, Wasnich RD. Predicting vertebral fracture incidence from prevalent fractures and bone density among non-black, osteoporotic women. *Osteoporosis Int* 1993; **3:** 120–6.

19. Gärdsell P, Johnell O, Nilsson BE, Gullberg B. Predicting various fragility fractures in women by forearm bone densitometry: a follow-up study. *Calcif Tissue Int* 1993; **52:** 348–53.

20. Gärdsell P, Johnell O, Nilsson BE. The predictive value of forearm bone mineral content measurements in men. *Bone* 1990; **11:** 229–32.

21. Cummings SR, Black DM, Nevitt MC et al. Bone density at various sites for prediction of hip fractures. *Lancet* 1993; **341**(8837): 72–5.

22. Black D, Cummings SR, Genant HK, Nevitt MC, Palermo L, Browner W. Axial and appendicular bone density predict fractures in older women. *J Bone Miner Res* 1992; **7:** 633–8.

23. Black D, Nevitt M, Palermo L, Ensrud K, Genant H. Prediction of new vertebral deformities. *J Bone Miner Res* 1993; **8**(suppl 1): S135.

24. Seeley DG, Kelsey J, Jergas M, Nevitt MC. Predictors of ankle and foot fractures in older women. *J Bone Miner Res* 1996; **11:** 1347–55.

25. Nguyen T, Sambrook P, Kelly P et al. Prediction of osteoporotic fractures by postural instability and bone density. *BMJ* 1993; **307:** 1111–15.

26. Cheng S, Suominen H, Era P, Heikkinen E. Bone density of the calcaneus and fractures in 75- and 80-year old men and women. *Osteoporosis Int* 1994; **4:** 48–54.

27. Torgerson DJ, Campbell MK, Thomas RE, Reid DM. Prediction of perimenopausal fracture by bone density and other risk factors. *J Bone Miner Res* 1996; **11:** 293–7.

28. Hui SL, Slemenda CW, Johnston CC. Age and bone mass as predictors of fracture in a prospective study. *J Clin Invest* 1988; **81:** 1804–9.

29. Gärdsell P, Johnell O, Nilsson BE. Predicting fractures in women by using forearm bone densitometry. *Calcif Tissue Int* 1989; **44:** 235–42.

30. Gärdsell P, Johnell O, Nilsson BE. The predictive value of bone loss for fragility fractures in women: a longitudinal study over 15 years. *Calcif Tissue Int* 1991; **49:** 90–4.

31. Marshall D, Johnell O, Wedel H. Meta-analysis of how well measures of bone mineral density predict occurrence of osteoporotic fractures. *BMJ* 1996; **312:** 1254–9.

32. Genant HK, Cann CE, Ettinger B, Gordan GS. Quantitative computed tomography of vertebral spongiosa: A sensitive method for detecting early bone loss after oophorectomy. *Ann Intern Med* 1982; **97:** 699–705.

33. Cann CE, Genant HK, Kolb FO et al. Quantitative computed tomography for prediction of vertebral fracture risk. *Metab Bone Dis Relat Res* 1984; **5:** 1–7.

34. Reinbold WD, Genant HK, Reiser UJ, Harris ST, Ettinger B. Bone mineral content in early-postmenopausal osteoporotic women and postmenopausal women: Comparison of measurement methods. *Radiology* 1986; **160:** 469–78.

35. Nordin BEC, Wishart JM, Horowitz M, Need AG, Bridges A, Bellon M. The relation between forearm and vertebral mineral density and fractures in postmenopausal women. *Bone Miner* 1988; **5:** 21–33.

36. Heuck A, Block J, Glüer CC, Steiger P, Genant HK. Mild versus definite osteoporosis: comparison of bone densitometry techniques using different statistical models. *J Bone Miner Res* 1989; **4:** 891–900.

37. Van Berkum FNR, Birkenhäger JC, Van Veen LCP et al. Noninvasive axial and peripheral assessment of bone mineral content: a comparison between osteoporotic women and normal subjects. *J Bone Miner Res* 1989; **5:** 679–85.

38. Pacifici R, Rupich R, Griffin M, Chines A, Susman N, Avioli LV. Dual energy radiography versus quantitative computer tomography for the diagnosis of osteoporosis. *J Clin Endocrinol Metab* 1990; **70:** 705–10.

39. Guglielmi G, Grimston SK, Fischer KC, Pacifici R. Osteoporosis: diagnosis with lateral and posteroanterior dual x-ray absorptiometry compared with quantitative CT. *Radiology* 1994; **192:** 845–50.

40. Ito M, Hayashi K, Ishida Y et al. Discrimination of spinal fracture with various bone mineral measurements. *Calcif Tissue Int* 1997; **60:** 11–15.

41. Nevitt M, Johnell O, Black DM, Ensrud K, Genant HK, Cummings SR. Bone mineral density predicts non-spine fractures in very elderly women. *Osteoporosis Int* 1994; **4:** 325–31.

42. Hansen MA, Overgaard K, Riis BJ, Christiansen C. Role of peak bone mass and bone loss in postmenopausal osteoporosis: 12 year study. *BMJ* 1991; **303:** 961–4.

43. Hui SL, Slemenda CW, Johnston CC. The contribution of bone loss to postmenopausal osteoporosis. *Osteoporosis Int* 1990; **1:** 30–4.

44. Porter R, Miller C, Grainger D, Palmer S. Prediction of hip fracture in elderly women: a prospective study. *BMJ* 1990; **301:** 638–41.

45. Heaney RP, Avioli LV, Chesnut CH III, Lappe J, Recker RR, Brandenburger GH. Ultrasound velocity through bone predicts incident vertebral deformity. *J Bone Miner Res* 1995; **10:** 341–5.

46. Hans D, Dargent-Molina P, Schott AM et al. Ultrasonographic heel measurements to predict hip fracture in the elderly. *Lancet* 1996; **348:** 511–14.

47. Stegman MR, Heaney RP, Recker RR. Comparison of speed of sound ultrasound with single photon absorptiometry for determining fracture odds ratios. *J Bone Miner Res* 1995; **10:** 346–52.

48. Stegman MR, Davies KM, Heaney RP, Recker RR, Lappe JM. The association of patellar ultrasound transmissions and forearm densitometry with vertebral fracture, number and severity: The Saunders county bone quality study. *Osteoporosis Int* 1996; **6:** 130–5.

49. Stewart A, Reid DM, Porter RW. Broadband ultrasound attenuation and dual energy x-ray absorptiometry in patients with hip fractures: which technique discriminates fracture risk. *Calcif Tissue Int* 1994; **54:** 466–9.

50. Bauer DC, Glüer CC, Genant HK, Stone K. Quantitative ultrasound and vertebral fracture in post menopausal women. *J Bone Miner Res* 1995; **10:** 353–8.

51. Turner CH, Peacock M, Timmerman L, Neal JM, Johnson CC Jr. Calcaneal ultrasonic measurements discriminate hip fracture independently of bone mass. *Osteoporosis Int* 1995; **5:** 130–5.

52. Schott AM, Weill-Engerer S, Hans D, Duboeuf F, Delmas PD, Meunier PJ. Ultrasound discriminates patients with hip fracture equally well as dual energy X-Ray absorptiometry and independently of bone mineral density. *J Bone Miner Res* 1995; **10:** 243–9.

53. Gonnelli S, Cepollaro C, Agnusdei D, Palmieri R, Rossi S, Gennari C. Diagnostic value of ultrasound analysis and bone densitometry as predictors of vertebral deformity in postmenopausal women. *Osteoporosis Int* 1995; **5:** 413–18.

54. Glüer CC, Cummings SR, Bauer DC et al. Osteoporosis: Association of recent fractures with quantitative ultrasound findings. *Radiology* 1996; **199:** 725–32.

55. Geusens P, Dequeker J, Verstraeten A, Nijs J. Age-, sex-, and menopause-related changes of vertebral and peripheral bone: population study using dual and single photon absorptiometry and radiogrammetry. *J Nucl Med* 1986; **27:** 1540–9.

56. Falch JA, Sandvik L. Perimenopausal appendicular bone loss: a 10-year prospective study. *Bone* 1990; **11:** 425–8.

57. Meema HE, Meindok H. Advantages of peripheral radiogrametry over dual-photon absorptiometry of the spine in the assessment of prevalence of osteoporotic vertebral fractures in women. *J Bone Miner Res* 1992; **7:** 897–903.

58. Jergas M, San Valentin R, Black D et al. Radiogrammetry of the metacarpals predicts future hip fractures. *J Bone Miner Res* 1995; **10**(suppl 1): S371.

59. Faulkner KG, McClung M, Cummings SR. Automated evaluation of hip axis length for predicting hip fracture. *J Bone Miner Res* 1994; **9:** 1065–70.

60. Faulkner KG, Cummings SR, Glüer CC, Palermo L, Black D, Genant HK. Simple measurement of femoral geometry predicts hip fracture: The Study of Osteoporotic Fractures. *J Bone Miner Res* 1993; **8:** 1211–17.

61. Faulkner KG. Hip axis length and osteoporotic fractures [letter to the editor]. *J Bone Miner Res* 1995; **10:** 506–8.

62. Geusens P. Geometric characterisics of the proximal femur and hip fracture risk. *Osteoporosis Int* 1996; **6**(suppl 3): S27–30.

63. Glüer CC, Cummings SR, Pressman A et al. Prediction of hip fractures from pelvic radiographs: The study of osteoporotic fractures. *J Bone Miner Res* 1994; **9:** 671–7.

64. Nakamura T, Turner CH, Yoshikawa T et al. Do variations of hip geometry explain differences in hip fracture risk between Japanese and white Americans. *J Bone Miner Res* 1994; **9:** 1071–6.

65. Cummings SR, Cauley JA, Palermo L et al. Racial differences in hip axis lengths might explain racial differences in rates of hip fractures. *Osteoporosis Int* 1994; **4:** 226–9.

66. Ross PD, Huang C, Davis JW, Wasnich RD. Vertebral dimension measurements improve prediction of vertebral fracture incidence. *Bone* 1995; **16:** 257S–62S.

67. Wasnich RD, Davis JW, Ross PD. Spine fracture risk is predicted by non-spine fractures. *Osteoporosis Int* 1994; **4:** 1–5.

68. Mallmin H, Ljunghall S, Persson I, Naessen T, Krusemo UB, Bergström R. Fracture of the distal forearm as a forecaster of subsequent hip fracture: a population based cohort study with 24 years of follow-up. *Calcif Tissue Int* 1993; **52:** 269–72.

69. Kotowicz MA, Melton LJ III, Cooper C, Atkinson EJ, O'Fallon WM, Riggs LB. Risk of hip fracture in women with vertebral fracture. *J Bone Miner Res* 1994; **9:** 599–605.

70. Burger H, van Daele PLA, Algra D et al. Vertebral deformities as predictors of non-vertebral fractures. *BMJ* 1994; **309:** 991–2.

71. Karlsson MK, Hasserius R, Obrant KJ. Individuals who sustain nonosteoporotic fractures continue to also sustain fragility fractures. *Calcif Tissue Int* 1993; **53:**229–31.

72. Ross PD, Davis JW, Vogel JM, Wasnich RD. A critical review of bone mass and the risk of fractures in osteoporosis. *Calcif Tissue Int* 1990; **46:** 149–61.

73. Cummings SR, Nevitt MC, Browner WS et al. Risk factors for hip fractures in white women. *N Engl J Med* 1995; **332:** 767–73.

74. Wasnich R. Fracture prediction with bone mass measurements. In: *Osteoporosis Update 1987* (Genant HK, ed.). San Francisco: Radiology Research and Education Foundation, 1987: 95–101.

75. Black DM, Palermo L, Genant HK, Cummings SR. Four reasons to avoid the use of BMD T-scores in treatment decisions for osteoporosis. *J Bone Miner Res* 1996; **11**(suppl 1): S118.

76. Looker AC, Wahner HW, Dunn WL et al. Proximal femur bone mineral levels of US adults. *Osteoporosis Int* 1995; **5:** 389–409.

77. Lehmann R, Wapniarz M, Randerath O et al. Dual-energy X-ray absorptiometry at the lumbar spine in German men and women: a cross-sectional study. *Calcif Tissue Int* 1995; **56:** 350–4.

78. Genant HK, Grampp S, Glüer CC et al. Universal standardization for dual x-ray absorptiometry: patient and phantom cross-calibration results. *J Bone Miner Res* 1994; **9:** 1503–14.

79. Genant HK, Lu Y, Mathur AK, Fuerst TP,

Cummings SR. Classification based on DXA measurements for assessing the risk of hip fractures. *J Bone Miner Res* 1996; **11**(suppl 1): S120.

80. Melton LJ III, Chrischilles EA, Cooper C, Lane AW, Riggs BL. How many women have osteoporosis? *J Bone Miner Res* 1992; **7:** 1005–10.

81. Black D, Bauer DC, Lu Y, Tabor H, Genant HK, Cummings SR. Should BMD be measured at multiple sites to predict fracture risk in elderly women? *J Bone Miner Res* 1995; **10**(suppl 1): S140.

82. Jergas M, Fuerst T, Grampp S, Uffmann M, Glüer CC, Genant HK. Assessment of spinal osteoporosis with dual x-ray absorptiometry of the spine and femur. *Radiology* 1995; **197**(suppl): 362.

83. Sheldon TA, Raffle A, Watt I. Department of Health shoots itself in the hip. Why the report of the advisory groups undermines evidence based purchasing. *BMJ* 1996; **312:** 296–7.

84. Barlow D, Cooper C, Reeve J, Reid D. Department of health is fair to patients with osteoporosis. *BMJ* 1996; **312:** 297–8.

85. Lange S, Richter K, Köbberling J. In: *Die Osteodensitometrie.* Biometrie, vol. 3 (Köhler W, Köpcke W, Naeve P, Weiß H, eds). Münster: Lit Verlag, 1994.

86. Glüer CC. Osteoporosediagnostik – ein radiologisches Problem? *Fortschr Röntgenstr* 1996; **165**(1): 1–3.

87. Neaton JD, Wentworth D. Serum cholesterol, blood pressure, cigarette smoking and death from coronary artery disease: overall findings and differences by age for 316 099 white men. *Arch Intern Med* 1992; **152:** 56–64.

88. Khaw K, Barrett-Connor E, Suarez L, Criqui MH. Predictors of stroke associated mortality in the elderly. *Stroke* 1984; **15:** 244–8.

89. Johnston CC Jr, Melton LJ III, Lindsay R, Eddy DM. Clinical indications for bone mass measurements. *J Bone Miner Res* 1989; **4**(suppl 2): 1–28.

90. Genant HK, Block JE, Steiger P, Glüer CC, Ettinger B, Harris ST. Appropriate use of bone densitometry. *Radiology* 1989; **170:** 817–22.

91. Jergas M, Genant HK. Current methods and recent advances in the diagnosis of osteoporosis. *Arthritis Rheum* 1993; **36:** 1649–62.

92. Compston JE, Cooper C, Kanis JA. Bone densitometry in clinical practice. *BMJ* 1995; **310**(6993): 1507–10.

93. Jönsson B, Christiansen C, Johnell O, Hedbrandt J. Cost-effectiveness of fracture prevention in established osteoporosis. *Osteoporosis Int* 1995; **5:** 136–42.

94. Melton LJ III, Kan SH, Wahner HW, Riggs BL. Lifetime fracture risk: and approach to hip fracture risk assessment based on bone mineral density and age. *J Clin Epidemiol* 1988; **41:** 985–94.

95. Black D, Cummings SR, Melton LJ. Appendicular bone mineral and a woman's lifetime risk of hip fracture. *J Bone Miner Res* 1992; **7:** 639–46.

96. Suman VJ, Atkinson EJ, W.M. OF, Black DM, Melton LJ. A nomogram for predicting lifetime hip fracture risk from radius bone mineral density and age. *Bone* 1993; **14:** 843–6.

97. Ettinger B, Miller P, McClung M. Use of bone densitometry results for decisions about therapy for osteoporosis [letter]. *Ann Intern Med* 1996; **125:** 623.

4

Ultrasonic evaluation of osteoporosis

D Hans, CC Glüer and CF Njeh

CONTENTS • **Quantitative ultrasonic parameters** • **Quantitative ultrasonic systems** • **What have we learned from in vitro studies?** • **What have we learned from in vivo studies?** • **Conclusions**

Osteoporosis represents a major worldwide public health problem and imposes a considerable financial burden on public health systems ($US10 billion in the USA in 1989).[1-3] It is a systematic skeletal disease characterized by low bone mass and microarchitectural deterioration of bone tissue, with a consequent increase in bone fragility and susceptibility to fracture.[4] It is manifested mostly as vertebral fractures resulting from a decrease in bone mineral density (BMD) and deterioration of structural properties of the bone. However, the most severe complications are hip fractures. Today the lifetime risk of hip fracture for a 50-year-old woman is about 18%[5] and the continuing rise in life expectancy is expected to cause a threefold rise in worldwide fracture incidence over the next 60 years.[5] It is well known that intrinsic bone fragility – together with falls – is the major determinant of hip fracture.[6-8] Melton et al[9] have shown that the incidence of hip fracture was inversely related to femoral bone density and, in a recent prospective study, a decrease of one standard deviation of the hip BMD was associated with a two- to threefold increase by the age of 65: the BMD-adjusted risk of hip fracture is multiplied by about a factor of two per decade.[10] Moreover, although patients with hip fracture have a lower bone density than controls, there is a large overlap between women with fracture and age- and sex-matched controls in terms of bone density.[1,9] In fact, BMD explains about 70–75% of the variance in

strength, whereas the remaining variance could be the result of the cumulative and synergistic effects of other factors, e.g. accumulated burden of fatigue damage, ineffective bone architecture, measurement artefacts and state of remodelling.[11,12] Bone architecture refers to the three-dimensional arrangement of trabecular struts; it may be defined by a combination of porosity (volume fraction), connectivity (degree of connection of trabecular fibres) and anisotropy (orientation dependence of connectivity).[13] Remodelling refers to the continuous formation and resorption of bone by the osteoblasts and the osteoclasts, respectively.

In the past 25 years, several non-invasive techniques based on the attenuation of ionizing radiation have been developed to quantify BMD in the axial and peripheral skeleton: single photon absorptiometry (SPA), single X-ray absorptiometry (SXA), dual X-ray absorptiometry (DXA) and quantitative computed tomography (QCT).[14] These techniques vary, not only in the source of energy, but also in the site and type of bone measured. They represent relatively expensive valid methods for the determination of BMD, but give limited information on bone structure and strength.[15] Consequently, most investigators from the academic institutions and the pharmaceutical industries are interested in new methodologies that may have a role in assessing skeletal status. An ideal screening tool should detect fragility, whatever its basis, and not just decreased bone mass, in addition, it should be inexpensive and free of ionizing radiation. As microfractures and bone architectural changes may also play a role in the process of bone weakening,[1,16] it is possible that a combination of information on bone elasticity, structure and density will provide a more sensitive tool for fracture prediction than DXA techniques, which measure only density.

Recently, ultrasonography (the technique involving use of ultrasound waves), which has long been used successfully to evaluate mechanical competence and detect the presence of damage in both materials and structures in non-destructive materials testing in industry, has been applied to bone assessment. Although indirect and/or in vitro experience has suggested that ultrasonography may give information not only about bone density but also about architecture and elasticity,[17,18] the clinical application of this technology, especially for fracture risk prediction, has still to be validated independently. In this regard, several new methods known as quantitative ultrasonography (QUS) have been developed for clinical use. Although several devices are now commercially available, registration with the US Food and Drug Administration (FDA) is still pending. Therefore, this technique is primarily used for research in the USA and most of the equipment in clinical use is distributed throughout Europe and Asia.

QUANTITATIVE ULTRASONIC PARAMETERS

Ultrasound is a mechanical vibration wave with a frequency range above the human audible range from 20 000 waves per second (20 kilohertz or kHz) to 100 000 000 waves per second (100 megahertz or MHz). One can imagine ultrasound hitting the bone like a hammer hitting a piece of iron (Figure 4.1). The mechanical energy is transmitted through the specimen and reaches the opposite side. When passing through bone, it causes both the cortex and the trabecular network to vibrate on a microscale, progressively altering the shape, intensity and speed of the propagating wave. The bone tissue may therefore be characterized in terms of velocity and attenuation of the ultrasound wave. The laws of physics provide the interrelationship of mechanical properties (in this case bone), three-dimensional bone architecture and velocity or attenuation of transmitted ultrasonic waves. An assessment of QUS parameters should allow the deduction of mechanical properties of cortical and trabecular bone which, in turn, are important determinants of whole bone stiffness, failure load and fracture risk.[20–24]

Velocity of ultrasound

The velocity of ultrasound wave propagation, or speed of sound (SOS), through bone is determined by dividing the distance traversed (e.g. bone diameter or length) by the transit time. The resulting velocity is expressed in metres per second (m/s). It depends on the material properties of the medium through which it is propagating and its mode of propagation.

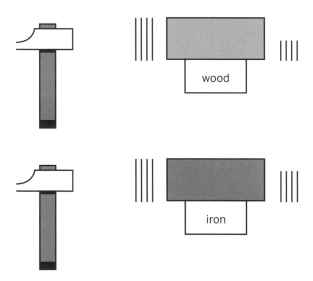

Figure 4.1 Diagrammatic representation of an ultrasound wave which is transmitted through the specimen and reaches the opposite site. When passing through the specimen it progressively alters the shape, intensity and speed of the propagating wave.

Longitudinal waves are the common mode of ultrasound propagation through tissue. High elastic modulus materials such as bone can support additional propagation modes such as shear waves. Bone is an anisotropic, heterogeneous and dispersive material, which means that it is not very easy to model the relationship between the mechanical properties of the bone and the velocity. Nevertheless, as a first approach and under certain conditions, SOS can be related to the mechanical properties of a material by the equation

$$SOS = (E/\rho)^{\frac{1}{2}} = \sqrt{\frac{E}{\rho}}$$

where E is the modulus of elasticity (a measure of resistance to deformation), and ρ is the bone density.[25–27]

Clinically, velocity measurement may be achieved by either reflection or transmission techniques using single large diameter piezoelectric transducers.[26,28] The reflection technique uses a single transducer to transmit and receive the signal. The generated ultrasound pulse travels through the sample and is reflected at an interface to be detected by the same transducer. In the transmission method, one transducer acts as the transmitter and the other as the receiver. For application to bone, the transmission technique is most commonly used.

In the clinical application of ultrasound velocity measurements, there is no convention for the use of terms or for the measurement method for velocity. For example, SOS, velocity of sound, apparent velocity of ultrasound (AVU) and ultrasound transmission velocity (UTV) all refer to the same generic ultrasound measurement. For the calcaneus, three different methods of calculating velocity have been utilized, resulting in the limb (heel) velocity (calcaneus plus soft tissue), bone velocity (calcaneus only) and time of flight velocity (TOF) (between transducers positioned at a fixed distance).

In clinical measurements, the TOF velocity method assumes a constant heel thickness and therefore the velocity measured is dependent upon heel width.[29,30] The three velocity calculations yield slightly different values but correlate strongly with each other. Miller et al[31] showed

that TOF had the optimum precision (coefficient of variation or CV = 0.7%), but the smallest dynamic range whereas bone velocity (CV = 2.7%) had the largest dynamic range, a factor that enhances its sensitivity. They recommended that TOF velocity should be performed for immersion techniques but limb (heel) velocity for contact measurements.

Attenuation and broadband ultrasound attenuation

As an ultrasonic beam interrogates a medium, some of its energy is lost, and this phenomenon is known as attenuation. The intensity of a plane wave propagating in the y-direction decreases with distance as:

$$I_y = I_0 e^{-\mu(f)y}$$

where $\mu(f)$ is the frequency (f)-dependent intensity attenuation coefficient (in dB/cm), I_0 is the incident intensity and I_y is the intensity at a distance y.

Factors contributing to attenuation include beam spreading (diffraction), scattering, absorption and mode conversion.[25,29] The predominant attenuation mechanism in cancellous bone is scattering whereas absorption predominates in cortical bone. Absorption is the dissipation of ultrasonic energy in the medium via conversion to heat, caused mainly by internal molecular friction. Scattering effects occur when particles absorb part of the ultrasonic energy and re-radiate it in all directions. The amount of scattering depends primarily on the ratio of ultrasound wavelength to the size of the scattering particle and on the acoustic impedance of the scattering particle.[25,27,28]

In the frequency range 0.1–1 MHz that is most useful for bone characterization, the total attenuation (expressed on a logarithmic scale) is linearly proportional to frequency. In clinical practice, the slope of attenuation as a function of frequency has become known as broadband ultrasound attenuation (BUA). In contrast to velocity, no theoretical relationship has been established between ultrasound attenuation and the mechanical properties of cancellous bone.

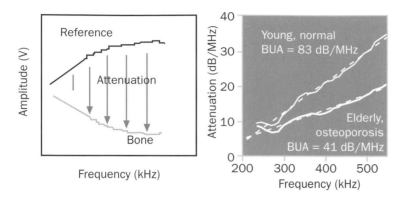

Figure 4.2 BUA measurement by the substitution method described by Langton et al.[19] The increase in attenuation as a function of frequency is measured by comparing the amplitude spectrum for a reference material with that for the measured sample. The slope of attenuation (BUA) in dB/MHz is given by linear regression of the spectral amplitude difference.

The clinical systems that measure BUA have adopted the substitution method described by Langton et al.[19] The increase in attenuation as a function of frequency is measured by comparing the amplitude spectrum for a reference material (e.g. degassed water using a surfactant) with that for the measured sample. The slope of attenuation (BUA) in dB/MHz is given by linear regression of the spectral amplitude difference (Figure 4.2).

Combined parameter

The manufacturers Lunar and Hologic also provide a calculated variable named 'stiffness' (which should not be confused with the biomechanical term) and quantitative ultrasound index (QUI) respectively, both of which are combinations of BUA and SOS. From the point of view of clinical interpretation, a single parameter such as 'stiffness' or QUI, which combines attenuation and velocity, can simplify interpretation.

QUANTITATIVE ULTRASONIC SYSTEMS (QUS)

Different machines have been developed since the late 1980s and continuing improvements have been made in recent years. The manufacturers are improving their systems by either enhancing hardware performance or optimizing analysis algorithms. The examination requires less time and the poor reproducibility of BUA –

still a main limitation in longitudinal studies – has already been improved. In general terms, the commercial QUS devices introduced show a greater technological diversity than bone densitometry equipment. Furthermore, different ultrasound technologies assess different parameters (BUA, SOS, Ad-SOS, etc.) and may not even assess the same anatomical site (heel, tibia, phalanges etc.). This may reflect a strength of QUS, but it also represents a challenge for the validation process. Results obtained on validated devices cannot necessarily be directly translated into performance statements of other technologically different QUS systems. The groups of approaches and equipment shown in Table 4.1 have been developed into commercially available systems.

Calcaneus

Calcaneal fixed point transmission
Calcaneal fixed single point transmission systems employing either water-based foot placement[32,33] or coupling by means of ultrasonic gel[34] have been used (Figure 4.3).

The calcaneus is the most popular measurement site for several reasons. The calcaneus is 90% cancellous bone, which, as a result of its high surface : volume ratio, has a higher metabolic turnover rate than cortical bone. Hence, cancellous bone will manifest bone metabolic changes before cortical bone.[35] The calcaneus is also easily accessible and the mediolateral surfaces are fairly flat and parallel, thus reducing

Table 4.1 Different approaches and types of equipment for bone assessment with quantitative ultrasonography

Device	Anatomical site	Coupling medium	Parameter	Precision (CV) (%)	Comments
Lunar Achilles Plus	Calcaneus	Water	BUA	0.8–2.5	Time of flight velocity
			SOS	0.2–0.4	
			Stiffness	1.0–2.0	
McCue CUBA Clinical	Calcaneus	Gel	BUA	1.5–4.0	Limb velocity
			SOS	0.2–0.6	
Walker Sonix UBA 575+	Calcaneus	Water	BUA	2.0–5.0	No longer in production
			SOS	0.2–0.6	Bone velocity
Hologic Sahara	Calcaneus	Gel	BUA	0.8–2.5	Limb velocity
			SOS	0.2–0.4	
			QUI	1.0–2.0	
DMS UBIS 3000	Calcaneus	Water	BUA	0.8–2.5	Imaging system
			SOS	0.2–0.4	
Osteometer DTU-1	Calcaneus	Water	BUA	0.8–2.5	Imaging system
			SOS	0.2–0.4	
Myriad Soundscan 2000	Midtibia	Gel	SOS	0.2–1.0	Cortical bone, soft tissue correction
IGEA DBM Sonic 1200	Phalanges	Gel	Ad-SOS	0.5–1.0	Amplitude-dependent velocity

CV, coefficient of variation.

repositioning errors. The choice of the calcaneus as the test site has been supported by Wasnich et al[36] and Black et al,[37] who reported that the calcaneus appeared to be the optimal BMD measurement site for routine screening of perimenopausal women for predicting the risk of any type of osteoporotic fractures.

Calcaneal imaging devices
Calcaneal imaging devices allow for flexible placement of regions of interest within the calcaneus[38,39] (Figure 4.3).

Ultrasonographic images are obtained in transmission mode by using a pair of broadband focused transducers immersed in a water bath at room temperature. The ultrasound beam is scanned across the heel in 1 mm steps to image the entire calcaneus. The advantage of the image is that it would allow the evaluation of standardized regions of interest in all patients; larger regions of interest can be used, potentially improving precision, and measurement artefacts can be clearly identified and avoided.

Finger phalanges

Single point QUS systems are used for measurements at the finger phalanges using gel coupling.[40–48] This technique uses the transmis-

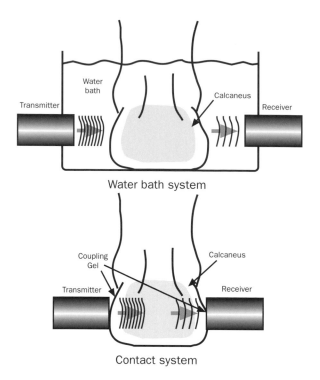

Figure 4.3 Calcaneal fixed single point transmission systems employing either water-based foot placement or coupling by means of ultrasonic gel.

sion technique to measure amplitude-dependent ultrasound speed of sound (Ad-SOS) through the proximal phalanges of the fingers (Figure 4.4).

The measurement site is the distal metaphysis of the first phalanx of the last four fingers. The mediolateral surfaces are approximately parallel, hence reducing scattering of ultrasound waves. In the metaphysis, both cortical and trabecular bone are present. Both types of bone tissue are extremely sensitive to age-related bone resorption. Anatomically, trabeculae decrease in number rather than thickness. Cortical bone usually becomes more porous with advancing age. Also, the cortices of long bone become thinner because the rate of endosteal resorption exceeds the rate of periosteal formation of bone. Taken together, the age-related losses of cortical and cancellous bone substantially increase the fragility of bone. In one study, the phalanges of old women had the highest deviation from peak adult bone mass compared with other techniques such as spine DXA, spine QCT, femoral neck DXA and forearm DXA.[49] They are, therefore, appropriate to evaluate the risk of fracture.

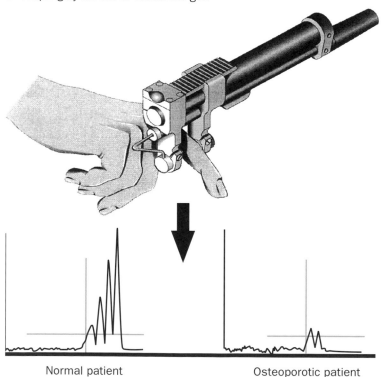

Figure 4.4 Single point QUS systems for measurements at the finger phalanges using gel coupling. This technique uses the transmission technique to measure amplitude-dependent ultrasound velocity through the proximal phalanges of the fingers.

Tibia

Assessment of ultrasound velocity measurements of the tibial cortex uses gel coupling.[50–53] The system differs from that previously mentioned, in that it measures velocity longitudinally along the middle third of the anterior tibia. The midtibia was chosen because of its long straight and smooth surface (Figure 4.5).

As 80% of the skeleton is cortical, and osteoporotic fracture may also involve cortical bone, it might be of clinical interest to measure a cortical bone such as the tibia. In addition, cortical bone loss may play an important role in determining whole bone strength. This device measures longitudinal ultrasound velocity along the anteromedial cortical border of midtibia, thereby taking advantage of a site that is easily accessible in most individuals.

Patella/Ulna

In addition, a number of other ultrasonographic approaches, including devices for measurements at the patella[54–56] or ulna (using a reflection technique),[57] have been described. However, they are not currently commercially marketed.

Quality control in the use of QUS

The application of a stringent quality control (QC) programme in the use of QUS in bone status assessment is very important. This is partly because changes in SOS and BUA caused by disease or treatment are relatively small. Therefore, measurements of bone status changes have to be very precise because procedural errors, malfunctioning equipment or erroneous data analysis may cause substantial interferences even if the data are erroneous by only a few percentage points. The QC protocols should be designed to ascertain that the equipment is functioning properly. Machine differences and lack of an absolute ultrasonographic bone phantom or of universally accepted cross-calibration procedures result in BUA and/or SOS variations when measuring the same subject on different systems.

The degree of complexity of the QC programme will depend on whether it is for an individual site or for a multicentre clinical trial. As an example, for an individual site two types of testing could be carried out: acceptance testing and routine testing.

1. Acceptance testing includes accuracy, in vivo and in vitro precision, and power output measurement. In vivo measurement should cover a wide age and body status range. This is because precision has been reported to vary between normal and osteoporotic subjects.
2. Routine testing includes regular measurement of a QC phantom to detect any drift in the machine and periodic graphical analysis of QC data. Ultrasonographic bone phantoms are not yet available but most manufacturers will provide system-specific ones.

Another aspect of QC is the proper training of the operator. Indeed, positioning error is one of the major sources of imprecision in QUS.[58] The manner of positioning the subjects is one of the main sources of error and the only one that depends on the working procedures of technicians.

WHAT HAVE WE LEARNED FROM IN VITRO STUDIES?

Although recent investigations in vivo have demonstrated the utility of QUS measurements

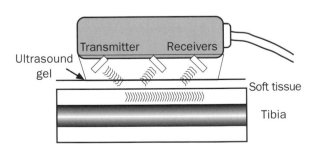

Figure 4.5 Assessment of ultrasound velocity measurements of the tibial cortex using gel coupling. The system measures velocity longitudinally along the middle third of the anterior tibia.

to provide information about bone that is relevant to the management of osteoporosis, the exact mechanisms of interaction of ultrasound with bone and the physical properties measured remain undetermined. It is currently believed that QUS parameters are influenced by the mechanical properties of bone which, in turn, are determined by the bone's material (e.g. BMD) and structural properties (e.g. bone architecture). Research continues to elucidate these relationships and some recent findings have at times provided conflicting information.

Early investigations of QUS showed a dependence of attenuation and velocity parameters on BMD. Recent reports continue to confirm these initial findings.[59–63] Wu et al[64] investigated the dependence of BUA on BMD in vitro. Using cubes of bovine trabecular bone, they measured BUA and BMD at various stages of demineralization achieved by formic acid attack. BUA was observed to decrease in a non-linear fashion with continuing decalcification, until all of the mineral had been removed. Tavakoli and Evans[65] had reported similar results, but did not observe the non-linear behaviour in the narrower range of density changes that they investigated. In another study, Wu et al[66] found significant correlations between site-matched measurements of BUA and BMD in vivo, but with a correlation coefficient of only $r = 0.74$. Thus only about half the variability of BUA was explained by BMD and it has been suggested that bone quality is its other primary determinant. In contrast, other studies of calcanei in vitro have demonstrated that BUA and SOS correlated very highly with BMD by QCT or DXA ($r^2 = 0.59–0.88$).[67–69] Correlations are generally higher in vitro than in vivo, and this perhaps results from the effects of soft tissue, acoustic coupling with the heel and differences in the regions of interest used for DXA and QUS. To varying degrees, these studies suggest that some component of the QUS measurement is not explained by BMD and could reflect other properties of bone.

Evidence that these other properties may be structure related is found in the anisotropy of QUS parameters.[64,70,71] It has been shown that BUA measured in trabecular bone cubes is dependent on trabecular orientation, being 50% higher along the axis of compressive trabeculae. This finding implies that attenuation is dependent on trabecular orientation, which suggests that structure also contributes to the ultrasonic properties of bone. Langton et al[72] measured cubes of equine bone in three orthogonal axes, and reported a significant variation between axes. This significant variation with orientation has also been reported by Nicholson et al[69] in human vertebrae and Njeh[25] in bovine femur. The density of an individual cube is independent of the axis studied, so any variation in ultrasonic properties with orientation will suggest a structural component. Tavakoli and Evans[65] used large static loads to modify the porosity of bovine femur samples, without changing the amount of bony tissue in the path of the ultrasound wave. They concluded that the observed changes in measured BUA were the result of structure rather than of the component material. Glüer et al[73] measured cubes in three orthogonal directions of cancellous bone, cut from fresh bovine proximal radii. The relative orientation of the trabeculae with respect to the direction of the ultrasound beam was evaluated on high-resolution conventional radiographs employing a semiquantitative 'alignment' score. They demonstrated that 'alignment' showed significant association with BUA, indicating that BUA depends on trabecular orientation. Other researchers such as Njeh[25] have used permeability (a parameter that determines the rate of flow of fluid or gas through a porous medium such as cancellous bone) to quantify the structure of bovine and human cancellous samples. However, in a recent investigation, Hans et al[74] reported results of a study of human calcanei in which they compared BMD, BUA and SOS with histomorphometric parameters, and found that, after adjustment for BMD, none of the histomorphometric measures was related to BUA or SOS. This is in contrast to earlier work by Glüer et al[73] who showed, in bovine bone, independent associations of SOS with trabecular separation and BUA with trabecular separation and connectivity. The use of a limited number of specimens, two-dimensional indices of bone architecture and the severity of the statistical test used are potential criticisms of Hans' study and additional investigation will be required. Bouxsein et al[75] have also demonstrated an association between QUS and morphology, but did not test for independence from BMD.

Clinical systems generally do not normalize attenuation to calcaneal thickness. As a result of the anatomical variations in human subjects, it would seem reasonable to attempt to normalize for heel thickness. The effect of normalization for calcaneal thickness has been investigated both in vitro[17,25,66,76,77] and in vivo.[66,78] Hans et al[29] investigated the relationship between QUS and various anthropometric parameters in 271 healthy women. After adjusting for age, only heel width remained a significant predictor for SOS and weight for BUA. Wu et al[66] measured BUA and the width of the calcaneus in 28 postmenopausal women, and found a positive but statistically insignificant correlation between BUA and bone size. Kotzki et al[30] found no significant correlation between heel width and BUA. Contrary to these findings, Serpe and Rho[76] and Njeh[25] reported a linear relationship between BUA and sample thickness in in vitro bovine and phantom studies respectively. However, there does not appear to be a large dependence of BUA on bone size over the range of heel widths typically found in women. Moreover, an earlier study showed no improvement in the ability to distinguish women with vertebral fracture when BUA was normalized for calcaneus width.[78] Although not demonstrated in vivo, it should be understood that BUA is dependent on bone width.

Wu et al[66] investigated the impact of bone size using specimens of bovine trabecular bone. Comparison of attenuation in a whole specimen (width = 24 mm) with the attenuation of the two halves (width = 12 mm) showed that BUA was 32–92% larger for the whole specimen than the mean of the corresponding halves. In addition, the BUA of the whole specimen was always less than the sum of the two halves, indicating that the association of bone size and BUA is complex and non-linear. These results suggest that normalization for bone width is non-trivial and perhaps clinically unnecessary. Indeed, the impact of bone size on BUA in the clinical setting should be small, except where there is a marked variability of calcaneal bone width, as in paediatric studies.

With regard to assessing osteoporotic fracture risk, the relationship between QUS and bone strength is a more interesting question. Several recent studies have investigated this relationship using mechanical testing.[26,75,79,80] The mechanical properties (elastic modulus and ultimate strength) of trabecular bone specimens measured in vitro are well correlated with both BUA and SOS. The empirical data fit reasonably with established theoretical relationships. Moreover, the anisotropy of bone structure, which is detectable with ultrasonography but not absorptiometry, is similarly reflected in the elastic modulus. In studies more applicable to the clinical use of ultrasound, Bouxsein et al[81] have shown that BUA and SOS in the calcaneus are strong predictors of femoral failure loads ($r^2 = 0.51$ and 0.40, respectively) compared with calcaneus BMD ($r^2 = 0.63$) and femoral neck BMD ($r^2 = 0.79$). These studies confirm the potential utility of QUS for bone assessment and fracture risk prediction.

WHAT HAVE WE LEARNED FROM IN VIVO STUDIES?

As an emerging alternative to photon absorptiometry techniques, there is a growing interest in the use of QUS measurements for the non-invasive assessment of osteoporotic fracture risk in the management of osteoporosis. Indeed the relationships of QUS with bone mass, structure and strength suggest that ultrasonography is a useful tool in the clinical assessment of osteoporosis. Measurements in vivo have established normative data and the patterns of changes in BUA and SOS with ageing. Studies have also been conducted to investigate the ability of ultrasonography to discriminate patients with osteoporotic fracture from age-matched controls, and the ability to monitor changes.

Precision and sensitivity

The measurement precision varies depending upon the parameter measured, the site and the system. Many authors have investigated the short-term precision of QUS measurements[50,81–86] (see Table 4.1). However, there is little information about long-term precision in vivo and only a few longitudinal studies on changes of QUS parameters over time have been published.[87–89] Although precision expressed as a percentage coefficient of variation (CV) looks excellent for some QUS parameters,[50,85,86] this may be misleading because it does not take into account the range of values of BUA and velocity across subjects and also whether sensitivity to skeletal change is low.[83–85] Sensitivity is affected by both the measurement technique and the measurement site. To assess the suitability for monitoring changes, the ratio of precision and sensitivity is important. This ratio can be expressed as standardized precision error, defined as the percentage CV of the precision error divided by the standard deviation of the variability across subjects.

The relatively modest precision can be explained, in part, by soft tissue, heel thickness, coupling and repositioning errors, and also the region of interest measured. One study of the factors influencing precision has shown that rotation of the foot about the axis of the leg and translation in the heel–toe direction have the largest impact on the BUA measurement.[90] Foot positioning was considered the primary source of error in the BUA measurement as a result of the inhomogeneity of the calcaneus. Other factors include immersion time of the foot in the water bath, water depth, water temperature, concentration and type of detergents. The authors proposed that the optimum measuring temperature of the water bath was $32 \pm 2°C$, because they demonstrated a decrease in BUA with temperature above $34°C$.

QUS and bone mineral density

Early investigations of QUS showed a dependence of attenuation and velocity parameters on BMD. Correlation coefficients have been reported from about 0.3 to 0.9 for both BUA and SOS.[59–63,89,91,92] Site-matched comparisons of BMD and QUS measurements have produced correlations of about 0.7.[91,92] Thus, only about 50% of the variability of QUS measurements can be explained by BMD. The remainder may be determined by other properties of bone related to bone strength, but this remains to be proven. The limited correlation may also result partly from measurement error. An interesting application of QUS is as a surrogate for BMD measurement by DXA or other radiation-based technique. However, it has been demonstrated that the error in predicting lumbar spine or femoral BMD from calcaneal QUS is large (15–30%) and consequently unreliable.[89] Estimation of bone mass is therefore an inappropriate application of QUS techniques. Furthermore, the relationship between ultrasonographic and absorptiometric parameters may not be linear and careful interpretation of these correlations is required. However, this does not mean that QUS is not useful for fracture risk estimation.

Age-related change

Numerous cross-sectional studies of ultrasonic normative data have been reported.[58,62,84,85,93] They all show that QUS parameters are inversely correlated with age, showing a significant decrease in both BUA and SOS, especially after the menopause. Before this age, both BUA and SOS are relatively stable, although two studies have shown steady declines from age 20.[86,93] Typical rates of change are 0.5–1.0 dB/MHz (0.5–1.0%) per year for BUA and 1–5 m/s (0.1–0.3%) per year for SOS at the heel, patella and tibia. However, there are substantial differences between different devices. The first longitudinal study has been performed by Schott et al[88] on 140 healthy postmenopausal women, measured at the calcaneus. The decrease that they observed over 2 years was $-1.0\% \pm 4.3\%$ for BUA, and $-0.8\% \pm 0.6\%$ for SOS. The decrease in SOS was significantly larger soon after menopause compared with later in life. A similar trend was observed for BUA, but this did not reach statistical significance. Similar results have been found by Krieg et al[94] in institutionalized elderly women.

Velocity and BUA diagnostic sensitivity

Cross-sectional[61,63,82,95] patient studies have demonstrated that QUS can be used to discriminate normal from osteoporotic subject groups, as well as traditional bone densitometry approaches. Moreover prospective studies[32,33,54,55,96] of osteoporotic fracture have shown the ability of calcaneal (and patella) QUS to predict fracture risk with the same power as, and in some cases independently of, measurements of bone mass.

Most investigations have been made with QUS at the calcaneus. Associations have been found with both vertebral and hip fractures as well as fractures of the forearm. Logistic regression analyses have found that risk of fracture (expressed as odds ratios) increases about 1.5–2.5 fold for each standard deviation decrease in BUA or SOS. This makes QUS comparable to, but slightly lower than, X-ray absorptiometry techniques which typically have odds ratios of 1.5–3.0 depending on the measurement site and the population studied. Recently reports have started to appear showing similar capabilities for ultrasonographic measurements at the patella, tibia and phalanges.[44,51,54–56,85,97] These cross-sectional studies are not as extensive as those done for calcaneal ultrasonography and need further investigations to strengthen the different findings. Association with prevalent spine fracture has been demonstrated for all three techniques. However, in some studies the association did not reach statistical significance.[55,62] Patella SOS has also been associated with incident non-spine fractures.[55] In one report of 11 women with hip fracture, tibial SOS was significantly lower in fractured cases than in age-matched controls.[85] Larger prospective studies are needed to evaluate these methods more thoroughly.

Schott et al[63] reported, on 43 hip-fractured

women and 86 age-matched controls, that the height- and weight-adjusted logistic regression coefficients associated with BUA, SOS, stiffness and BMD were all significant ($p < 0.0001$), demonstrating the association of all ultrasonic and DXA parameters with the risk of hip fracture. To assess sensitivity and specificity, the area under the receiver operating characteristic (ROC) curves (AUC) of these parameters was calculated and compared. No statistical difference was, however, found. Similarly, Turner et al[82] reported that velocity measured at the calcaneus (AUC = 0.85) and BUA (AUC = 0.79) had sensitivity comparable to femoral neck BMD (AUC = 0.78) in hip fracture prediction and better than spine BMD (AUC = 0.53). Both studies found that, after adjusting the logistic regressions for femoral neck BMD, ultrasonic parameters were still significant independent predictors of hip fracture.[60,61,63,82,95] In two cross-sectional studies of hip fractures, the association of BUA with the type of fracture (trochanteric versus cervical) was investigated.[63,98] Both studies performed measurements within 2 weeks of the fracture event. In one study,[63] significantly lower BUA was found in cases of trochanteric fracture whereas the other showed no difference, suggesting that the two types of fracture might correspond to different processes. As the calcaneus is composed primarily of trabecular bone, a better association with trochanteric fractures may be expected. However, two prospective studies confirmed the results of Schott et al.[33,99] Hans et al[99] found, in the EPIDOS study population (5662 elderly women aged 75 and older; 115 hip fractures including 62 cervical and 53 trochanteric), that the relative risk (RR) associated with BMD or with the ultrasonic parameters was significantly higher for inter-trochanteric than for cervical fractures, except for the femoral neck BMD where the RR was not significantly higher than that for cervical fracture (Table 4.2). Controlling for femoral neck or trochanteric BMD did not affect the significance of the associations between BUA parameters and the risk of cervical or trochanteric fracture, whereas SOS was no longer significant for the cervical fracture. Furthermore, they

Table 4.2 Relative risk (RR) of hip fracture for a 1 standard deviation reduction in ultrasonic and densitometric parameters according to the type of fracture

	RR (95% CI)[a]		
	All hip fractures	Cervical hip fractures	Trochanteric hip fractures
BUA (dB/MHz)	**2.0** (1.6–2.4)	**1.6** (1.2–2.2)	**2.9** (2.1–4.0)
SOS (m/s)	**1.7** (1.4–2.1)	**1.3** (1.0–1.7)	**2.5** (1.8–3.5)
Femoral neck BMD (g/cm²)	**1.9** (1.6–2.4)	**2.0** (1.5–2.7)	**2.4** (1.7–3.4)

	RR after adjustment for			
	Cervical HF		Trochanteric HF	
	fnBMD	Troch BMD	fnBMD	Troch BMD
BUA (dB/MHz)	1.4	1.3	2.4	2.0
SOS (m/s)	n.s.	n.s.	2.0	1.6

[a] 95% CI, 95% confidence interval; $p < 0.001$.
HF, hip fracture; Troch, trochanteric; fn, femoral neck.

combined calcaneal BUA with femoral neck BMD. It appears that combination of both femoral neck BMD and BUA does not improve the detection of women at high risk of cervical fracture, whereas this combination makes sense for the trochanteric fracture. They concluded that the predictive value of QUS parameters is strongly influenced by the type of hip fracture: BUA – but not SOS – predicts cervical hip fracture independently of hip BMD, whereas both BUA and SOS predict trochanteric hip fracture independently of hip BMD; the use of both methods increases the identification of women at very high risk only of trochanteric hip fracture[99] (Figure 4.6). This confirmed the earlier studies of Bauer et al.[33]

Porter et al[96] demonstrated for the first time the predictive power of BUA in a prospective study on hip fractures in postmenopausal women. However, the statistical analysis did not quantify the fracture risk associated with the decrease of BUA. The first large prospective study of hip fractures (7598 very elderly women), by Hans et al,[32] reported that velocity and BUA measured at the calcaneus had the same diagnostic sensitivity as femoral neck BMD in predicting hip fractures in an age- and weight-adjusted model (Figure 4.7). The increased risk associated with a decrease of one standard deviation of ultrasonography and DXA was estimated as about 2.0 for both velocity and BMD of the femoral neck and 2.2 for BUA. After adjusting BUA and SOS for neck BMD, the logistic regressions showed that both ultrasonic parameters were still significant independent predictors of hip fractures. Similarly, Bauer et al,[33] in another large prospective study conducted in the USA on 6183 elderly women, found an adjusted relative risk of 2.0, 2.2 and 2.6 for os calcis BUA, os calcis BMD and femoral neck BMD, respectively, in hip fracture prediction (Figure 4.7). The associations between BUA and hip fracture remained significant after adjustment for hip BMD, but were no longer

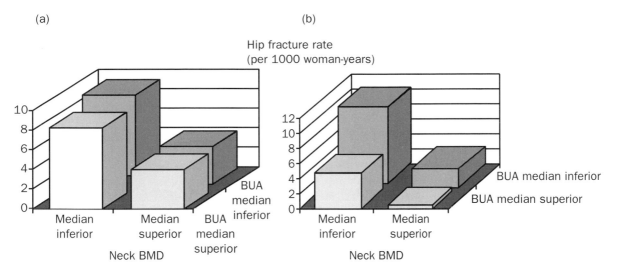

Figure 4.6 Incidence of hip fracture (per 1000 woman-years) as a function of calcaneal BUA and femoral neck BMD median according to the type of fracture: (a) cervical hip fracture; (b) trochanteric hip fracture.

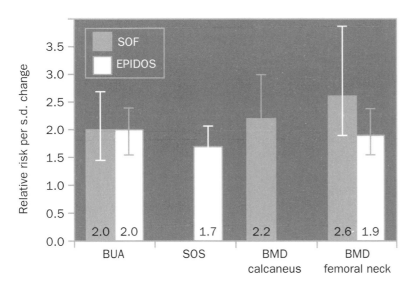

Figure 4.7 Relative risks per standard deviation decrease for the ultrasonic and bone density parameters from two large prospective studies of hip fractures: EPIDOS[32] and SOF[33] studies.

significant after adjustment for calcaneal BMD. It is worth noting that these two studies were carried out using two different ultrasonography systems – the Lunar Achilles for the French study and Walker Sonix UBA575 for the American study – and two different DXA sys-

tems. Recently Glüer et al[100] reported that the odds ratios for hip fracture discrimination vary between ultrasonography systems. This could explain the discrepancies reported between the two studies.

With the exception of the report by Stewart

et al,[101] BUA and velocity have been reported to be as sensitive as spine or forearm BMD to discriminate between normal subjects and patients with vertebral fracture.[55,60,61,82,95,102,103] The association was independent of BMD.[60,95] Heaney et al[54] confirmed the ability of ultrasound velocity at the patella to predict vertebral fractures in a 2-year prospective study.

The associations of QUS parameters with Colles' fractures were not as strong as the association found for hip fractures. Nevertheless, velocity at the patella has been reported to work as well as at the spine or forearm BMD for discriminating patients with Colles' fractures.[104,105]

Stegman et al[55] demonstrated that apparent ultrasound velocity at the patella was as good as forearm BMD for discriminating between normal and low trauma fractures.

QUS and longitudinal monitoring

Jones et al[106] reported that active and sedentary groups of volunteers could be distinguished using BUA ($p < 0.001$). Volunteers were included in the active group if they performed at least 6 hours per week of weight-bearing active exercise, and in the sedentary group if they did less than one hour of weight-bearing activity per fortnight. They observed an increase in BUA ($p < 0.05$) after a year of brisk walking (16–18 km/week).

To date few studies have reported drug effects[87,107–110] or addressed the usefulness of ultrasonography for monitoring treatment of osteoporosis. Hence further longitudinal studies are required (Figure 4.8). Four studies with 2-year follow-up measurements have shown positive changes in QUS parameters between controls and women treated with calcitonin (+4.2% for BUA and +0.8% for SOS),[87] hormone replacement therapy (HRT) (+3.6% for BUA and +0.7% for SOS)[110] and bisphosphonates (estimated +18% for BUA).[108,109] These changes were statistically significant for treatment with calcitonin and HRT but not with bisphosphonate. The power of the bisphosphonate study was limited by the very small sample

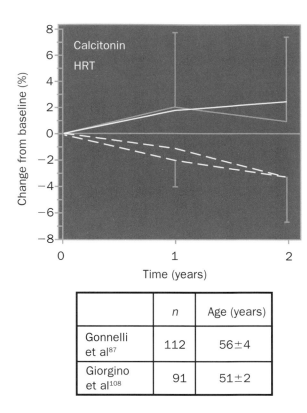

	n	Age (years)
Gonnelli et al[87]	112	56±4
Giorgino et al[108]	91	51±2

Figure 4.8 Two examples of the potential usefulness of ultrasonography for monitoring treatment of osteoporosis: calcitonin and hormone replacement therapy (HRT).

size ($n = 12$). These results suggest some utility for QUS in monitoring patients longitudinally. However, the imprecision of the measurement will make evaluation of changes in the individual more difficult.

CONCLUSIONS

The early scepticism about the role of ultrasonography in osteoporosis is decreasing as a result of the growing body of evidence, particularly from prospective studies, that quantitative ultrasonography is useful for the assessment of bone. Although some in vitro studies have demonstrated that both ultrasound velocity and BUA give structural information, further studies are still necessary to quantify this structural information. Therefore, there is a need to determine which features of ultrasound velocity and attenuation are related to bone density, which reflect changes in architecture independent of density, and how they correlate with mechanical competence. This can be achieved by establishing a theoretical interrelationship of BUA, velocity, architecture and the mechanical properties of cancellous bone.

BUA and SOS are associated with all types of osteoporotic fractures and the associations seem to be partly independent of BMD. In addition, the associations with hip fractures tended to be stronger than with other types of fracture. However, as Glüer et al[100] reported the estimated odds ratios for osteoporotic fracture may vary between ultrasonographic systems. Thus comparison of results across studies may not be valid.

Although osteoporosis is a widespread disease with a substantial impact on the individual, as well as on society, a general screening for this disease is still controversial and must be evaluated based on cost-effectiveness. Bone density is a major risk factor for osteoporosis, with individuals having a low bone density being more likely to have an osteoporotic fracture. However, all established methods for bone density measurements are afflicted with some radiation risk, and they are also relatively expensive. The absence of ionizing radiation, the portability of the equipment and its cost-effectiveness make ultrasonography assessment an attractive option for managing osteoporosis and may be suited as a screening tool for osteoporosis. However, as a result of the ambiguities in assessing accuracy of QUS and the moderate correlation of densitometric and ultrasonic results, currently there is no agreement on how results of QUS devices should be interpreted in order to diagnose osteoporosis. In the near future, it may be possible to find criteria similar to those used for bone densitometry based on the *t*-score and proposed by a WHO study group. However, a general clinical consensus still remains to be established.

REFERENCES

1. Cummings SR, Kelsey JL, Nevitt MC, O'Dowd KJ. Epidemiology of osteoporosis and osteoporotic fractures. *Epidemiol Rev* 1985; **7**: 178–208.
2. Cummings SR, Rubin MPH, Black D. The future of hip fractures in the United States. *Clin Orthop Rel Res* 1990; **252**: 163–6.
3. Cooper C, Campion G, Melton LJ III. Hip fractures in the elderly: a worldwide projection. *Osteoporosis Int* 1992; **2**: 285–9.
4. Consensus Development Conference: Diagnosis, Prophylaxis, and treatment of Osteoporosis. *Am J Med* 1993; **94**: 646–50.
5. Melton LJ, Chrischilles EA, Cooper C, Lane AW, Riggs BL. Perspective: how many women have osteoporosis? *J Bone Miner Res* 1992; **7**: 1005–10.
6. Chevalley T, Rizzoli R, Nydegger V et al. Preferential low bone mineral density of the femoral neck in patients with a recent fracture of the proximal femur. *Osteoporosis Int* 1991; **1**: 147–54.
7. Duboeuf F, Braillon P, Chapuy MC et al. Bone mineral density of the hip measured with dual-energy X-ray absorptiometry in normal elderly women and in patients with hip fracture. *Osteoporosis Int* 1991 **1**: 242–9.
8. Cummings SR, Black DM, Nevitt MC et al. Bone density at various sites for prediction of hip fractures. *Lancet* 1993; **341**: 72–5.
9. Melton LJ, Wahner HW, Richelson LS et al. Osteoporosis and the risk of hip fracture. *Am J Epidemiol* 1986; **124**: 254–61.
10. Cummings SR, Black DM, Nevitt MC et al. Appendicular bone density and age predict hip fracture in women. *JAMA* 1990; **263**: 665–8.
11. Kleerekoper M, Villaneuva AR, Stanciu J, Rao DS, Parfit AM. The role of three-dimensional trabecular microstructure in the pathogenesis of vertebral compression fracture. *Calcif Tissue Int* 1985; **37**: 594–7.
12. Mosekilde L. Sex differences in age-related loss of vertebral trabecular bone mass and structure – biomechanical consequences. *Bone* 1989; **10**: 425–32.
13. Langton CM. Recent advances in the ultrasonic

assessment of bone. *Proceedings of Current Research in Osteoporosis and Bone Mineral Measurement II*, Bath, 1992: 44.

14. Genant HK, Engelke K, Fuerst T et al. Noninvasive assessment of bone mineral and structure: State of the art. *J Bone Miner Res* 1996; **11:** 707–30.

15. Mosekilde L, Bentzen SM, Ortoft G, Jorgensen J. The predictive value of quantitative computed tomography for vertebral body compressive strength and ash density. *Bone* 1989; **10:** 465–70.

16. Melton LJ, Riggs BL. Risk factors for injury after a fall. *Clin Ger Med* 1985; **1:** 525–36.

17. Kaufman JJ, Einhorn TA. Perspective: ultrasound assessment of bone. *Osteoporosis Int* 1993; **8:** 517–25.

18. Hans D, Schott AM, Meunier PJ. Ultrasonic assessment of bone: A review. *Eur J Med* 1993; **2:** 157–63.

19. Langton CM, Palmer SB, Porter RW. The measurement of broadband ultrasound attenuation in cancellous bone. *Eng Med* 1984; **13:** 89–91.

20. Glüer CC for the International Quantitative Ultrasound Consensus Group. Quantitative ultrasound techniques for the assessment of osteoporosis: expert agreement on current status. *J Bone Miner Res* 1997, **12:** 1280–8.

21. Abendschein W, Hyatt GW. Ultrasonics and selected physical properties of bone. *Clin Orthop Rel Res* 1970; **69:** 294–301.

22. Ashman RB, Corin JD, Turner CH. Elastic properties of cancellous bone: Measurement by an ultrasonic technique. *J Biomechanics* 1987; **20:** 979–86.

23. Grimm MJ, Williams JL. Use of ultrasound attenuation and velocity to estimate Young's modulus in trabecular bone. *Proceedings of the IEEE 19th Northeast Bioengineering Conference,* 1993: 62–3.

24. Ashman B, Cowin SC, Van Buskirk WC, Rice JC. A continuous wave technique for the measurement of the elastic properties of cortical bone. *J Biomech* 1984; **17:** 349–61.

25. Njeh CF. The dependence of ultrasound velocity and attenuation on the material properties of cancellous bone. PhD thesis. Sheffield Hallam University, 1995.

26. Rho JY, Ashman RB, Turner CH. Young's modulus of trabecular and cortical bone material: ultrasonic and microtensile measurements. *J Biomech* 1993; **26:** 111–19.

27. Kinsler LE, Frey AR, Coppens AB, Sanders JV. *Fundamentals of Acoustics.* New York: Wiley, 1992.

28. Bamber JC, Tristam M. Diagnostic ultrasound. In: *The Physics of Medical Imaging* (Webb S, ed.). Bristol: Adam Hilger, 1988: 319–86.

29. Hans D, Schott AM, Arlot ME, Sornay E, Delmas PD, Meunier PJ. Influence of anthropometric parameters on ultrasound measurements of Calcaneus. *Osteoporosis Int* 1995; **5:** 371–6.

30. Kotzki PO, Buyck D, Hans D et al. Influence of fat on ultrasound measurements of the calcaneus. *Calcif Tissue Int* 1994; **54:** 91–5.

31. Miller CG, Herd RJM, Ramalingarn T, Fogelman I, Blake GM. Ultrasonic velocity measurements through the calcaneus: which velocity should be measured? *Osteoporosis Int* 1993; **3:** 31–5.

32. Hans D, Dargent P, Schott AM et al. Ultrasonographic heel measurements to predict hip fracture in elderly women: The EPIDOS prospective study. *Lancet* 1996; **348:** 511–14.

33. Bauer DC, Glüer CC, Cauley JA et al. Bone ultrasound predicts fractures strongly and independently of densitometry in older women: A prospective study. *Arch Intern Med* 1997; **157:** 629–34.

34. Langton CM, Ali AV, Riggs CM, Evans GP, Bonfield W. A contact method for the assessment of ultrasonic velocity and broadband attenuation in cortical and cancellous bone. *Clin Phys Physiol Metab* 1990; **11:** 243–9.

35. Vogel JM, Wasnich RD, Ross PD. The clinical relevance of calcaneus bone mineral measurements: a review. *Bone Miner* 1988; **5:** 35–58.

36. Wasnich RD, Ross PD, Heilbrun LK, Vogel JM. Selection of the Optimal skeletal site for fracture prediction. *Clin Orthop Rel Res* 1987; **216:** 262–9.

37. Black DM, Cummings SR, Genant HK, Nevitt MC, Palermo L, Browner W. Axial and appendicular bone density predict fractures in older women. *J Bone Miner Res* 1992; **7:** 633–8.

38. Laugier P, Giat P, Berger G. Broadband ultrasonic attenuation imaging: A new imaging technique of the os calcis. *Calcif Tissue Int* 1994; **54:** 83–6.

39. Roux CH, Fournier B, Laugier P et al. Ultrasound bone imaging: Clinical evaluation of skeletal status. *Osteoporosis Int* 1996; **6:** 84.

40. Guglielmi G, Giannantempo GM, Scillitani A, Chiodini I, Liuzzi A, Cammisa M. Phalangeal QUS and computed X-ray images of hand radiographs. *Osteoporosis Int* 1996; **6:**(suppl 1): 207.

41. Cadossi R, Cané V. Pathways of transmission of ultrasound energy through the distal metaph-

ysis of the second phalanx of pigs: an in vitro study. *Osteoporosis Int* 1996; **6**: 196–206.

42. Mauloni M, Mura M, Paltrinieri F, Ventura V, Isani R. Bone health evaluated in the female population by an ultrasound instrument on proximal phalanxes. *J Bone Miner Res* 1995; **10**(suppl 1): S471.

43. Duboeuf F, Hans D, Dchott A, Giraud S, Delmas PD, Meunier PJ. Ultrasound velocity measured at the proximal phalanges: precision and age related changes in normal females. *Rev Rheum* 1996; **63**: 427–34.

44. Alenfeld FE, Wüster C, Beck C, Meeder P-J, Ziegler R. Quantitative Ultrasound at the phalanges: separation of osteoporotic and non-osteoporotic fractures. *J Bone Miner Res* 1995; **10**(suppl 1): S273.

45. Benitez CL, Schneider DL. QUS assessment of bone in normal and osteoporotic subjects: ability to distinguish between those with and without HRT. *Osteoporosis Int* 1996; **6**(suppl 1): 129.

46. Alenfeld FE, Eggens U, Diessel et al. Quantitative ultrasound and bone mineral density measurements at the proximal phalanges in rheumatoid arthritis. *Osteoporosis Int* 1996; **6**(suppl 1): 170.

47. Ventura V, Mauloni M, Mura M, Patrinieri F, de Aloysio D. Ultrasound velocity changes at the proximal phalanges of the hand in pre-, prei-, and postmenopausal women. *Osteoporosis Int* 1996; **6**: 368–75.

48. Rico H, Aguado F, Revilla M e Coll. Ultrasound bone velocity and metacarpal radiogrammetry in hemodialyzed patients. *Miner Electrolyte Metab* 1994; **20**: 103–6.

49. Kleerekoper M, Nelson DA, Flynn MJ, Pawluszka AS, Jacobsen G, Peterson EL. Comparison of radiographic absorptiometry with dual-energy x-ray absorptiometry and quantitative computed tomography in normal older white and black women. *J Bone Miner Res* 1994; **9**: 1745–9.

50. Orgee JM, Foster H, McCloskey EV, Khan S, Coombes G, Kanis JA. A precise for the assessment of tibial ultrasound velocity. *Osteoporosis Int* 1996; **6**: 1–7.

51. Foldes AJ, Rimon A, Keinan DD, Popovtzer MM. Quantitative ultrasound of the tibia: a novel approach for assessment of bone status. *Bone* 1995; **17**: 363–7.

52. Fan B, Zucconi F, Fuerst T, Glüer CC, Genant HK. Precision assessment: ultrasonic velocity measurement of the mid-tibia versus other techniques. *J Bone Miner Res* 1995; **10**(suppl 1): S368.

53. Stegman MR, Heaney RP, Travers-Gustafson D, Leist J. Cortical ultrasound velocity as an indicator of bone status. *Osteoporosis Int* 1995; **5**: 349–53.

54. Heaney RP, Avioli LV, Chesnut CH, Lappe J, Recker RR, Brandenburger GH. Ultrasound velocity through bone predicts incident vertebral deformity. *J Bone Miner Res* 1995; **10**: 341–5.

55. Stegman MR, Heaney RP, Recker RR. Comparison of speed of sound ultrasound with single photon absorptiometry for determining odds ratio. *J Bone Miner Res* 1995; **10**: 346–52.

56. Lehmann R, Wapniarz M, Kvasnicka HM, Klein K, Allolio B. Velocity of ultrasound at the patella: Influence of age, menopause and estrogen replacement therapy. *Osteoporosis Int* 1993; **3**: 308–13.

57. Zerwekh JE, Antich PP, Sakhaee K, Gonzales J, Gottschalk F, Pak CYC. Assessment by reflection ultrasound method of the effect of intermittent slow-release sodium fluoride–calcium citrate therapy on material strength of bone. *J Bone Miner Res* 1991; **6**: 239–44.

58. Heaney RP, Avioli LV, Chesnut CH, Lappe J, Rescker RR, Brandenburger GH. Osteoporotic bone fragility, detection by ultrasound transmission velocity. *JAMA* 1989; **261**: 2986–90.

59. Gnudi S, Malavolta N, Ripamonti C, Caudarella R. Ultrasound in the evaluation of osteoporosis: a comparison with bone mineral density at distal radius. *Br J Radiol* 1995; **68**: 476–80.

60. Ross P, Huang C, Davis J et al. Predicting vertebral deformity using bone densitometry at various skeletal sites and calcaneus ultrasound. *Bone* 1995; **16**: 325–32.

61. Funke M, Kopka L, Vosshenrich R et al. Broadband ultrasound attenuation in the diagnosis of osteoporosis: correlation with osteodensitometry and fracture. *Radiology* 1995; **194**: 77–81.

62. Rosenthall L, Tenenhouse A, Caminis J. A correlative study of ultrasound calcaneal and dual-energy x-ray absorptiometry bone measurements of the lumbar spine and femur in 100 women. *Eur J Nucl Med* 1995; **22**: 402–6.

63. Schott AM, Weill-Engerer S, Hans D, Duboeuf F, Delmas PD, Meunier PJ. Ultrasound discriminates patients with hip fracture equally well as dual energy x-ray absorptiometry and independently of bone mineral density. *J Bone Miner Res* 1995; **10**: 243–9.

64. Wu C, Glüer CC, Fuerst T, Gindele A, Genant

HK. Ultrasound characterization of bone demineralization. *J Bone Miner Res* 1995; **10**(suppl 1): S374.

65. Tavakoli MB, Evans JA. Dependence of the velocity and attenuation of ultrasound in bone on the mineral content. *Phys Med Biol* 1991; **36**: 1529–37.

66. Wu C, Glüer CC, Jergas M, Bendavid E, Genant HK. The impact of bone size on broadband ultrasound attenuation. *Bone* 1995; **16**: 137–41.

67. Smeets AJ, Kuiper JW, Slis HW. A comparison of site-matched ultrasound, QDR and DXA measurements in the os calcis in vitro: a pilot study. *Osteoporosis Int* 1995; **5**: 303.

68. Droin P, Laugier P, Laval-Jeantet AM, Berger G. Relationships between acoustic parameters and BMD assessed in vitro ultrasound parametric imaging. *Program and Abstracts of the 11th International Bone Densitometry Workshop*, 1995: 28.

69. Nicholson PHF, Haddaway MJ, Davie MW. The dependence of ultrasonic properties on orientation in human vertebral bone. *Phys Med Biol* 1994; **39**: 1013–24.

70. Bouxsein ML, Radloff SE, Hayes WC. Quantitative ultrasound reflects the anistropy of calcaneal trabecular bone. *Program and Abstracts of the 11th International Bone Densitometry Workshop*, 1995: 29.

71. Glüer CC, Wu CY, Jergas M, Goldstein SA, Genant HK. Three quantitative ultrasound parameters reflect bone structure. *Calcif Tissue Int* 1994; **55**: 46–52.

72. Langton CM, Evans GP, Hodgskinson R, Riggs CM. Ultrasonic, elastic and structural properties of cancellous bone. In: *Current Research in Osteoporosis and Bone Miner Measurement* (Ring EFG, ed.). Bath: British Institute of Radiology, 1990.

73. Glüer CC, Wu CY, Genant HK. Broadband ultrasound attenuation signals depend on trabecular orientation: an in vitro study. *Osteoporosis Int* 1993; **3**: 185–91.

74. Hans D, Arlot ME, Schott AM, Roux JP, Kotzki PO, Meunier PJ. Do ultrasound measurements on the os calcis reflect more the bone microarchitecture than the bone mass?: A two-dimensional histomorphometric study. *Bone* 1995; **16**: 295–300.

75. Bouxsein ML, Radloff SE, Hayes WC. Quantitative ultrasound of the calcaneus reflects trabecular bone strength, modulus, and morphology. *J Bone Miner Res* 1995; **10**(suppl 1): S175.

76. Serpe L, Rho J. Broadband ultrasound attenuation values depend on bone path length: An in vitro study. *J Bone Miner Res* 1994; **9**(suppl 1): S278.

77. Bouxsein ML, Radloff SE, Toledano TR, Hayes WC. Calcaneal ultrasound measurements are moderately correlated with trabecular bone density and independent of foot geometry. *J Bone Miner Res* 1994; **9**(suppl 1): S208.

78. Blake GM, Herd RJM, Miller CG, Fogelman I. Should broadband ultrasonic attenuation be normalized for width of the calcaneus? *Br J Radiol* 1994; **67**: 1206–9.

79. Bouxsein ML, Courtney AC, Hayes WC. Ultrasound and densitometry of the calcaneus correlate with the failure loads of cadaveric femurs. *Calcif Tissue Int* 1995; **56**: 99–103.

80. Njeh CF, Langton CM. Prediction of bone strength from ultrasound velocity and apparent density. *Program and Abstracts of the 11th International Bone Densitometry Workshop*, 1995: 30.

81. Mautalen C, Vega E, Gonzales D et al. Ultrasound and dual x-ray absorptiometry densitometry in women with hip fracture. *Calcif Tissue Int* 1995; **57**: 165–8.

82. Turner CH, Peacock M, Tirnmerrnan L, Neal JM, Johnston CC Jr. Calcaneal ultrasonic measurements discriminate hip fractures independently of bone mass. *Osteoporosis Int* 1995; **5**: 400–5.

83. Naessen T, Mallmin H, Ljunghall S. Heel ultrasound in women after long-term ERT compare with bone densities in the forearm, spine and hip. *Osteoporosis Int* 1995; **5**: 205–10.

84. Van Daele PLA, Burger H, Algra D et al. Age-associated changes in ultrasound measurements of the calcaneus in men and women: the Rotterdam study. *J Bone Miner Res* 1994; **9**: 1751–7.

85. Funck C, Wuster C, Alenfeld FE et al. Ultrasound velocity of the tibia in the normal German women and hip fracture patients. *Calcif Tissue Int* 1996; **58**: 390–4.

86. Moris M, Peretz A, Tjeka R, Negaban N, Wouters M, Bergmann P. Quantitative ultrasound bone measurements: normal values and comparison with bone mineral density by dual x-ray absorptiometry. *Calcif Tiss Int* 1995; **57**: 6–10.

87. Gonnelli S, Cepollaro C, Pondrelli C, Martini S, Rossi S, Gennari C. Ultrasound parameters in Osteoporotic patients treated with salmon calci-

tonin: a longitudinal study. *Osteoporosis Int* 1996; **6:** 303–7.

88. Schott AM, Hans D, Garnero P, Sornay E, Delmas PD, Meunier PJ. Age-related changes in os calcis ultrasonic indices: a two-year prospective study. *Osteoporosis Int* 1995; **5:** 478–83.

89. Faulkner KG, McClung MR, Coleman LJ, Kingston-Sandahl E. Quantitative ultrasound of the heel: correlation with densitometric measurements at different skeletal sites. *Osteoporosis Int* 1994; **4:** 42–7.

90. Evans WD, Jones EA, Owen GM. Factors affecting the in vivo precision of broadband ultrasonic attenuation. *Phys Med Biol* 1995; **40:** 407–51.

91. Glüer CC, Vahlensieck M, Faulkner KG, Engelke K, Black D, Genant HK. Site-matched calcaneal measurement of broadband ultrasound attenuation and single X-ray absorptiometry: Do they measure different skeletal properties? *J Bone Miner Res* 1992; **7:** 1071–9.

92. Salamone LM, Krall EA, Harris S, Dawson-Hughes B. Comparison of broadband ultrasound attenuation to single x-ray absorptiometry measurements at the calcaneus in postmenopausal women. *Calcif Tissue Int* 1994; **54:** 87–90.

93. Schott AM, Hans D, Sornay-Rendu E, Delmas PD, Meunier PJ. Ultrasound measurements in os calcis: precision and age-related changes in a normal female population. *Osteoporosis Int* 1993; **3:** 249–54.

94. Krieg MA, Thiebaud D, Burckhardt P. Quantitative Ultrasound of bone in institutionalized elderly women: a cross-sectional and longitudinal study. *Osteoporosis Int* 1996; **6:** 189–95.

95. Bauer DC, Glüer CC, Genant HK, Stone K. Quantitative ultrasound and vertebral fracture in postmenopausal women. *J Bone Miner Res* 1995; **10:** 353–8.

96. Porter RW, Miller CG, Grainger D, Palmer SB. Prediction of hip fracture in elderly women: a prospective study. *BMJ* 1990; **301:** 638–41.

97. Alenfeld F, Wüster C, Goetz M, Beck C, Ziegler R. Diagnostic value of ultrasound measurements of bone mineral density on the metacarpals in healthy and osteoporotic subjects. *Bone* 1995; **16:** 147S.

98. Dretakis EK, Kontakis GM, Steriopoulos K, Dretakis K, Kouvidis G. Broadband ultrasound attenuation of the os calcis in female postmenopausal patients with cervical and trochanteric fracture. *Calcif Tissue Int* 1995; **57:** 419–21.

99. Hans D, Dargent P, Schott AM, Breart G, Meunier PJ, and the EPIDOS Group. Ultrasound parameters are better predictors of trochanteric than cervical hip fracture: The Epidos Prospective Study. *Osteoporosis Int* 1996; **6**(suppl 1): 89.

100. Glüer CC, Fuerst T, Wu CY et al. Diagnostic sensitivity of various quantitative ultrasound and dual x-ray absorptiometry approaches. *J Bone Miner Res* 1995; **10**(suppl 1): S373.

101. Stewart A, Felsenberg D, Kalidis L, Reid DM. Vertebral fractures in men and women: how discriminative are bone mass measurements? *Br J Radiol* 1995; **68:** 614–20.

102. Stegman MR, Heaney RP, Travers-Gustafson D, Leist J. Cortical ultrasound velocity as an indicator of bone status. *Osteoporosis Int* 1995; **5:** 349–53.

103. Wuster C, Paetzold W, Scheidt-Nave C, Brandt K, Ziegler R. Equivalent diagnostic validity of ultrasound and dual x-ray absorptiometry in a clinical case-comparison study of women with vertebral osteoporosis. *J Bone Miner Res* 1994; **9**(suppl 1): S211.

104. Dretakis EC, Kontakis GM, Steriopoulos CA, Dretakis CE. Decreased broadband ultrasound attenuation of the calcaneus in women with fragility fracture. *Acta Orthop Scand* 1994; **65:** 305–8.

105. Kroger H, Jurvelin J, Amala I et al. Ultrasound attenuation of the calcaneus in normal subjects and in patients with wrist fracture. *Acta Orthop Scand* 1995; **66:** 47–52.

106. Jones PRM, Hardman AE, Hudson A, Norgan NG. Influence of brisk walking on the broadband ultrasonic attenuation of the calcaneus in previously sedentary women aged 30–61 years. *Calcif Tissue Int* 1991; **49:** 112–15.

107. Acotto C, Schott AM, Hans D, Njepomniszeze H, Mautalen CA, Meunier PJ. Hyperthyroidism influences ultrasound bone measurements of the calcaneus. *J Bone Miner Res* 1995; **10**(suppl 1): S400.

108. Giorgino R, Paparella P, Lorusso D, Mancuso S. Effects of oral alendronate treatment and discontinuance on ultrasound measurements of the heel in postmenopausal osteoporosis. *J Bone Miner Res* 1996; **11**(suppl 1): M639 (abstract).

109. Ryan P, Herd R, Blake CC, Fogelman I. Calcaneal BUA changes in a 2 year placebo controlled study of pamidronate in post menopausal osteoporosis. *Osteoporosis Int* 1996; **6**(suppl 1): 212.

110. Giorgino R, Lorusso D, Paparella P. Ultrasound bone densitometry and 2-year hormonal replacement therapy efficacy in the prevention of early postmenopausal bone loss. *Osteoporosis Int* 1996; **6**(suppl 1): 226.

5

Clinical usefulness of markers of bone remodelling in osteoporosis

P Garnero and PD Delmas

Bone metabolism is characterized by two opposite activities: the formation of new bone by osteoblasts and the degradation (resorption) of old bone by the osteoclasts. Both activities are tightly coupled in time and space in a sequence of events that define the same remodelling unit. Bone mass depends on the balance between resorption and formation within a remodelling unit and on the number of remodelling units that are activated within a given period of time in a defined area of bone.

Invasive techniques measuring bone turnover have provided useful information, but all have their limitations. Histomorphometry of the iliac crest provides unique information on the rate of formation both at the cell and the tissue levels, and allows the measurement of the activation frequency of remodelling units, although the assessment of bone resorption is less accurate. In addition, measurement of bone turnover is limited to a small area of the cancellous and the corticoendosteal envelope which may not always reflect bone turnover of other sites of the skeleton.[1] Calcium kinetic studies have allowed the quantification of the increase of bone turnover after the menopause, but measurement of calcium accretion rate – an index of bone formation – may be inaccurate in elderly women.[2] Finally, whole body retention (WBR)

of labelled bisphosphonates, a marker of bone turnover and bone formation, has not proved to be very sensitive.[3] These limitations, in addition to the need for non-invasive techniques that can be applied more widely and repeated several times in a single patient, explain the development of markers of bone turnover that are measured in blood and urine.

Osteoporosis is a disease characterized by a low bone mass and architectural deterioration of bone tissue; both are related to abnormalities of bone turnover. However, and in contrast to metabolic bone diseases such as Paget's disease and renal osteodystrophy which are characterized by large changes in bone turnover, osteoporosis is a disease in which subtle modifications of bone remodelling can result in a substantial loss of bone over a prolonged period of time. This explains why data generated with conventional markers such as total alkaline phosphatase activity and urinary hydroxyproline are, most of the time, in the normal range for osteoporotic patients. Consequently, there has recently been a major effort to develop more specific and sensitive biochemical markers of bone turnover.

The rate of bone formation or degradation can be assessed either by measuring an enzymatic activity of the osteoblastic or osteoclastic

---

Table 5.1 Biochemical markers of bone turnover

Formation	Resorption
Serum	**Plasma**
Osteocalcin (bone gla protein)	Tartrate-resistant acid phosphatase
Total and bone-specific	Free pyridinoline and deoxypyridinoline and
alkaline phosphatase	type 1 collagen N- and C-telopeptide breakdown products
Procollagen I carboxy- and N-terminal	
extension peptides	
	Urine
	Urinary pyridinoline and deoxypyridinoline (collagen cross-links) and type I collagen N- and C-telopeptide breakdown products
	Fasting urinary calcium and hydroxyproline
	Urinary hydroxylysine glycosides

---

cells – such as alkaline and acid phosphatase activity – or by measuring components of the bone matrix released into the circulation during formation or resorption, such as osteocalcin and pyridinoline cross-links (Table 5.1). Biochemical markers have been separated into markers of formation and resorption, but in disease states, where both events are coupled and change in the same direction, either of these markers will reflect the overall rate of bone turnover. This chapter reviews the new developments of biochemical markers of bone turnover and their potential uses for the clinical investigation of osteoporosis.

BIOCHEMICAL MARKERS OF BONE FORMATION

Serum total and bone alkaline phosphatase

Serum total alkaline phosphatase activity, usually measured by an automated procedure based on the enzymatic hydrolysis of *p*-nitrophenyl phosphate, is the most commonly used marker of bone formation, but it lacks sensitivity and specificity, especially in patients with osteoporosis. Nevertheless, several studies have shown that its activity increases with ageing in adults, especially in women after the menopause.[4] In patients with vertebral osteoporosis, values are either normal or slightly elevated, and correlate poorly with bone formation determined by iliac crest histomorphometry.[5,6] In addition, a moderate increase of serum alkaline phosphatase is ambiguous because it may reflect a mineralization defect in elderly patients, or the effect of one of the numerous medications that have been shown to increase the hepatic isoenzyme of alkaline phosphatase. To improve the specificity of serum total alkaline phosphatase measurement, techniques have been developed to differentiate the bone and the liver isoenzymes. These techniques rely on the use of differentially effective activators and inhibitors (heat, phenylalanine and urea), wheat germ lectin or concanavalin-A precipitation, separation by electrophoresis and indirect separation by liver-specific antibodies.[7–9] In general, these assays have slightly enhanced the sensitivity of this marker, but most of them are indirect, technically cumbersome, not always specific and their long-term precision is somewhat variable.

A real improvement has been obtained recently by using monoclonal antibodies that recognize preferentially the bone isoenzyme[10] and immunoassays using these antibodies have been developed.[11,12] In normal serum, bone and liver alkaline phosphatase isoenzymes each account for about 50% of the total activity and their structure only differs by post-translational modifications because they are coded by a single gene; it is therefore important to determine the liver cross-reactivity of such immunoassays. These immunoassays have been found to have a low liver cross-reactivity of about 15–20%[11] (Garnero and Delmas, unpublished data). Bone alkaline phosphatase levels obtained by such a direct immunoassay are highly correlated with the electrophoretic assessment of the bone isoenzyme in patients with Paget's disease.[11,12] Immunoassays for bone alkaline phosphatase represent a sensitive marker of the increased bone turnover in postmenopausal women and are an accurate index of the effects of antiresorptive drugs on bone turnover, as discussed below.

Serum osteocalcin

Osteocalcin, also called bone Gla protein (BGP), is a small non-collagenous protein that is specific for bone tissue and dentin, but its precise function remains unknown.[13] However, a recent study showed an increased bone formation without impairment of bone resorption or mineralization in osteocalcin-deficient mice, suggesting that osteocalcin could limit in vivo bone formation.[14] Osteocalcin is predominantly synthesized by the osteoblasts and incorporated into the extracellular matrix of bone, but a fraction of neosynthesized osteocalcin is released into the circulation where it can be measured by radioimmunoassay.[15–17] Osteocalcin mRNA has also been detected in bone marrow

megakaryocytes and peripheral blood platelets, but the protein itself was undetectable in human platelets,[18] suggesting that platelet osteocalcin is unlikely to contribute significantly to either serum or plasma levels. Circulating osteocalcin has a short half-life and is rapidly cleared by the kidneys.[16,19] Serum osteocalcin correlates with skeletal growth at the time of puberty, and is increased in a variety of conditions characterized by increased bone turnover, such as primary and secondary hyperparathyroidism, hyperthyroidism, Paget's disease and acromegaly. Conversely, it is decreased in hypothyroidism and hypoparathyroidism, and in glucocorticoid-treated patients and some with multiple myeloma and malignant hypercalcaemia (reviewed in Delmas[20]). Comparisons of serum osteocalcin with iliac crest histomorphometry and calcium kinetics data have shown that, in most conditions, serum osteocalcin is a valid marker of bone turnover when resorption and formation are coupled, and is a specific marker of bone formation whenever formation and resorption are uncoupled.[21–25]

Radioimmunoassays for circulating human osteocalcin most often utilize bovine osteocalcin as a tracer, standards and immunogen for the production of antibodies, because human and bovine osteocalcin differ by only five amino acids out of a total of 49. The precise antigenic determinants of the osteocalcin molecule have not been clearly identified, but most antisera used in conventional bovine radioimmunoassays recognize the carboxy-terminal region of the molecule, which has been shown to be identical in both human and bovine osteocalcins.[13] Whatever the epitope recognized by these antisera, most – if not all – of these assays do not exhibit a 100% cross-reactivity with human osteocalcin, resulting in poor dilution curves with some serum samples. In plasma, some immunoreactive but not characterized osteocalcin fragments have been found in normal people,[26] in patients with chronic renal failure[27] and in patients with Paget's disease.[26] The disparity between osteocalcin fragments reported by several studies may result from the different ability of various antibodies to detect osteocalcin-related

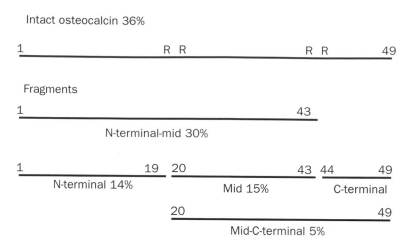

Figure 5.1 Circulating immunoreactive forms of human osteocalcin: the fragments shown on the diagram can be released in vitro by trypsin digestion, because of the Arg–Arg bonds in positions 19–20 and 43–44. In vivo studies using specific monoclonal antibodies recognizing different epitopes on the osteocalcin molecule have confirmed the existence of such fragments in serum. However, the C-terminal fragment has not been detected, probably because of rapid in vivo degradation and clearance from the circulation. (Adapted from Garnero et al.[29])

peptides. Fragments detected in the serum of patients with high bone turnover have been speculated to be released into the circulation during osteoclastic resorption of the bone matrix[27] and a Paget's disease-specific fragment has recently been reported.[26] Nevertheless, the most abundant of these osteocalcin peptides does not seem to be related to bone resorption[28] and the significance of these fragments remains unclear.

Using a battery of monoclonal antibodies directed against the various epitopes of the human osteocalcin molecule, we have found that the intact molecule represents about a third of the immunoreactivity in the adult serum (or plasma). A third is represented by several small fragments and another third by a large N-terminal mid-molecule fragment (N-mid-fragment)[29] (Figure 5.1). This large fragment (about 43 amino acids compared with 49 for the intact molecule), which has not so far been identified by standard chromatographic techniques, is not released from degradation of bone matrix, because its circulating level does not change after acute treatment with bisphosphonate, a potent and specific inhibitor of bone resorption. It has been shown that, after a few hours at room temperature, a significant fraction of plasma intact osteocalcin is rapidly converted into the large N-mid-fragment, resulting in a significant loss of immunoreactivity with

most polyclonal antibodies. We believe that this pattern could account for some of the discrepancies reported in the literature[30–32] and for the surprisingly wide scatter of individual values observed in several studies. From a practical point of view, measuring both the intact molecule and the N-mid-fragment with an assay using appropriate antibodies results in a more robust and sensitive assay. In addition, such an assay reduces, by 50%, the long-term precision error when osteocalcin measurement is repeated over months in a single patient (Garnero and Delmas, unpublished data) and the sensitivity to detect changes in bone turnover is enhanced.[33]

Procollagen I extension peptides

During the extracellular processing of type I collagen, there is a cleavage of the amino-terminal (PINPs) and carboxy-terminal (PICPs) extension peptides before fibril formation. These peptides circulate in the blood where they might represent useful markers of bone formation, because collagen is by far the most abundant organic component of the bone matrix. It has been shown that a single dose of 30 mg prednisone suppresses serum PICPs measured by radioimmunoassay without decreasing urinary hydroxyproline;[34] this suggests that, indeed, circulating PICPs reflect bone formation. Serum PICPs are weakly correlated with histological bone formation, with *r* values ranging from 0.36 to 0.50, in patients with vertebral osteoporosis.[35] The menopause induces a significant, but marginal (+20%), increase in serum PICPs, which is not correlated with the subsequent rate of bone loss measured by densitometry.[36]

Recently, immunoassays for serum PINPs, using different synthetic peptides, have been developed.[37,38] The serum concentration of PINPs may vary 100-fold according to the assay used, suggesting a heterogeneity of the circulating forms of PINPs. Although serum PINPs correlate with serum osteocalcin and alkaline phosphatase activity, it is generally less sensitive than these two other bone formation markers at assessing abnormalities of bone turnover in patients with metabolic bone disease.[37] However a recent study suggests that PINPs are a more sensitive test than PICPs for detecting increased bone turnover in metabolic bone diseases, such as Paget's disease, and for following the decrease in bone turnover after oestrogen replacement therapy.[39]

The reasons for the lack of sensitivity of procollagen extension propeptides are not clear. One important limitation is that these markers reflect not only bone collagen synthesis, but also synthesis in other sites, although the amount of type I collagen produced in bone probably exceeds that produced in all other tissues in adults. Another drawback of these propeptides is that the antigen detected in serum could also result from collagen degradation, because both PICPs and PINPs have been shown to be partially incorporated into collagen fibres.[40] In addition, the metabolism of these peptides is unknown in humans, although it has been shown in the rat that PICPs are bound and internalized by the endothelial cells of the liver through the mannose receptor,[41] and serum concentrations may be affected by degradation and excretion. Characterization of the circulating immunoreactive forms of PICPs and PINPs may help to clarify these uncertainties.

BIOCHEMICAL MARKERS OF BONE RESORPTION

Fasting urinary calcium, hydroxyproline and hydroxylysine glycosides

Fasting urinary calcium measured on a morning sample and corrected by creatinine excretion is certainly the cheapest marker of bone resorption. It is useful for detecting a marked change of bone resorption, but it lacks sensitivity, especially in conditions characterized by subtle alterations of bone turnover such as osteoporosis. Fasting urinary calcium reflects the amount of calcium released during resorption, but also the renal handling of calcium that is influenced by calcium-regulating hormones and oestrogens. Hydroxyproline is found mainly in collagens and represents about 13% of the amino acid content of the molecule.[42] Hydroxyproline is derived from proline by a post-translational hydroxylation occurring within the peptide chain. As free hydroxyproline released during degradation of collagen cannot be reutilized in collagen synthesis, most of the endogenous hydroxyproline present in biological fluids is derived from the degradation of various forms of collagen.[43] As half of human collagen resides in bone, where its turnover is probably faster than in soft tissues, excretion of hydroxyproline in urine is regarded as a marker of bone resorption, although the C1q fraction of the complement contains significant amounts of hydroxyproline and could account for up to 40% of the total urinary excretion of hydroxyproline.[44]

Hydroxyproline is highly metabolized before being excreted and the urinary total hydroxyproline represents only about 10% of total collagen catabolism. Hydroxyproline is present in urine under three forms: free hydroxyproline, small hydroxyproline-containing peptides that can be dialysed and represent over 90% of the total urinary excretion of this amino acid, and a small number of non-dialysable polypeptides containing hydroxyproline.[42] Colorimetric assay of hydroxyproline is usually performed on a hydrolysed urine sample, which therefore reflects the total excretion of the amino acid. As a consequence of its tissue origin and metabolism pattern, urinary hydroxyproline is poorly correlated with bone resorption assessed by calcium kinetics or bone histomorphometry.[19] The sensitivity of the assay can be improved by high-pressure liquid chromatography (HPLC), but there is an obvious need for a more convenient and sensitive marker of bone resorption.

Hydroxylysine is another amino acid unique to collagen and proteins containing collagen-like sequences. Like hydroxyproline, hydroxylysine is not reutilized for collagen biosynthesis and, although it is much less abundant than hydroxyproline, it is a potential marker of collagen degradation.[44] Hydroxylysine is present in part as galactosyhydroxylysine (GHYL) and in part as glucosylgalactosylhydroxylysine (GGHYL). The relative proportion and total content of GHYL and GGHYL vary in bone and soft tissues – the ratio GGHYL : GHYL being 1.6 : 1 in skin and 1 : 7 in bone[44] – which suggests that their urinary excretion might be a more sensitive marker of bone resorption than urinary hydroxyproline. Urinary GHYL increases with ageing,[45] and in patients with Paget's disease, and is more sensitive than hydroxyproline in patients with postmenopausal osteoporosis.[46,47] The recent development of monoclonal antibodies specific for GHYL should be useful for confirming the clinical usefulness of this marker in osteoporosis.[48,49]

Plasma tartrate-resistant acid phosphatase

Acid phosphatase is a lysosomal enzyme that is present primarily in bone, prostate, platelets, erythrocytes and spleen. These different isoenzymes can be separated by electrophoretic methods, which lack sensitivity and specificity. The bone acid phosphatase is resistant to L(+)-tartrate, whereas the prostatic isoenzyme is inhibited by this compound.[50] Acid phosphatase circulates in blood and shows higher activity in serum than in plasma, because of the release of platelet phosphatase activity during the clotting process. In normal plasma, tartrate-resistant acid phosphatase (TRAP) corresponds to plasma isoenzyme 5, which originates partly from bone,

because osteoclasts contain TRAP that is released into the circulation.[51] Plasma TRAP is increased in a variety of metabolic bone disorders with increased bone turnover,[52] and elevated after oophorectomy[53] and in vertebral osteoporosis,[54] but it is not clear whether this marker is actually more sensitive than urinary hydroxyproline.[53] The lack of specificity of plasma TRAP activity for the osteoclast, its instability in frozen samples and the presence of enzyme inhibitors in serum are potential drawbacks which will limit the development of enzymatic assays of TRAP in osteoporosis. Conversely, the development of new immunoassays using antibodies specifically directed against the bone isoenzyme of TRAP[55,56] should be valuable in assessing the ability of this marker to predict osteoclast activity in osteoporosis.

Collagen pyridinium cross-links and type I collagen telopeptide breakdown products

Pyridinoline (Pyr) and deoxypyridinoline (D-Pyr), also called respectively hydroxylysylpyridinoline (HP) and lysylpyridinoline (LP), are two non-reducible pyridinium cross-links present in the mature form of collagen.[57] This posttranslational covalent cross-linking generated from lysine and hydroxylysine residues is unique to collagen and elastin molecules. It creates interchain bonds which stabilize the molecule within the extracellular matrix. The concentration of Pyr and D-Pyr in connective tissues is very low and varies dramatically with tissue type.[58] The highest concentration of Pyr (expressed in moles/mole of collagen) is found in articular cartilage, whereas D-Pyr is present in minute amounts in this tissue.[59,60] Pyr and D-Pyr are present in tendons and the aorta, but absent from the skin, an abundant source of type I collagen.[61] As bone is by far the most abundant source of collagen matrix and because its rate of turnover is markedly higher than some other connective tissues such as cartilage, Pyr and D-Pyr concentrations in biological fluids are likely to be predominantly derived from bone. The relative proportion of Pyr and D-Pyr in bone matrix is variable according to the species. In human bone the ratio Pyr : D-Pyr is 3. Pyr and D-Pyr are released from bone matrix during its degradation by the osteoclasts. As both cross-links result from a post-translational modification of collagen molecules, they cannot be reutilized during collagen synthesis. Pyr and D-Pyr are excreted in urine in a free form (about 40%) and a peptide-bound form (60%). The total amount can be measured by fluorimetry after reversed phase HPLC of a cellulose-bound extract of hydrolysed urine.[59,62]

Total urinary Pyr and D-Pyr are markedly higher in children than in adults,[60] increased by 50–100% at the time of menopause, and go down to premenopausal levels under oestrogen ther-

apy.[63] In patients with vertebral osteoporosis, the urinary cross-link levels, especially of D-Pyr, are correlated with bone turnover measured by calcium kinetics[64] and bone histomorphometry,[65,66] contrasting with poor correlations obtained with urinary hydroxyproline. In pagetic patients treated with intravenous pamidronate, Pyr and D-Pyr – but not markers of bone formation – fall rapidly (within 2 days), indicating that this marker is specific for bone resorption.[67] In contrast to hydroxyproline, Pyr and D-Pyr contained in gelatin are not absorbed by the gut, which allows the collection of urine without any food restriction.[68]

So far, most of the data have been obtained

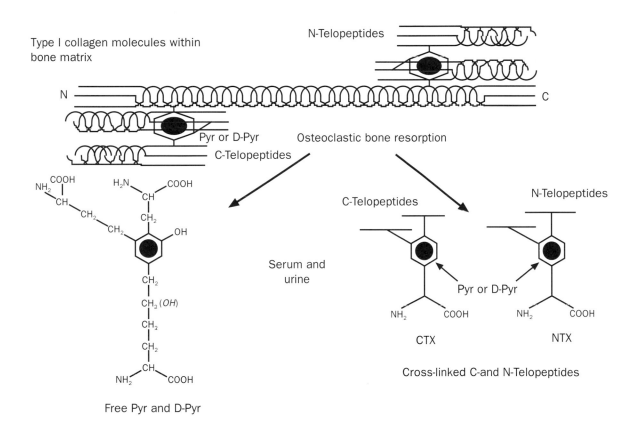

Figure 5.2 Type I collagen breakdown products as markers of bone resorption: type I collagen molecules in bone matrix are linked by pyridinoline cross-links (pyridinoline or deoxypyridinoline) in the region of N- and C-telopeptides. Pyridinoline (Pyr) differs from deoxypyridinoline (D-Pyr) by the presence of a hydroxyl residue, shown in italic. During osteoclastic bone resorption, pyridinoline cross-links are released into the circulation and then excreted in urine as a free form or linked to C- (CTX) or N-telopeptides (NTX) of type I collagen. Free Pyr, free D-Pyr, CTX and NTX can be measured in urine using specific immunoassays.

using the HPLC assay of total Pyr and D-Pyr excretion. More convenient techniques are required for a broad clinical use of this marker. Immunoassays have recently been developed, using antibodies directed against either free Pyr and/or free D-Pyr[69,70] or against peptides in the cross-linking domains of type I collagen. Assays have been developed with antibodies raised against the N-telopeptide to helix domain,[71] the C-telopeptide to helix[72] and against a sequence of the C-telopeptide of an α1 chain[73] (Figure 5.2). These immunoassays are based on antibodies recognizing different moieties, the metabolic clearance of which remains largely unknown. They are likely to have different clinical significance and need to be characterized in various metabolic bone diseases.

Urinary free Pyr is highly correlated with the total Pyr excretion measured by HPLC, and increases significantly after the menopause and in patients with active Paget's disease of bone.[74] The enzyme-linked immunosorbent assay (ELISA) of free D-Pyr, using a monoclonal antibody that does not cross-react with free Pyr, is highly correlated with total D-Pyr measured by HPLC and provides fivefold higher values in children than in normal adults. It is also increased in osteoporotic patients compared with age-matched controls and in diseases characterized by increased bone turnover, such as primary and secondary hyperparathyroidism, Paget's disease and bone metastases from breast cancer.[70]

The urinary ELISA developed against the N-telopeptide to helix (NTX) and against breakdown products of type I collagen C-telopeptide (CTX) show a circadian rhythm similar to that of total pyridinoline excretion, with peak excretion in the early morning and a nadir in the afternoon. The mean amplitude (peak to trough) could reach 100%,[75–78] suggesting that timing of urine collection should be standardized. Bone resorption assessed by NTX and CTX levels markedly increases after the menopause and returns to the premenopausal range after hormone replacement therapy; it is elevated in patients with hyperthyroidism, primary hyperparathyroidism and Paget's disease.[75,79–81]

The fraction of free and peptide-bound pyridinoline cross-links does not appear to be constant. Increased bone turnover, as reflected by the total urinary excretion of pyridinoline cross-links, is associated with a preferential

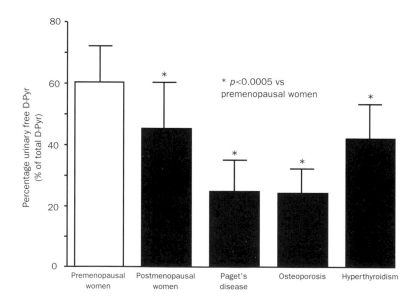

Figure 5.3 Urinary fraction of free deoxypyridinoline (free D-Pyr) in premenopausal and postmenopausal women and in patients with metabolic bone disease. Free D-Pyr is measured by HPLC without hydrolysis of urine samples and the results are expressed as the fraction of the total cross-link excretion measured after hydrolysis of urine. With increasing bone turnover after the menopause and in bone disease states, the fraction of free cross-link decreases. Bars represent the mean + 1 s.d. (Adapted from Garnero et al.[81])

increase of the peptide bound/total fraction and a decrease of the free/total fraction, although the absolute values of both free and peptide-bound cross-links are increased. This observation applies to the normal range of bone turnover in pre- and postmenopausal women, as well as in diseases with high turnover rates such as Paget's disease and hyperthyroidism[81] (Figure 5.3). Recently, it has been shown that the proportion of free cross-links is about twofold lower in serum than in urine (16–20% vs 40%) and that the renal clearance is about fourfold higher for free than for peptide-bound cross-links.[82] These findings could be related to the cleavage of peptide-bound cross-links to free forms in the kidney. If this conversion of peptide-bound to free cross-links is saturable, this could explain part of the inverse relationship between increased bone turnover and decreased free cross-link fraction in urine, an intriguing possibility that should be investigated further. Clearly, for a correct clinical interpretation of the results, it should be borne in mind that each of these new immunoassays for free pyridinoline and related peptides may reflect different aspects of bone resorption.

Urinary assays for bone resorption have several drawbacks. As a result of the marked diurnal variation, collection needs to be controlled and standardized. Values obtained from urinary measurements have to be corrected for urinary creatinine, which adds to the imprecision of the results. In addition, it would be more convenient to measure both markers of bone formation and resorption in a single serum sample. Recently, immunoassays for serum free Pyr, free D-Pyr, NTX and CTX have been developed.[72,82–86] Although preliminary clinical data obtained with some of these new serum assays seem promising (Table 5.2), they clearly deserve further elevation in osteoporosis. An important finding in this field is probably the recent demonstration that the Asp–Gly sequence within C-telopeptides of α1 chains of type I collagen within bone matrix can undergo a β isomerization (Figure 5.4), which is believed in other proteins to reflect ageing of molecules.[87] Thus, in bone matrix, C-telopeptides of α1 chains of type I collagen are present in two forms: linear (α) and isomeric (β) (Figure 5.4).[87,88]

During bone resorption, breakdown products of these two forms, so-called α CTX and β CTX, respectively, are released into the circulation and excreted in urine where they can be specifically measured by immunoassays.[73,89] We have recently found that, in Paget's disease – a disease characterized by a marked increase of bone remodelling in localized areas of bone resulting in a woven bone structure with an irregular and patchy arrangement of collagen fibres[90] – the urinary excretion of α CTX was markedly increased compared with β CTX,

Table 5.2 Serum type I collagen C-telopeptide breakdown products (CTX) in normal individuals and patients with metabolic bone disease

Subjects	n	Serum CTX (ng/ml)	p (vs premenopausal women)
Premenopausal women	22	69 ± 24	
Postmenopausal women	46	125 ± 43	<0.001
Paget's disease	15	234 ± 95	<0.001
Primary hyperparathyroidism	10	335 ± 82	<0.001

Adapted from Bonde et al.[85]

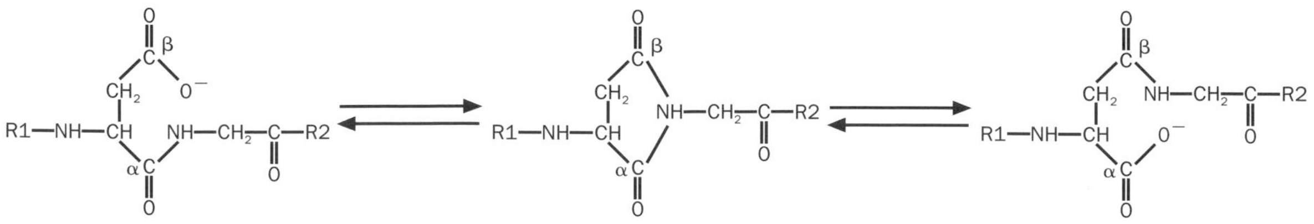

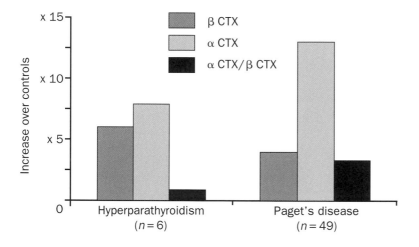

R1-Asp-Gly-R2   R1-Asp-Succinimidyl-R2   R1-β Asp-Gly-R2

Figure 5.4 Spontaneous isomerization of the Asp–Gly sequence within C-telopeptides of α_1 chains of type I collagen. The attack by a peptide backbone nitrogen on the side chain carbonyl group of an adjacent aspartyl residue may result in the formation of a succinimide ring. This ring is prone to further hydrolysis producing β-Asp. The Asp–Gly sequence is present in the C-telopeptides of α chains of type I collagen. Two forms of C-telopeptides of type I collagen are present in bone matrix: the native form (Asp linked to Gly via the α-carbonyl group) and the isomeric form (Asp linked to adjacent Gly residue via the β-carbonyl group). With increasing age of type I collagen molecules, the proportion of the isomeric form within bone matrix increases. Degradation products of these two isomeric forms can be distinguished and measured in urine using specific ELISAs.

Figure 5.5 Increased urinary levels of linear (α CTX) and isomeric (β CTX) forms of type I collagen C-telopeptide breakdown products in patients with metabolic bone disease. For each biochemical marker in each group of patients, results are expressed as the increase over the mean of 97 sex- and age-matched controls.

leading to a urinary ratio α CTX : β CTX three-fold higher than in controls (Figure 5.5). In contrast, in other bone diseases with an increased bone turnover, but with no defect of bone matrix such as primary hyperparathyroidism, the α CTX : β CTX ratio remains normal.[89] These results suggest that the newly synthe-sized collagen fibres found in the woven pagetic bone are characterized by a marked decrease in the degree of isomerization. These exciting findings open new perspectives for the clinical use of bone markers, not only to measure quantitative changes of bone turnover, but also to assess bone quality.

BONE MARKERS IN THE PROGNOSTIC ASSESSMENT OF OSTEOPOROSIS

Bone turnover, postmenopausal bone loss and osteoporosis

Oophorectomy induces a sharp increase of bone turnover markers which peaks one year later and is sustained for at least 10 years.[53] Similarly, several cross-sectional studies indicate that bone turnover increases rapidly after the menopause, with a 50–100% increase of serum osteocalcin and bone alkaline phosphatase, a 50–150% increase of urinary cross-link excretion, and a less pronounced but significant increase of plasma TRAP and urinary hydroxyproline. In contrast with what was originally thought, this increase has been shown, in both bone formation and bone resorption, to be sustained long after the menopause, even in elderly women (Figure 5.6). Hence the age-related bone loss, which has been shown to persist at a significant rate at the hip until the ninth decade,[92] results primarily from the increased bone turnover, although the osteoblastic activity at the level of a remodelling unit declines with age as indicated by histomorphometric studies.[93,94] This pattern has also been documented by the increase of bone formation and resorption measured on iliac crest biopsy in normal women in their late 60s compared with women in their 30s.[2] Markers of bone turnover are negatively correlated with bone mass measured by dual energy X-ray absorptiometry (DXA) at several skeletal sites, and the correlation becomes much stronger with advancing age (Figure 5.7).[91] These cross-sectional data suggest that a sustained increase of bone turnover induces a faster bone loss and thus a

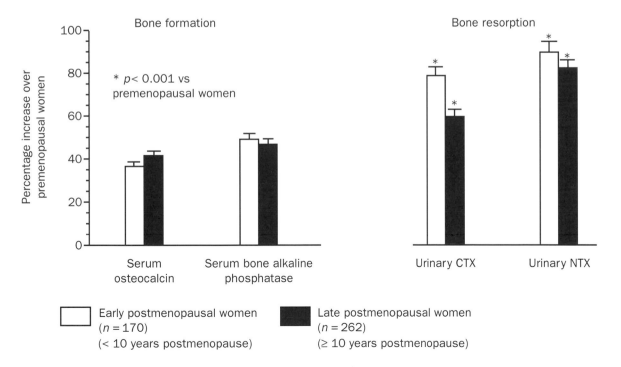

Figure 5.6 Increased bone turnover in early and late postmenopausal women. Bars represent levels of biochemical markers of bone turnover in early and late postmenopausal women expressed as a percentage increase from the mean of 134 healthy premenopausal women. The marked increase of bone formation and bone resorption after the menopause is sustained long after menopause. (Adapted from Garnero et al.[91])

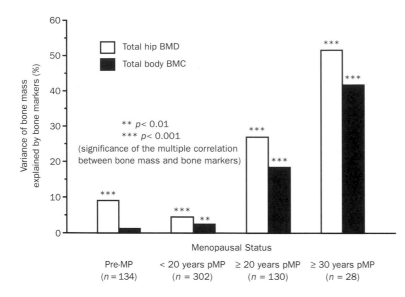

Figure 5.7 Contribution of bone turnover rate to the variance of bone mass as a function of menopausal status and skeletal site. Each bar represents the square of the multiple correlation coefficient between bone markers (osteocalcin, bone alkaline phosphatase, urinary CTX and NTX) and bone mineral density (BMD) at the hip or total body bone mineral content (BMC) measured with DXA. In premenopausal women (pre-MP) and in early postmenopausal women (pMP), within 20 years of menopause (mean age 59 years), bone turnover explained less than 10% of the variance of bone mass assessed. With advancing postmenopausal age, the contribution of bone turnover rate to bone mass variance increases, explaining up to 55% of bone mass in women at more than 30 years after the menopause. (Adapted from Garnero et al.[91])

lower bone mass in elderly women, whereas a relatively low turnover is associated with a lower rate of bone loss in postmenopausal women.

Several studies have shown that, in untreated postmenopausal women followed for 2–4 years, bone marker levels are correlated with the spontaneous rate of bone loss assessed by repeated measurements of the bone mineral content of the radius and the lumbar spine, i.e. the higher the bone turnover rate, the higher the rate of bone loss.[95–97] A combination of a single measurement of serum osteocalcin, urinary hydroxyproline and D-Pyr in early postmenopausal women can predict the rate of bone loss over 2 years with an r value of 0.77.[63] A long-term study suggests that the rate of bone loss measured over 12 years is increased in postmenopausal women classified as rapid

losers from the initial bone marker measurements.[98] Indeed, despite identical bone mass at baseline, women who were diagnosed as fast losers at the initial biochemical measurement had lost 50% more bone 12 years later than those diagnosed as slow losers (total bone loss 26.6% vs 16.6%, $p < 0.001$). Recently, it has been shown that, in those elderly women with high baseline levels of bone markers, the rate of hip bone loss measured prospectively over 4 years was significantly greater than in those with lower levels (Figure 5.8).[99] Although these findings have not been confirmed in all studies,[100] the combination of bone mass measurement and assessment of bone turnover by a battery of specific markers is likely to be helpful in the future for the assessment of the risk of osteoporosis in those postmenopausal women with equivocal bone mass value.

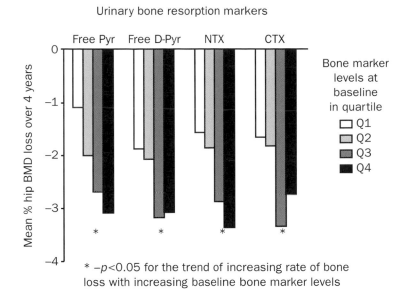

Urinary bone resorption markers

Figure 5.8 Prediction of bone loss by biochemical markers of bone resorption in elderly women. In this study, 410 healthy women, aged 67 years and over, were followed prospectively for an average of 3.8 years. Women were categorized according to baseline levels of urinary markers of bone resorption expressed in quartiles. Higher levels of every bone resorption marker were associated with more rapid bone loss at the hip during the subsequent 4 years. (Adapted from Cummings et al.[99])

* −p<0.05 for the trend of increasing rate of bone loss with increasing baseline bone marker levels

Bone turnover and the risk of osteoporotic fractures

Despite the importance of hip fracture as a major health problem, few studies have investigated potential bone turnover abnormalities in those patients. Histological studies suggest an increased bone resorption as a consequence of secondary hyperparathyroidism. Serum osteocalcin and urinary hydroxyproline have been reported to be either low or normal,[101–103] but the acute changes of body fluid – and perhaps of bone turnover – related to the trauma might obscure subtle changes of bone remodelling. In a large group of patients studied immediately after hip fractures, increased urinary cross-links excretion were found compared with age-matched healthy elderly people, suggesting that increased bone resorption might be a determinant of the low bone mass that characterizes patients with hip fracture.[103] The cross-sectional data are supported by recent prospective studies. Riis et al[104] reported that women within 3 years of menopause classified as 'fast bone losers', i.e. with a high bone turnover rate, had

a twofold higher risk of sustaining vertebral and peripheral fractures, during a 15-year follow-up, than women classified as 'normal' or 'slow' losers. In addition, women with both a low bone mass and a fast rate of bone loss just after the menopause had a higher risk for subsequently sustaining fractures than women with only one of the two risk factors.

Concordant results have recently been obtained in a prospective study of risk factors for hip fractures conducted in a large cohort of elderly healthy women in France.[105] In those women who had a hip fracture during a 2-year follow-up, baseline measurements of urinary CTX and free D-Pyr were higher than in non-fractured controls; increased CTX and free D-Pyr above the normal range of premenopausal women was associated with a twofold increase of the risk of hip fracture, which was still significant after adjusting for hip bone mineral density and mobility status. Thus, the combination of bone mass and bone turnover measurements should be useful for improving the risk assessment of osteoporotic fractures (Figure 5.9). Another interesting result

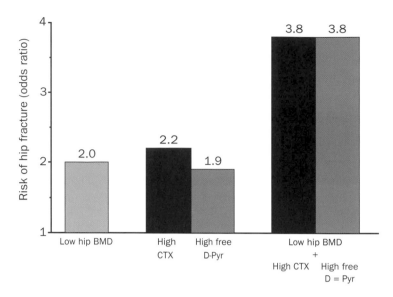

Figure 5.9 Combination of the assessment of bone mineral density (BMD) and bone resorption rate to predict hip fracture risk in elderly women followed prospectively for 2 years: the EPIDOS study. Low BMD was defined as values in the lowest quartile of elderly women. High bone resorption was defined by CTX or free D-Pyr values higher than the upper limit (mean $\pm$ 2 s.d.) of the premenopausal range. Women with both low hip BMD *and* high bone resorption at baseline were at higher risk of subsequently sustaining a hip fracture than women with either low hip BMD *or* high bone resorption. For details concerning the EPIDOS study see the footnotes to Table 5.3. (Adapted from Garnero et al.[105])

of that study was that the susceptibility of hip fracture was not proportionally associated with an increase of absolute levels of bone resorption markers, a finding that contrasts with the progressive increase of hip fracture risk with the decrease in bone mass (Table 5.3). Actually, levels of urinary CTX and free D-Pyr levels above – but not lower than – the upper limit of the premenopausal range was associated with increased hip fracture risk, suggesting that bone resorption becomes deleterious for bone strength, only when it exceeds the normal physiological threshold (mean $\pm$ 2 s.d. for the premenopausal population). For clinical use of bone markers as a predictor of fractures, measurements have to be reliable and reproducible for the correct identification of patients at risk, i.e. those women with a high level of bone turnover. To address this issue, a large group of postmenopausal women was followed over 3 years with four consecutive measurements of bone markers, including serum osteocalcin and bone-specific alkaline phosphatase and the urinary excretion of CTX.[106] According to the marker considered, from 85% to 92% of women classified at baseline as high or low turnover,

i.e. with bone marker levels above and below the upper limit of the premenopausal range respectively, remained similarly classified 3 years later using a different measurement (Figure 5.10). Thus, a single measurement of biochemical markers should be useful to classify reliably postmenopausal women at high- or low-bone turnover.

Vitamin K deficiency has been found in elderly patients with hip fracture.[107] As osteocalcin contains three residues of γ-carboxyglutamic acid (GLA), a vitamin K-dependent amino acid, it was postulated that impaired γ-carboxylation of osteocalcin could be a marker of osteoporosis in elderly people. The level of circulating under-carboxylated osteocalcin, which can be indirectly measured after incubation with hydroxyapatite, is significantly increased in elderly women and decreases with vitamin K treatment.[108,109] In a prospective study in a cohort of elderly institutionalized women followed for 3 years, it was shown that serum under-carboxylated osteocalcin measured at baseline was significantly higher in those who subsequently sustained a hip fracture, whereas other biochemical parameters, including total

Table 5.3 Relationship of decreased bone mass, increased resorption and risk of hip fracture in elderly women

Quartile	Risk of hip fracture: OR (95% CI)	
	Femoral neck BMD	Urinary CTX
I	4.5 (2.1–9.6)	1
II	3.8 (1.7–8.1)	1.8 (0.9–3.5)
III	1.8 (0.8–4.1)	1.0 (0.5–2.1)
IV	1	2.7 (1.4–5.2)

Elderly women belong to the EPIDOS prospective study (7500 healthy independently living women, >75 years of age). During an average of 2 years of follow-up, 109 women sustained a hip fracture. Each hip fractured patient was age matched with three controls who did not sustain a fracture during the same period (nested case-control study). At baseline we measured femoral neck bone mineral density (BMD) using dual X-ray absorptiometry and the urinary excretion of type I collagen C-telopeptide breakdown products (CTX).

Elderly women were stratified in quartiles of femoral neck BMD or quartiles of urinary CTX levels. The risk of hip fracture for women in quartiles I, II and III of BMD was compared with those in the highest quartile. For CTX, the risk of hip fracture for women in quartiles II, III and IV was compared with those in the lowest quartile.

OR, odds ratio; 95% CI, 95% confidence interval.

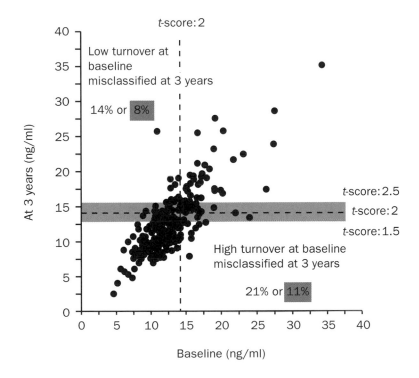

Figure 5.10 Concordance between two measurements of serum bone alkaline phosphatase (BAP) at a 3-year interval in 228 postmenopausal women. At baseline, high bone turnover was defined as BAP levels 2 s.d. above the premenopausal mean, i.e. a t-score > 2 (dotted line). At 3 years, according to the 10% analytical interassay variation, the cut-off point between high and low turnover may vary from 1.5 to 2.5 (grey zone). Patients were considered to be misclassified if they changed classification between the baseline and the 3-year assessment.

osteocalcin, and hormonal measurements showed no differences in the groups.[110,111] In those women with a subnormal level of circulating under-carboxylated osteocalcin, the relative risk of hip fracture was increased.[110,111] In addition, serum under-carboxylated osteocalcin may reflect vitamin D status.[110] Thus, the level of the γ-carboxylation of osteocalcin appears to reflect the poor nutritional status of elderly institutionalized patients with hip fracture and its significance deserves further investigation in the general population of elderly people.

Recently, the authors developed a direct immunoassay for under-carboxylated osteocalcin using human recombinant non-carboxylated osteocalcin as a standard, and a monoclonal antibody that is specific for the non-carboxylated mid-region of human osteocalcin.[112] It was shown that this assay exhibits only a 5% cross-reactivity with carboxylated human osteocalcin and that values measured by this immunoassay are highly correlated with those obtained by the conventional hydroxyapatite method. Using this direct assay, recently the authors found that increased under-carboxylated osteocalcin levels, although not total osteocalcin, was associated with increased hip fracture risk independently of bone mass in a large cohort of elderly women living at home and followed prospectively for 2 years. Thus, this immunoassay should represent a valuable alternative – with possibly increased sensitivity – to the cumbersome and indirect hydroxyapatite assay.

BONE MARKERS FOR MONITORING TREATMENT OF OSTEOPOROSIS

In patients with osteoporosis, there is a wide scatter of individual values of biochemical markers of bone turnover beyond the normal range, which reflects the histological heterogeneity of bone turnover in this disease. The subgroup of osteoporotic patients with high turnover – characterized by increased osteocalcin and hydroxyproline – showed a significant

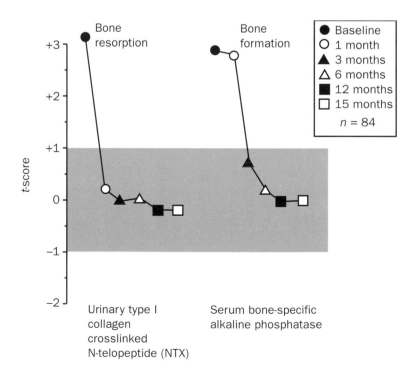

Figure 5.11 Response of markers of bone turnover to treatment with alendronate in late postmenopausal women with a low bone mass. Bone formation and bone resorption markers were measured at baseline and then subsequently after 1, 3, 6, 12 and 15 months of treatment with 10 mg/day of oral alendronate in women (mean age 65 years) with a low bone mass (>2 s.d. below the mean of young adults). Results are shown as t-score, i.e. as number of standard deviations from the mean of premenopausal women. Before treatment both bone formation and bone resorption were markedly increased compared with premenopausal women. After treatment, resorption and formation decreased, earlier for bone resorption than for bone formation, and levels returned to the normal premenopausal range within 3–6 months.

increase of spinal bone mineral density after one year of calcitonin therapy, although those with low turnover had no increase of bone mass despite the same therapy.[113] The authors suggested that patients with high turnover are more likely to benefit from calcitonin therapy. A larger effect on bone mass in high than in low turnover patients with other antiresorptive therapy, such as oestrogen and bisphosphonates, remains controversial.

Antiresorptive therapies, such as oestrogen and bisphosphonate, induce a significant decrease of markers of resorption and formation which fall within the premenopausal range within 3–6 months – earlier for resorption than formation markers (Figure 5.11). In a study comparing various doses of the bisphosphonate alendronate,[114] there was a clear dose-dependent decrease of serum osteocalcin and urinary pyridinoline at the end of the 6-week treatment which reflected the dose-dependent prevention of postmenopausal bone loss observed at 9 months by bone mass measure-

ment.[114] These results, along with other data from various clinical trials, suggest that bone turnover markers could be used to monitor bone mass response to antiresorptive therapy. Given the precision of bone mass measurement by DXA of the lumbar spine and the expected change in bone mass induced by antiresorptive treatment, it is usually necessary to wait up to 2 years after initiating therapy to determine, in a single patient, if treatment is effective, i.e. increases bone mass significantly. Conversely, repeating bone marker measurement within 3–6 months is likely to provide the same information on treatment effectiveness. As shown in Table 5.4, the significant decrease of bone turnover after 3 months of bisphosphonate treatment in osteoporotic women was significantly correlated with an increase of BMD at the lumbar spine at 2 years, with a low rate of false-positive and false-negative results.[115] Thus, repeating the measurement of a sensitive and specific marker of either bone formation or resorption 3–6 months after initiation of oestro-

Table 5.4 Use of bone markers to monitor the long-term effect of bisphosphonate therapy on bone mass

Bone marker	n	Correlation coefficient[a]	p
Osteocalcin	75	−0.67	0.0001
Bone alkaline phosphatase	75	−0.67	0.0001
Total D-Pyr	74	−0.48	0.0001
Type 1 collagen cross-linked N-telopeptide (NTX)	71	−0.53	0.0001

Adapted from Garnero et al.[107]
Late postmenopausal women (mean age: 63 years) with low bone mass at baseline (>2 s.d. below the mean of premenopausal women) were treated with oral alendronate (5 or 10 mg/day) for 2 years. Bone markers were measured at baseline and after 1, 3, 6, 12 and 15 months of treatment (see Figure 5.11).
[a] Between percentage change from baseline of bone markers at 3 months and percentage change from baseline of spine BMD at 2 years.

gen or bisphosphonate therapy is likely to be useful in the management of osteoporotic patients.

CONCLUSION

The immunoassays of osteocalcin and bone alkaline phosphatase represent so far the most effective markers of bone formation in osteoporosis. The measurement of pyridinium crosslinks, and of some type I collagen breakdown products, is the most sensitive marker of bone resorption, and well-characterized immunoassays are valuable alternatives to the HPLC technique. Several cross-sectional and longitudinal studies performed in postmenopausal women strongly suggest that increased bone turnover is associated with increased bone loss and lower bone mass in elderly people and eventually more osteoporotic fractures. Bone markers are likely to improve the efficacy of assessing the risk of osteoporosis by bone mass measurement, but those postmenopausal women who should be targeted for such a combined approach need to be defined. As a result of the small and relatively small change of bone mass (as compared with its long-term precision error) in patients treated with antiresorptive therapy, monitoring treatment efficacy by DXA in the individual patient is a challenge. Clearly, repeated bone marker measurement during treatment is likely to improve the management of osteoporotic patients.

REFERENCES

1. Delmas PD. Biochemical markers of bone turnover in osteoporosis. In: *Osteoporosis: Etiology, Diagnosis and Management* (Riggs BL, Metton LJ, eds). New York: Raven Press, 1988: 297.
2. Eastell R, Delmas PD, Hodgson SF et al. Bone formation rate in older normal women: concurrent assessment with bone histomorphometry, calcium kinetics and biochemical markers. *J Clin Endocrinol Metab* 1988; **67:** 741–8.
3. Thomsen K, Rodbro P, Christiansen C. Bone turnover determined by urinary excretion of [^{99m}Tc] disphosphonate in the prediction of post-menopausal bone loss. *Bone Miner* 1987; **2:** 125–31.
4. Crilly RG, Jones MM, Horsman A et al. Rise in plasma alkaline phosphatase at the menopause. *Clin Sci* 1980; **53:** 341–2.
5. Brown JP, Delmas PD, Arlot M et al. Active bone turnover of the corticoendosteal envelope in postmenopausal osteoporosis. *J Clin Endocrinol Metab* 1987; **64:** 954–9.
6. Podenphant J, Johansen JS, Thomsen K et al. Bone turnover in spinal osteoporosis. *J Bone Miner Res* 1987; **2:** 497–503.
7. Moss DW. Alkaline phosphatase isoenzymes. *Clin Chem* 1982; **28:** 2007–16.
8. Farley JR, Chesnut CJ, Baylink DJ. Improved method for quantitative determination in serum alkaline phosphatase of skeletal origin. *Clin Chem* 1981; **27:** 2002–7.
9. Onica D, Sundblad L, Waldenlind L. Affinity electrophoresis of human isoenzymes in agarose gel containing lectin. *Clin Chim Acta* 1986; **155:** 285–94.
10. Hill CS, Wolfert RL. The preparation of monoclonal antibodies which react preferentially with human bone alkaline phosphatase and not liver alkaline phosphatase. *Clin Chim Acta* 1986; **186:** 315–20.
11. Garnero P, Delmas PD. Assessment of the serum levels of bone alkaline phosphatase with a new immunoradiometric assay in patients with metabolic bone disease. *J Clin Endocrinol Metab* 1993; **77:** 1046–53.
12. Gomez B, Haugen S, Ardakani S et al. Measurement of bone specific alkaline phosphatase activity in serum using a monoclonal antibody. *J Bone Miner Res* 1994; **9**(suppl 1): S348.
13. Price PA. Vitamin K-dependent bone proteins. In: *Calcium Regulation and Bone Metabolism. Basic and Clinical Aspects* (Cohn DV, Martin TJ, Meunier PJ, eds). Oxford: Elsevier Science, 1987: 419–26.
14. Ducy P, Desbois C, Boyce B et al. Increased bone formation in osteocalcin-deficient mice. *Nature* 1996; **382:** 448–52.

15. Price PA, Parthemore JG, Deftos LJ. New biochemical marker for bone metabolism. *J Clin Invest* 1980; **66:** 878–83.

16. Price PA, Williamson MK, Lothringer JW. Origin of vitamin K-dependent bone protein found in plasma and its clearance by kidney and bone. *J Biol Chem* 1981; **256:** 12760–6.

17. Delmas PD, Stenner D, Wahner HW et al. Serum bone gla-protein increases with aging in normal women: implications for the mechanism of age-related bone loss. *J Clin Invest* 1983; **71:** 1316–21.

18. Thiede MA, Smock SL, Petersen DN, Grasser WA, Thompson DD, Nishimoto SK. Presence of messenger of ribonucleic acid encoding osteocalcin, a marker of bone turnover, in bone marrow megakaryocytes and peripheral blood platelets. *Endocrinology* 1994; **135:** 929–37.

19. Delmas PD, Wilson DM, Mann KG et al. Effect of renal function on plasma levels of bone gla-protein. *J Clin Endocrinol Metab* 1983; **57:** 1028–30.

20. Delmas PD. Biochemical markers of bone turnover for the clinical assessment of metabolic disease. *Endocrin Metab Clin N Am* 1990; **19:** 1–18.

21. Brown JP, Delmas PD, Malaval L et al. Serum bone Gla-protein: A specific marker for bone formation in postmenopausal osteoporosis. *Lancet* 1984; **i:** 1091–3.

22. Charles P, Poser JW, Mosekilde L, Jensen FT. Estimation of bone turnover evaluated by 47 calcium kinetics. Efficiency of serum bone gamma-carboxyglutamic acid containing protein, serum alkaline phosphatase and urinary hydroxyproline excretion. *J Clin Invest* 1985; **76:** 2254–8.

23. Delmas PD, Malaval L, Arlot ME, Meunier PJ. Serum bone gla-protein compared to bone histomorphometry in endocrine diseases. *Bone* 1985; **6:** 329–41.

24. Delmas PD, Demiaux B, Malaval L et al. Serum bone gla-protein (osteocalcin) in primary hyperparathyroidism and in malignanat hypercalcemia. Comparison with bone histomorphometry. *J Clin Invest* 1986; **77:** 985–91.

25. Bataille R, Delmas P, Sany J. Serum bone gla-protein in multiple myeloma. *Cancer* 1987; **59:** 329–34.

26. Taylor AK, Linkart S, Mohan S, Chrinstenson RA, Singer FR, Baylink D. Multiple osteocalcin fragments in human urine and serum as detected by a midmolecule osteocalcin radioim-

munoassay. *J Clin Endocrinol Metab* 1990; **70:** 467–72.

27. Gundberg C, Weinstein RS. Multiple immunoreactive forms in uremic serum. *J Clin Invest* 1986; **77:** 1762–7.

28. Tracy RP, Andrianorivo A, Riggs BL, Mann KG. Comparison of monoclonal and polyclonal antibody-based immunoassays for osteocalcin. A study of sources of variation in assay results. *J Bone Miner Res* 1990; **5:** 451–61.

29. Garnero P, Grimaux M, Seguin P, Delmas PD. Characterization of immunoreactive forms of human osteocalcin generated in vivo and in vitro. *J Bone Miner Res* 1994; **9:** 255–64.

30. Delmas PD, Christiansen C, Mann KG, Price PA. Bone gla-protein (osteocalcin) assay standardization report. *J Bone Miner Res* 1990; **1:** 5–11.

31. Blumsohn A, Hannon RA, Eastell R. Apparent instability in serum osteocalcin as measured with different commercially available immunoassays. *Clin Chem* 1995; **41:** 318–19.

32. Hellman J, Käkönen SM, Matikainen M-T et al. Epitope mapping of nine monoclonal antibodies against osteocalcin: combinations into two-site assays affect both specificity and sample stability. *J Bone Miner Res* 1996; **11:** 1165–75.

33. Garnero P, Grimaux M, Demiaux B, Preaudat C, Seguin P, Delmas PD. Measurement of serum osteocalcin with a human-specific two-site immunoradiometric assay. *J Bone Miner Res* 1992; **7:** 1389–98.

34. Simon LS, Krane SMK. Procollagen extension peptides as markers of collagen synthesis. In: *Clinical Disorders of Bone and Miner Metabolism* (Frame B, Potts JT Jr, eds). Amsterdam: Excerpta Medica, 1983: 108–11.

35. Parfitt AM, Simon LS, Villanueva AR et al. Procollagen Type I carboxy-terminal extension peptide in serum as a marker of collagen biosynthesis in bone. Correlation with iliac bone formation rates and comparison with total alkaline phosphatase. *J Bone Miner Res* 1987; **2:** 427–36.

36. Hassager C, Fabbri-Mabelli G, Christiansen C. The effect of the menopause and hormone replacement therapy on serum carboxyterminal propeptide of type I collagen. *Osteoporosis Int* 1993; **3:** 50–2.

37. Ebeling PR, Peterson JM, Riggs BL. Utility of type I procollagen propeptide assays for assessing abnormalities in metabolic bone diseases. *J Bone Miner Res* 1992; **7:** 1243–50.

38. Linkhart SG, Linkhart TA, Taylor AK, Wergedal JE, Bettica P, Baylink DJ. Synthetic peptide-based immunoassay for amino-terminal propeptide of type I procollagen: Application for evaluation of bone formation. *Clin Chem* 1993; **39:** 2254–8.

39. Naylor KE, Blumshon RA, Hannon NFA, Eastell R. Different responses of carboxy and amino terminal propeptides of type I procollagen in three clinical models of high bone turnover. *J Bone Miner Res* 1996; **11**(suppl 1): S194.

40. Fleischmajer R, Perlish JS, Olsen BR. Amino and carboxy propeptides in bone collagen fibrils during embryogenesis. *Cell Tissue Res* 1987; **247:** 105–9.

41. Smedsrod B, Melkko J, Ristelli L, Ristelli J. Circulating C-terminal propeptide of type I procollagen is cleared mainly via the mannose receptor in liver endothelial cells. *Biochem J* 1990; **271:** 345–50.

42. Prockop OJ, Kivirikko KI. Hydroxyproline and the metabolism of collagen. In: *Treatise on Collagen* (Gould BS, ed.). New York: Academic Press, 1968: 215–46.

43. Prockop OJ, Kivirikko KI, Tuderman K et al. The biosynthesis of collagen and its disorders. *N Engl J Med* 1979; **301:** 13–23.

44. Krane SM, Kantrowitz FG, Byrne M, Pinnel SR, Singer FR. Urinary excretion of hydroxylysine and its glycosides as an index of collagen degradation. *J Clin Invest* 1977; **59:** 819–27.

45. Moro L, Mucelli RSP, Gazzarrini C et al. Urinary β-1-galactosyl-*O*-hydroxylysine (GH) as a marker of collagen turnover of bone. *Calcif Tissue Int* 1988; **42:** 87–90.

46. Bettica P, Moro L, Robins SP et al. Bone-resorption markers galactosyl hydroxylysine, pyridinium crosslinks, and hydroxyproline compared. *Clin Chem* 1992; **38:** 2313–18.

47. Bettica P, Taylor AK, Talbot J, Moro L, Talamini R, Baylink DJ. Clinical performances of galactosyl hydroxylysine, pyridinoline, and deoxypyridinoline in postmenopausal osteoporosis. *J Clin Endocrinol Metab* 1996; **81:** 542–6.

48. MacFarlane, Sinykin C, Wang J, Hillam R, Obrisch J. Generation and initial characterization of monoclonal antibodies against synthetic galactosylhydroxylysine. *J Bone Miner Res* 1996; **11**(suppl 1): S192

49. Ju J, Leigh SD, Lundgard RP, Daniloff Gy, Liu V. Development of an immunoassay for galactosylhydroxylysine. *J Bone Miner Res* 1996; **11**(suppl 1): S191.

50. Li CY, Chuda RA, Lam WKW et al. Acid phosphatase in human plasma. *J Lab Clin Med* 1973; **82:** 446–60.

51. Minkin C. Bone acid phosphatase: Tartrate-resistant acid phosphatase as a marker of osteoclast function. *Calcif Tissue Int* 1982; **34:** 285–90.

52. Stepan JJ, Silinkova-Malkova E, Havrenek T et al. Relationship of plasma tartrate-resistant acid phosphatase to the bone isoenzyme of serum alkaline phosphatase in hyperparathyroidism. *Clin Chim Acta* 1983; **133:** 189–200.

53. Stepan JJ, Pospichal J, Presl J et al. Bone loss and biochemical indices of bone remodeling in surgically induced postmenopausal women. *Bone* 1987; **8:** 279–84.

54. Piedra C, Torres R, Rapado A et al. Serum tartrate resistant acid phosphatase and bone mineral content in postmenopausal osteoporosis. *Calcif Tissue Int* 1989; **45:** 58–60.

55. Kraenzlin M, Lau KHW, Liang L. Development of an immunoassay for human serum osteoclastic tartrate-resistant acid phosphatase. *J Clin Endocrinol Metab* 1990; **71:** 442–51.

56. Cheung CK, Panesar NS, Haines C, Masarei J, Swaminathan R. Immunoassay of tartrate-resistant acid phosphatase in serum. *Clin Chem* 1995; **41:** 679–86.

57. Fujimoto D, Morigachi T, Ishida T, Hayashi H. The structure of pyridinoline, a collagen crosslink. *Biochem Biophys Res Commun* 1978; **84:** 52–7.

58. Eyre DR. Collagen crosslinking amino-acids. *Methods Enzymol* 1987; **144:** 115–39.

59. Eyre DR, Koob TJ, Van Ness KP. Quantitation of hydroxypyridinium crosslinks in collagen by high-performance liquid chromatography. *Anal Biochem* 1984; **137:** 380–8.

60. Beardsworth LJ, Eyre DR, Dickson I. Changes with age in the urinary excretion of lysyl- and hydroxylysylpyridinoline, two new markers of bone collagen turnover. *J Bone Miner Res* 1990; **5:** 671–6.

61. Eyre DR, Dickson IR, Van Ness KP. Collagen cross-linking in human bone and articular cartilage. Age-related changes in the content of mature hydroxypyridinium residues. *Biochem J* 1988; **252:** 495–500.

62. Black D, Duncan A, Robins SP. Quantitative analysis of the pyridinium crosslinks of collagen in urine using ion-paired reversed-phase high-performance liquid chromatography. *Anal Biochem* 1988; **169:** 197–203.

63. Uebelhart D, Schlemmer A, Johansen J, Gineyts

E, Christiansen C, Delmas PD. Effect of menopause and hormone replacement therapy on the urinary excretion of pyridinium crosslinks. *J Clin Endocrinol Metab* 1991; **72:** 367–73.

64. Eastell R, Hampton L, Colwell A. Urinary collagen crosslinks are highly correlated with radio isotopic measurements of bone resorption. In: *Proceedings of the Third International Symposium on Osteoporosis* (Christiansen C, Overgaard K, eds). Aalborg, Denmark: Osteopress, 1990: 469–70.

65. Delmas PD, Schlemmer A, Gineyts E, Riis B, Christiansen C. Urinary excretion of pyridinoline crosslinks correlates with bone turnover measured on iliac crest biopsy in patients with vertebral osteoporosis. *J Bone Miner Res* 1991; **6:** 639–44.

66. Roux JP, Arlot ME, Gineyts E, Meunier PJ, Delmas PD. Automated interactive measurement of resorption cavities in transiliac bone biopsies and correlation with deoxypyridinoline. *Bone* 1995; **17:** 153–6.

67. Uebelhart D, Gineyts E, Chapuy MC, Delmas PD. Urinary excretion of pyridinium crosslinks: a new marker of bone resorption in metabolic bone disease. *Bone Miner* 1990; **8:** 87–96.

68. Colwell A, Eastell R, Assiri AMA, Russell RGG. Effect of diet on deoxypyrinoline excretion. In: *Osteoporosis* (Christiansen C, Overgaard K, eds). Aalborg, Denmark: Osteopress APS, 1990: 520–91.

69. Seyedin S, Zuk R, Kung V, Daniloff Y, Shepard K. An immunoassay to urinary pyridinoline: the new marker of bone resorption. *J Bone Miner Res* 1993; **8:** 635–42.

70. Robins SP, Woitge H, Hesley R, Ju J, Seyedin S, Seibel MJ. Direct, enzyme-linked immunoassay for urinary deoxypyridinoline as a specific marker for measuring bone resorption. *J Bone Miner Res* 1994; **9:** 1643–9.

71. Hanson DA, Weiss MAE, Bollen AM, Maslan SL, Singer FR, Eyre DR. A specific immunoassay for monitoring human bone resorption: quantitation of type I collagen cross-linked N-telopeptides in urine. *J Bone Miner Res* 1992; **7:** 1251–8.

72. Ristelli J, Elomaa I, Niemi S, Novamo A, Ristelli L. Radioimmunoassay for the pyridinoline cross-linked carboxy-terminal telopeptide of type I collagen: a new serum marker of bone collagen degradation. *Clin Chem* 1993; **39:** 635–40.

73. Bonde H, Quist P, Fidelins C, Riss BJ, Christiansen C. Immunoassay for quantifying type I collagen degradation products in urine evaluated. *Clin Chem* 1994; **40:** 2022–5.

74. Delmas PD, Gineyts E, Bertholin A, Garnero P, Marchand F. Immunoassay of pyridinoline crosslink excretion in normal adults and in Paget's disease. *J Bone Miner Res* 1993; **5:** 643–8.

75. Schlemmer A, Hassager C, Jensen SB, Christiansen C. Marked diurnal variation in urinary excretion of pyridinium cross-links in premenopausal women. *J Clin Endocrinol Metab* 1992; **74:** 476–80.

76. Eastell R, Calvo MS, Burritt MF, Offord KP, Russell RGG, Riggs BL. Abnormalities in circadian patterns of bone resorption and renal calcium conservation in type I osteoporosis. *J Clin Endocrinol Metab* 1992; **74:** 487–94.

77. Blumsohn A, Herrington K, Hannon RA, Shao P, Eyre DR, Eastell R. The effect of calcium supplementation on the circadium rhythm of bone resorption. *J Clin Endocrinol Metab* 1994; **79:** 730–5.

78. Alexandersen P, Schlemmer A, Riis BJ, Christiansen C. Circadian variation in Crosslaps™. A new marker of bone resorption. *J Bone Miner Res* 1994; **9**(suppl 1): S190.

79. Garnero P, Gineyts E, Riou JP, Delmas PD. Assessment of bone resorption with a new marker of collagen degradation in patients with metabolic bone disease. *J Clin Endocrinol Metab* 1994; **3:** 780–5.

80. Bonde B. Qvist P, Fledelius C, Riis BJ, Christiansen C. Applications of an enzyme immunoassay for a new marker of bone resorption (Crosslaps™): Follow-up of hormone replacement therapy and osteoporosis risk. *J Clin Endocrinol Metab* 1995; **80:** 864–8.

81. Garnero P, Gineyts E, Arbault P, Christiansen C, Delmas PD. Different effects of bisphosphonate and estrogen therapy on free and peptide-bound crosslinks excretion. *J Bone Miner Res* 1995; **10:** 641–9.

82. Colwell A, Eastell R. Renal clearance of free and conjugated pyridinium crosslinks of collagen. *J Bone Miner Res* 1996; **11:** 1976–80.

83. Visor J, Freeman K, Cerelli MJ, Stringer M, Liu V. An immunoassay for the quantitation of pyrdidinoline in serum. *J Bone Miner Res* 1996; **11**(suppl 1): S191.

84. Cheung P, Ju J, Brown B, Cerelli MJ, Liu V. The development of an ELISA for deoxypyridinoline in serum. *J Bone Miner Res* 1996; **11**(suppl 1): S191.

85. Bonde M, Garnero P, Fledelius C, Qvist P, Delmas PD, Christiansen C. Measurement of bone degradation products in serum using antibodies reactive with an isomerized form of an 8 amino acid sequence of the C-telopeptide of type I collagen. *J Bone Miner Res* 1997; **12**: 1028–34.

86. Clemens D, Herrick M, Singer F, Eyre D. Monitoring bone resorption by immunoassay of cross-linked N-telopeptides of type I collagen (NTX) in serum. *J Bone Miner Res* 1996; **11**(suppl 1): S156.

87. Fledelius C, Johsen AH, Cloos P, Bonde M, Qvist P. Characterization of urinary degradation products derived from type I collagen. Identification of a β-isomerized aspartyl residue within the C-telopeptide (α1) region. *J Biol Chem* 1997; in press.

88. Garnero P, Fledelius C, Bonde M, Christiansen C, Delmas PD. Impaired isomerization of type I collagen C-telopeptide in Paget's disease: an index of bone quality. *J Bone Miner Res* 1996; **11**(suppl 1): S370.

89. Bonde M, Fledelius C, Qvist P, Christiansen C. A coated tube radioimmunoassay (α crosslaps RIA) for the assessment of bone resorption. *Clin Chem* 1997; in press.

90. Meunier PJ, Coindre J, Edouard C, Arlot M. Bone histomorphometry in Paget's disease. *Arthritis Rheum* 1981; **23**: 1073–234.

91. Garnero P, Sornay-Rendu E, Chapuy MC, Delmas PD. Increased bone turnover in late postmenopausal women is a major determinant of osteoporosis. *J Bone Miner Res* 1996; **11**: 337–49.

92. Jones G, Nguyen T, Kelly PJ, Eisman JA. Progressive loss of bone in the femoral neck in elderly people: longitudinal findings from the Dubbo osteoporosis epidemiology study. *BMJ* 1994; **309**: 691–5.

93. Lips P, Courpron P, Meunier PJ. Mean wall thickness of trabecular bone packets in the human iliac crest: changes with age. *Calcif Tissue Res* 1978; **26**: 13–17.

94. Parfitt AM, Mathews CHE, Villanueva AR, Kleerekoper M, Frame B, Rao DS. Relationship between surface, volume and thickness of iliac trabecular bone in aging and in osteoporosis. *J Clin Invest* 1983; **72**: 1396.

95. Slemenda C, Hui SL, Longcope C et al. Sex steroids and bone mass. A study of changes about the time of menopause. *J Clin Invest* 1987; **80**: 1261–9.

96. Johansen JS, Riis BJ, Delmas PD et al. Plasma BGP: an indicator of spontaneous bone loss and effect of estrogen treatment in postmenopausal women. *Eur J Clin Invest* 1988; **18**: 191–5.

97. Mole PA, Walkinshaw MH, Robins SP, Paterson CR. Can urinary pyrdidinium crosslinks and urinary oestrogens predict bone mass and rate of bone loss after the menopause. *Eur J Clin Invest* 1992; **22**: 767–71.

98. Hansen MA, Kirsten O, Riss BJ, Christiansen C. Role of peak bone mass and bone loss in postmenopausal osteoporosis: 12 years study. *BMJ* 1991; **303**: 961–4.

99. Cummings SR, Black D, Ensrud K et al. Urine markers of bone resorption predict hip bone loss and fractures in older women: The study of osteoporotic fractures. 1996. *J Bone Miner Res* 1996; **11**(suppl 1): S128.

100. McClung MR, Faulkner KG, Ravn et al. Inability of biochemical markers to predict bone density changes in early postmenopausal women. *J Bone Miner Res* 1996; **11**(suppl 1): S127.

101. Thompson SP, White DA, Hosking DJ, Wilton TJ, Pawley E. Changes in osteocalcin after femoral neck fracture. *Ann Clin Biochem* 1989; **26**: 487–91.

102. Delmi M, Rapin CH, Bengoa JM et al. Dietary supplementation in elderly patients with fractured neck of femur. *Lancet* 1990; **335**: 1013–16.

103. Akesson K, Vergnaud P, Gineyts E, Delmas PD, Obrant K. Impairment of bone turnover in elderly women with hip fracture. *Calcif Tissue Int* 1993; **53**: 162–9.

104. Riis SBJ, Hansen AM, Jensen K, Overgaard K, Christiansen C. Low bone mass and fast rate of bone loss at menopause-equal risk factors for future fracture. A 15 year follow-up study. *Bone* 1996; **19**: 9–12.

105. Garnero P, Hausher E, Chapuy MC et al. Markers of bone resorption predict fractures in elderly women: The Epidos prospective study. *J Bone Miner Res* 1996; **11**(10): 1531–8.

106. Garnero P, Sornay-Rendu E, Delmas PD. Classification of postmenopausal women with markers of bone turnover: A longitudinal study. *J Bone Miner Res* 1996; **11**(suppl 1): S157.

107. Hodges SJ, Pilkington MJ, Stam TCB et al. Depressed levels of circulating menaquinones in patients with osteoporotic fractures of the spine and femoral neck. *Bone* 1991; **12**: 387–9.

108. Knapen MHJ, Hamulyak K, Vermeer C. The effect of vitamin K supplementation on circulating osteocalcin (bone gla protein) and urinary calcium excretion. *Ann Intern Med* 1989; **111**: 1001–5.

109. Plantalech L, Guillaumont M, Leclercq M, Delmas PD. Impaired carboxylation of serum osteocalcin in elderly women. *J Bone Miner Res* 1991; **6:** 1211–16.

110. Szulc P, Chapuy MC, Meunier PJ, Delmas PD. Serum undercarboxylated osteocalcin is a marker of the risk of hip fracture in elderly women. *J Clin Invest* 1993; **91:** 1769–74.

111. Szulc P, Chapuy MC, Meunier PJ, Delmas PD. Serum undercarboxylated osteocalcin is a marker of the risk of hip fracture: a three year follow-up study. *Bone* 1996; **5:** 487–8.

112. Vergnaud P, Katayama M, Delmas PD. A direct and specific immunoassay for undercarboxylated osteocalcin. *J Bone Miner Res* 1993; **8**(suppl 1): S179.

113. Civitelli R, Gonnelli S, Zacchei F et al. Bone turnover in postmenopausal osteoporosis. Effect of calcitonin treatment. *J Clin Invest* 1988; **82:** 1268–74.

114. Harris ET, Gertz BJ, Genant HK et al. The effect of short term treatment with alendronate on vertebral density and biochemical markers of bone remodeling in early postmenopausal women. *J Clin Endocrinol Metab* 1993; **76:** 1399–403.

115. Garnero P, Shih WJ, Gineyts E, Karpf DB, Delmas PD. Comparison of new biochemical markers of bone turnover in late post-menopausal osteoporotic women in response to alendronate treatment. *J Clin Endocrinol Metab* 1994; **79:** 1693–700.

6

Distal forearm and humerus fractures: events that reveal osteoporosis

O Johnell

DISTAL FOREARM FRACTURES

Distal forearm fractures are mainly of two types. The one most related to osteoporosis is Colles' fracture with a dorsal angulation (Figure 6.1). The more unusual and less osteoporotic type is Smith's fracture with a volar angulation.

Treatment

The main treatment for these fractures is, if necessary, reduction, plaster of Paris over a period of 3–4 weeks and rehabilitation training.[1] In recent years there has been a trend towards a more aggressive operative approach, with both open surgery and transfixation to stabilize the fracture. However, few randomized controlled trials have studied the effect of operative treatment. A new approach is to inject biomaterials that will serve as a scaffold for bone cells to invade the material, resorb it and change it to bone. In these biomaterials bone active macromolecules could be added to enhance healing.

Natural course

There are few studies that have followed up patient. One by Frykman,[2] followed 431

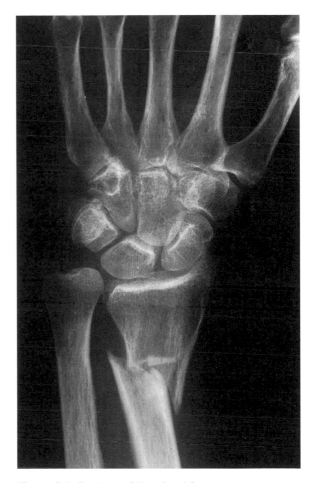

Figure 6.1 Fracture of the distal forearm.

patients for almost 3 years and found that about 6% were recorded as poor, 19% as fair and 75% as good or excellent. The result seemed to be slightly worse with increasing age. Kopylov et al[3] followed younger (30–50 years) patients for 30 years and found that very few had major problems and few developed osteoarthritis. The main problem occurred among those with intra-articular fracture and a step in the joint space of over 1 mm. Bickerstaff and Kanis[4] found that algodystrophy was common in a prospective study of 274 patients with Colles' fracture; six months after the injury, pain and swelling occurred in 20–30%, vascular instability and tenderness in 50% and stiffness in 80%. By one year the problem had decreased; pain occurred in 14% but there was still stiffness in 50%. From this it can be concluded that the morbidity of a fracture of the forearm is low but not unimportant. At least 10% had problems after 2–3 years.

Mortality

The hip fracture is known to have a high morbidity and mortality. The fracture of the forearm has no increased mortality compared with the general population,[5] and Olsson and Hägglund[6] found that patients with fracture of the distal end of the forearm had a better survival than the general population (standardized mortality ratio, or SMR = 0.76).

Incidence of forearm fractures

Forearm fractures are very common. In Malmö, Sweden, they were the most common out of fractures of the hip, the proximal end of the humerus and the radius, and clinical vertebral fractures. In the USA, Melton et al[7] showed similar lifetime risk: hip fracture 18% in women and 6% in men, forearm fracture 16% and 3%, respectively, and vertebral fractures 16% and 5%, respectively. A study from Trondheim, Norway,[8] found that the forearm fracture was the most common fracture admitted to the university hospital there. The incidence is also dif-

ferent in different races. Baron et al[9] showed that black people had a lower risk than white people of sustaining fracture of the hip, distal forearm, proximal humerus and ankle.

The incidence of fracture of the distal end of the radius is hard to calculate because only a minority are hospitalized. Most will, however, probably attend the health care system. The incidence shows that Swedish data, both from Malmö[10] and Uppsala,[11] have the highest incidence, together with Norwegian data,[12] whereas data from the USA[7] and Finland[13] are slightly lower, lower in the UK[14,15] and even lower in a study from Africa.[16]

There has been a trend in Malmö where an increasing incidence was found from 1950 to 1982.[10] This increasing trend seems to have changed and levelled out or it is slightly lower.[17]

The incidence data on fracture of the distal end of the forearm follows the pattern of hip fracture, with the highest incidence in Scandinavia, lower in the rest of Europe and lowest in Africa. The secular trend in Sweden showed an increase until the 1980s and thereafter a levelling out.

RISK FACTORS FOR FRACTURE OF THE DISTAL FOREARM

Bone mineral density

Several studies using patients with fracture of the distal end of the forearm and controls found lower bone mineral density (BMD) values in these patients.[18–21] Nilsson and Westlin[18] found a 7% difference measured at the forearm and expressed a standard deviation (s.d.) of 0.42. Mallmin et al[19] found an 11% reduction in BMD measured at the forearm and expressed an s.d. of 0.48. Krølner et al[20] found a 9% reduction in lumbar BMD and the difference depended on what work capacity the women had. They also found a non-significant difference in forearm BMC of 5%. Wong and Pun[21] measured Colles' fractures in Hong Kong with the dual energy X-ray absorptiometry (DEXA) technique and found a significant difference (8%) in the femoral region, 7% in the pelvis and 9% in the spine. The hip showed an s.d. of about 0.5. From cross-sectional data the difference between individuals with a fracture of the distal end of the forearm and controls is therefore about half a standard deviation, which is less than that for hip fractures in case-control studies[22] where the difference measured at the femoral neck or trochanter was between 0.9 and 1 s.d. from the controls.

In a prospective study, Kelsey et al[23] showed that a strong predictor of fractures was low BMD. When comparing the highest quartile of BMD with the lowest, the risk ratio was 4.1 and for fracture of the proximal end of the humerus it was 7.5. For a standard deviation change of 1 in bone mass, the relative risk was estimated to be 1.7 for forearm fractures and 2.0 for humerus fractures. The Study of Osteoporotic Fractures (SOF) also showed that BMD measurement had a slightly less predictive value for fracture of the proximal end of the radius compared with hip fractures, thus indicating that fracture of the proximal end of the radius is less osteoporotic but is still a fragility fracture. Other risk factors are poor visual acuity, number of falls and frequent walking. These data support fracture of the distal end of the forearm occurring as a result of a fall in relatively healthy women with low BMD of the forearm. Gärdsell et al[24] showed that the predictive value of bone mineral density in a 13-year prospective study was less for fracture of the proximal end of the radius compared with hip fractures and clinical vertebral fractures; for −1 standard deviation of BMD the relative risk for forearm fracture was 1.70.

Conclusion
Most studies have shown that, compared with controls, individuals with fracture of the distal end of the forearm have lower bone mass. In case-control studies the s.d. is about 0.5; two prospective studies measuring the relative risk at the forearm for a 1 standard deviation decrease in bone mass gave a value of 1.70. These data indicate that fracture of the distal end of the radius is osteoporotic, although slightly less osteoporotic than the hip fracture.

Risk factors

Falling is also an important risk factor.[15] O'Neill et al[25] could not explain the variation in the incidence of distal forearm fractures in women with variations in fall frequency. Mallmin et al[26] showed that heredity for fractures and nulliparity were risk factors, and that protective factors were late menopause and postmenopausal osteoporosis therapy. Hemmenway et al[27] found that smoking and alcohol consumption were not related to the risk of wrist or hip fractures in women. They also examined the risk of distal forearm fractures in men:[28] smoking, alcohol consumption, body height and relative height were not related to risk of wrist fractures. Handedness was significantly associated with wrist fractures with left-handers having a multivariate relative risk of wrist fractures that was 1.56 times that of right-handers. Alderman et al[29] examined the postmenopausal risk of hip and forearm fractures, and found that relative weight and duration of oestrogen use were significantly related, but not smoking, parity or lactation. Hernandez-Avila et al[30] found that alcohol was a risk factor for hip fractures and forearm fractures, and was more pronounced in hip fractures, whereas caffeine consumption was significant for hip fractures but not for forearm fractures.

Forearm fractures as a predictor of later osteoporotic fractures

Peel et al[31] examined bone density and distal forearm fracture and concluded that it might be worthwhile measuring bone density in women with distal forearm fractures in the sixth decade because they seem to be at a high risk of vertebral fractures. Bengnér and Johnell[10] found that men and women with radial fracture had a higher risk of having a hip fracture than the total population of Malmö – twice the expected risk. If only those fractures that did not occur simultaneously were included, the values were 1.4 times the expected number of hip fractures. Gärdsell et al[32] found that previous fractures are important predictors of later fractures. A previous fracture of the distal forearm could predict any fragility fracture that will occur later with a relative risk of 1.54 (1.11–2.09) at age 50–59 and 1.75 (1.20–2.56) at age over 70. This is slightly less than the predictive ability of trochanteric or vertebral fractures. In a subgroup analysis of a younger cohort, it was found that, in the age group 40–49 years, the relative risk was 2.67 (1.02–6.94) whereas in the 50–59 group it was 2.32 (1.21–4.44), indicating that, in the younger cohort, it is important to detect the forearm fractures. Mallmin et al[33] studied a population-based cohort over 24 years and found that fracture of the distal end of the forearm in women had a relative hazard of sustaining a subsequent hip fracture of 1.54 and of 2.27 in men.

Lauritzen et al[34] studied radial and humeral fractures as predictors of subsequent fractures and found that women aged 60–79 years who had had a fracture of the distal end of the radius had a relative risk (RR) of sustaining a hip fracture of 1.9 (1.3–2.6); for those who had a fracture of the proximal end of the humerus the value was 2.5 (1.3–3.6). They also found that, when the fracture had occurred in snow or icy weather, the risk for a subsequent hip fracture was only marginally increased – RR = 1.3. They also calculated that a 50-year-old woman with a radial or humeral fracture had an estimated residual lifetime risk of sustaining a subsequent hip fracture of 17% or 16%, respectively, compared with 11% for the background population.

The average relative risk for subsequent hip fractures in those who had had a forearm fracture is 1.5. Thus, selection of patients for a BMD could be considered in those who had had a forearm fracture. This is a large group of people. However, treatment based on a forearm fracture as the sole indicator is probably not necessary at present. If the effect of treating all women with fracture of the distal end of the forearm were calculated, there would be one positive factor: you do not have to screen these women, because they are already there and have visited a doctor. If we use the model proposed by Cummings,[35] his equation is

$$\text{Preventable risk} = I \times p \times \text{RR} \times k \times (A).$$

Where, I = the incidence of fractures in those without the risk factor; P = prevalence of the risk factor; RR = relative risk of fracture due to the risk factor; K = the proportional reduction of the fracture due to an intervention; A = applicability of the treatment. This gives the annual reduction – using the Swedish data for the annual incidence of hip fracture for a 50-year-old woman, the value is 0.00062, the annual incidence for fracture of the distal end of the radius is 0.0077, and the RR is calculated as 1.5 for those with wrist fracture having a subsequent hip fracture; the fracture reduction resulting from the treatment is 0.5.

As a result of the low number of both hip fractures and fractures of the distal end of the radius, the effect in 1000 women would be the prevention of 0.0035 hip fractures in the next year (total hip fractures of 0.62). At the age of 60, there is a higher incidence; the corresponding figures for 1000 women are 0.02 (2.23) and, for 70-year-old women the figures are 0.64 (6.89). Comparing this with other selection mechanisms, and selecting a hip fracture incidence of 0.01, if the prevalence of fracture of the distal end of the radius was 10%, then the corresponding figures would be 0.75 saved hip fractures (total of 10 hip fractures in 1000 women) in the next year. If the selection was those with an s.d. of bone mass of less than −1, and an RR of 2.6, 2.08 hip fractures (10) would be saved the next year; if there was a higher incidence of fractures of the distal end of the radius, such as 34%, then the figures would be 2.25 (10). The effect is of course much greater when calculating for a 10–20 year effect. It might be interesting in the future to discuss selection of specific treatment in this group, using this calculation.

To summarise, patients with fractures of the distal end of the radius could be offered a BMD measurement either at the age 50–70 years if they have one or more risk factors for fractures (such as low bodyweight, maternal history of fracture, previous fracture after 50 years, early menopause, loss of height, glycocorticoid treatment etc.), or at the age of 70 years with none or one risk factor.

Patients with fractures of the distal end of the radius are in the health care system and can

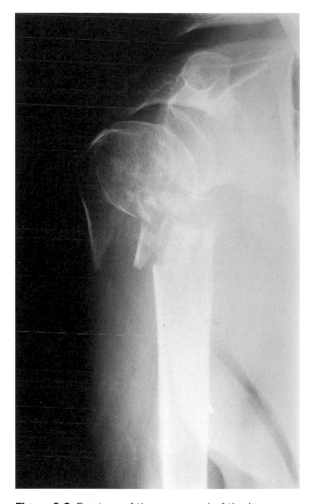

Figure 6.2 Fracture of the upper end of the humerus.

easily be detected and no screening is necessary.

FRACTURE OF THE UPPER END OF THE HUMERUS

This fracture is defined as occurring in different types, according to Neer[36] (Figure 6.2). Far fewer data are available about this fracture, compared with fractures of the distal end of the forearm.

The incidence of fracture of the upper end of the humerus has, consequently, been presented to a lesser extent than for hip fractures or fractures of the distal end of the forearm. In Malmö, Sweden, the fracture is less common, but the incidence is increasing much more steeply with increasing age than fracture of the distal end of the radius; it has approximately the same shape as the incidence curve for hip fracture.[37] There has been an increasing incidence of fracture of the upper end of the humerus, similar to that found for hip fractures and fractures of the distal end of the radius. Nordqvist and Petersson[38] carried out a follow-up from 1987 and they found approximately the same incidence as that at the start of the 1980s. Similar data were presented from the USA.[39]

Fracture of the upper end of the humerus seems to be an osteoporotic fracture rather more than the wrist fracture and is fairly frequent.

Natural course

Einarsson[40] published data from his study in which he followed patients with fracture of the proximal end of the humerus; he found that 10% had problems after 4 years. Clifford[41] found that 81% had a satisfactory result after a year, so this is a fracture with a slightly higher morbidity than fracture of the distal end of the radius.

Incidence

The most common area is the northern parts of Europe. These fractures have a higher cost than the fracture of the distal end of the radius – the patients are older, hospitalized more and more sickly.

Risk factors

These were studied by Kelsey et al.[23] The risk factor pattern showed that patients have a recent decline in health status, including insulin-dependent diabetes mellitus, infrequent walking and several indicators of neuromuscular weakness, such as an inability to stand with the feet in a tandem position for more than a few seconds. The hypothesis that distal forearm fractures occurred more often as a result of falls in relatively healthy and active women with low BMD who have a good neuromuscular function, whereas fractures of the proximal end of the humerus tend to occur as a result of a fall in less healthy and active women with low BMD, who have poor muscular function was supported.

Few studies have been presented on the subsequent fractures after fracture of the proximal end of the humerus, but M. Gunnes and colleagues (personal communication) showed that this fracture was one of the best predictors for vertebral and later hip fractures. Lauritzen et al[34] showed similar findings: at the age of 60–79 years, a woman with a humeral fracture had a relative risk of 2.5 of sustaining a hip fracture.

In summary, patients with fracture of the upper end of the humerus could be offered a BMD measurement in the same way as for the patients with a fracture of the distal end of the radius.

REFERENCES

1. Jupiter JB. Fractures of the distal radius. *Instructional Course Lectures* 1992; **41:** 13–23.

2. Frykman G. Fracture of the distal radius including sequelae – shoulder–hand–finger syndrome, disturbance in the distal radio-ulnar joint and impairment of nerve function. *Acta Orthop Scand* 1967; suppl 108.

3. Kopylov PH, Johnell O, Redlund-Johnell I. Fractures of the distal end of the radius in adults: a 30-year follow-up. *J Hand Surg* 1993; **18B:** 45–9.

4. Bickerstaff DR, Kanis JK. Algodystrophy: an under-recognized complication of minor trauma. *Br J Rheumatol* 1994; **33:** 240–8.

5. Cooper C, Atkinson EJ, Jacobsen SJ, O'Fallon WM, Melton III LJ. Population-based study of survival after osteoporotic fractures. *Am J Epidemiol* 1993; **137:** 1001–5.

6. Olsson H, Hägglund G. Reduced cancer morbidity and mortality in a prospective cohort of women with distal forearm fractures. *Am J Epidemiol* 1992; **136:** 422–7.

7. Melton III LJ, Chrischilles EA, Cooper C, Lane AW, Riggs BL. How many women have osteoporosis? *J Bone Miner Res* 1992; **7:** 1005–10.

8. Sahlin Y. Occurrence of fractures in a defined population: a 1-year study. *Injury* 1990; **21:** 158–60.

9. Baron JA, Barrett J, Malenka D et al. Racial differences in fracture risk. *Epidemiology* 1994; **5:** 42–7.

10. Bengnér U, Johnell O. Increasing incidence of forearm fractures. *Acta Orthop Scand* 1985; **56:** 158–60.

11. Mallmin H, Ljunghall S. Incidence of Colles' fracture in Uppsala. *Acta Orthop Scand* 1992; **63:** 213–15.

12. Falch JA. Epidemiology of fractures of the distal forearm in Oslo, Norway. *Acta Orthop Scand* 1983; **54:** 291–5.

13. Kaukonen J-P. Fractures of the distal forearm in the Helsinki district. *Ann Chir Gynaecol* 1985; **74:** 19–21.

14. Miller SWM, Grimley Evans J. Fractures of the distal forearm in Newcastle: an epidemiological survey. *Age Ageing* 1985; **14:** 155–8.

15. Winner SJ, Morgan CA, Grimley Evans J. Perimenopausal risk of falling and incidence of distal forearm fracture. *BMJ* 1989; **298:** 1486–8.

16. Adebajo AO, Cooper C, Gimley Evans J. Fractures of the hip and distal forearm in West Africa and the United Kingdom. *Age Ageing* 1991; **20:** 435–8.

17. Jónsson B, Bengnér U, Redlund-Johnell I, Johnell O. Changes in the incidence of forearm fractures in Malmö. *Acta Orthop Scand* 1996 **67**(suppl 270): 67.

18. Nilsson BE, Westlin NE. The bone mineral content in the forearm of women with Colles' fracture. *Acta Orthop Scand* 1974; **45:** 836–44.

19. Mallmin H, Ljunghall S, Naessén T. Colles' fracture associated with reduced bone mineral content. *Acta Orthop Scand* 1992; **63:** 552–4.

20. Krølner B, Tondevol E, Toft B, Berthelsen B, Pors Nielsen S. Bone mass of the axial and the appendicular skeleton in women with Colles' fracture: its relation to physical activity. *Clin Physiol* 1982; **2:** 147–57.

21. Wong FHW, Pun KK. Total and regional bone mineral densities in women with Colles' frac-

tures: a comparative study with normal matched controls. *Singapore Med J* 1993; **34**: 229–32.

22. Marshall D, Johnell O, Wedel H. Meta-analysis of how well measures of bone mineral density predict occurrence of osteoporotic fractures. *BMJ* 1996; **312**: 1254–9.

23. Kelsy JL, Browner WS, Seeley DG, Nevitt MC, Cummings SR. Risk factors for fractures of the distal forearm and proximal humerus. *Am J Epidemiol* 1992; **135**: 477–89.

24. Gärdsell P, Johnell O, Nilsson BE, Gullberg B. Predicting various fragility fractures in women by forearm bone densitometry: a follow-up study. *Calcif Tissue Int* 1993; **52**: 348–53.

25. O'Neill TW, Varlow J, Reeve J et al. Fall frequency and incidence of distal forearm fracture in the UK. *J Epidemiol Commun Health* 1995; **49**: 597–8.

26. Mallmin H, Ljunghall S, Persson I, Bergström R. Risk factors for fractures of the distal forearm: a population-based case-control study. *Osteoporosis Int* 1994; **4**: 298–304.

27. Hemenway D, Colditz GA, Willet WC, Stampfer MJ, Speizer FE. Fractures and lifestyle: effect of cigarette smoking, alcohol intake, and relative weight on the risk of hip and forearm fractures in middle-aged women. *Am J Public Health* 1988; **78**: 1554–7.

28. Hemenway D, Azrael DR, Rimm EB, Feskanich D, Willett WC. Risk factors for wrist fracture: effect of age, cigarettes, alcohol, body height, relative weight, and handedness on the risk for distal forearm fractures in men. *Am J Epidemiol* 1994; **140**: 361–7.

29. Alderman BW, Weiss NS, Daling JR, Ure CI, Ballard JH. Reproductive history and post-menopausal risk of hip and forearm fracture. *Am J Epidemiol* 1986; **124**: 262–7.

30. Hernandez-Avila M, Colditz GA, Stampfer MJ, Rosner B, Speizer FE, Willet WC. Caffeine, moderate alcohol intake, and risk of fractures of the hip and forearm in middle-aged women. *Am J Clin Nutr* 1991; **54**: 157–63.

31. Peel NFA, Barrington NA, Smith TWD, Eastell R. Distal forearm fracture as risk factor for vertebral osteoporosis. *BMJ* 1994; **308**: 1544–5.

32. Gärdsell P, Johnell O, Nilsson BE, Nilsson JÅ. The predictive value of fracture, disease, and falling tendency for fragility fractures in women. *Calcif Tissue Int* 1989; **45**: 327–30.

33. Mallmin H, Ljunghall S, Persson I, Naessén T, Krusemo U-B, Bergström R. Fracture of the distal forearm as a forecaster of subsequent hip fracture: a population-based cohort study with 24 years of follow-up. *Calcif Tissue Int* 1993; **52**: 269–72.

34. Lauritzen JB, Schwarz P, McNair P, Lund B, Transbøl I. Radial and humeral fractures as predictors of subsequent hip, radial or humeral fractures in women, and their seasonal variation. *Osteoporosis Int* 1993; **3**: 133–7.

35. Cummings SR. Prevention of osteoporotic fractures: what we need to know. In: *Osteoporosis 1990* (Christiansen C, Overgaard K, eds). Copenhagen: Osteopress ApS, 14–20 October 1990.

36. Neer CS. Displaced proximal humerus fracture. *J Bone Joint Surg* 1970; **52A**: 1077–89.

37. Bengnér U, Johnell O, Redlund-Johnell I. Changes in the incidence of fracture of the upper end of the humerus during a 30-year period. *Clin Orthop* 1988; **231**: 179–82.

38. Nordqvist A, Petersson CJ. Incidence and causes of shoulder girdle injuries in an urban population. *J Shoulder Elbow Surg* 1995; **4**: 107–12.

39. Rose SH, Melton III LJ, Morrey BF, Ilstrup DM, Riggs BL. Epidemiologic features of humeral fractures. *Clin Orthop* 1982; **168**: 24–30.

40. Clifford PC. Fractures of the neck of the humerus: a review of the late results. *Injury* 1980; **12**: 91.

41. Einarsson F. Fracture of the upper end of the humerus. *Acta Orthop Scand* 1958; suppl 32.

7

Oestrogens and anti-oestrogens for the prevention and treatment of osteoporosis

CP Spencer and JC Stevenson

Osteoporosis can be defined as a metabolic bone disorder that results in low bone mass and microarchitectural deterioration of bone structure, leading to an increase in bone fragility and, consequently, an increase in fracture risk. These fractures can occur almost anywhere in the body but the most common sites are the hip, lumbar spine and wrist. The most important clinical site for osteoporotic fracture is the femoral neck because morbidity and mortality is highest in women who have this type of fracture. The risk of osteoporosis development is higher in women than in men – 75% of osteoporotic fractures occur in women – and there is also a geographical variation with the highest incidence of osteoporosis being in Asia.[1] In North America and northern Europe, the lifetime risk of osteoporotic fracture in 50-year-old postmenopausal women is at least 40%.

Although women may begin to lose bone from the proximal femur by the age of 30, it is the onset of the menopause that results in major bone loss from all sites, as a result of a reduction in circulating oestrogens.[2] After the menopause, bone loss accelerates and as much as 5%, or more, of trabecular and 1.5% of cortical bone are lost annually. After 5–10 years, this rate may slow but continued bone loss persists into old age. This reduction in bone mass seen at the menopause is related to a decline in ovarian function and, consistent with this, a similar loss of bone density is observed in women who undergo a premature menopause. Oestrogen replacement therapy is effective in reducing the risk of osteoporotic fractures in later life and in addition, according to epidemiological studies, reduces the risk of coronary heart disease by as much as 50%.[3,4] Nevertheless, there are several disadvantages to hormone replacement therapy (HRT) which include side effects from therapy as well as a possible increased risk of breast cancer after many years of treatment. In addition, in non-hysterectomized women it is necessary to administer a progestogen for at least 12 days of each month to reduce the risk of endometrial hyperplasia/carcinoma development.

Anti-oestrogens are a class of drugs that were originally developed as postcoital contraceptives but have been extensively used in the treatment of breast cancer and anovulatory infertility. These compounds exert an oestrogen agonist effect on bone and may hold promise as future agents in the treatment of osteoporosis without the disadvantages of conventional HRT. Other oestrogen analogues include tibolone which has oestrogenic, progestogenic and androgenic properties, and also has a bone-conserving effect.[5–7]

OESTROGENS FOR THE TREATMENT OF OSTEOPOROSIS

Hormone replacement therapy is a well-established mode of treatment for osteoporosis and results not only in arresting bone loss but also in an improvement in bone density and a reduced risk of osteoporotic fracture. Epidemiological[8-15] as well as clinical data[16-21] support this effect consistently. Synthetic oestrogens, such as ethinyl oestradiol used in the combined oral contraceptive pill, also act as bone conservers.[22] Bone density has been shown to increase by up to 10% in post-menopausal women treated with a year of HRT and fracture risk is reduced by as much as 60% if HRT is taken for 6 years or longer.[11] Despite these positive effects on bone mineral density, there appears to be a group of women who do not conserve bone while on oestrogen replacement.[16,23] Assessing the precise number of these women is difficult because the precision error of bone density measurements may be of the same magnitude as normal postmenopausal bone loss in the short term. Furthermore, the site of bone loss seems to be important in assessing non-responders to HRT: in the distal forearm it is about 1%,[24] 12% in the femoral neck and 2% in the lumbar spine.[16] Cessation of

HRT results in a resumption of normal post-menopausal bone loss but if treatment is taken for 5 years the incidence of hip fracture could be reduced by 50%.[25]

There are several types of oestrogens currently used in HRT formulations: commonly used ones include conjugated equine oestrogens, oestradiol valerate, 17β-oestradiol and oestrone sulphate. These can be administered orally, subcutaneously and percutaneously; Table 7.1 summarizes these formulations and the dosages needed for the preservation of bone density. In general, the oral and transdermal routes appear to be equally effective in conserving bone.[29] Women who experience a premature menopause, as a result of either surgery or medical reasons, may need a higher dose of oestrogens for bone conservation. Those who are many years from the menopause may experience fewer oestrogenic side effects – particularly mastalgia – if started on a low dose of oestrogen replacement: 25 μg transdermal oestradiol or 1 mg oestradiol valerate daily. This can then be increased if necessary after a period of about 3 months, although some older women may conserve bone on the lower doses. Sequential HRT formulations include 12 days of a progestational agent to ensure adequate endometrial protection but 'bleed-free' continuous

Table 7.1 Formulations and dosages of oestrogens needed to preserve bone density	
Oestrogen	**Bone-conserving dose**
Oral oestradiol valerate[26]/ 17β-oestradiol[27]	1–2 mg daily
Transdermal 17β-oestradiol[16]	50 μg daily
Percutaneous 17β-oestradiol[28]	1.5 mg daily
Conjugated equine oestrogens[29]	0.625 mg daily
Subcutaneous 17β-oestradiol[30-32]	25–50 mg every 6 months

combined preparations are becoming more popular and these may be suited to women who are many years beyond the menopause. Continuous combined HRT consists of an oestrogen and progestogen formulation given on a daily basis to produce endometrial atrophy. These HRT regimens maintain bone density adequately[33,34] and there is some evidence that they do so to a greater extent than sequential regimens.[35,36]

Androgens, specifically nandrolone decanoate, increase spinal bone mineral density in postmenopausal women[37] and there is some evidence to suggest that the addition of subcutaneous testosterone to oestrogen implant therapy confers a greater bone-conserving effect than oral oestrogen alone.[38] Furthermore, the addition of testosterone in subcutaneous implant form to subcutaneous oestrogen replacement therapy is advocated by some because the former not only improves libido but may have a greater effect than oestrogen implants alone,[39] although other investigators have not been able to demonstrate this.[40]

MECHANISM OF OESTROGEN'S BONE-CONSERVING ACTION

Bone metabolism is regulated by the activity of two types of cell which affect bone remodelling: osteoblastic cells responsible for bone formation and osteoclastic cells which increase bone resorption. Both of these cell types are regulated by local humoral factors (cytokines, prostaglandins, growth factors, etc.) and systemic hormones (calcitonin, oestrogens, corticosteroids, thyroxine, etc.). Cytokines that increase osteoclastic activity include granulocyte–macrophage colony-stimulating factor (GM-CSF), macrophage colony-stimulating factor (M-CSF), tumour necrosis factor α (TNFα), interleukin-1 (IL-1) and interleukin-6 (IL-6). Local tissue factors that increase osteoblastic activity include IL-4 and transforming growth factor β (TGFβ). The precise mechanism of oestrogen's antiresorptive effects are not fully understood, but oestrogens exert a direct effect on bone as well as indirectly affecting local humoral mechanisms.

Direct actions

Oestrogen receptors have been identified in normal osteoblastic cells,[41] osteoblast-like osteosarcoma cell populations[42] and osteoclastic cells.[43,44] These receptors are, however, found in relatively low concentrations when compared with other oestrogen cell targets, which implies that additional indirect antiresorptive mechanisms may also play an important role in bone conservation. In vitro studies have shown that 17β-oestradiol acts directly on osteoblasts by increasing mRNA levels encoding the α1 chain of procollagen type I[45] and this effect seems to be negated by anti-oestrogens. In addition, 17β-oestradiol increases insulin-like growth factor 1 (IGF-1) mRNA levels and reduces parathyroid hormone (PTH) stimulated adenylate cyclase activity in laboratory studies[46] which may also contribute to oestrogens's bone-conserving action.

Local indirect actions

Bone monocytes and macrophages may also be important in the local regulation of resorptive and antiresorptive mechanisms. Interleukin-1 and TNF are potent cytokines that increase osteoblastic stimulation of osteoclastic development and maturation from bone marrow precursors.[47] Both of these cytokines also potentiate the release of other humoral agents that are responsible for osteoclast maturation – these include IL-6, M-CSF and GM-CSF. Experimental studies have demonstrated that oestradiol inhibits the release of TNF from monocytes in postmenopausal women[48] and the interleukins IL-1 to IL-6 are increased in postmenopausal women who undergo oophorectomy.[49] Conversely, oestrogen has been shown to inhibit IL-6 cytokine production in both osteoclasts and bone marrow stromal cells.[50] Transcription factors NF-κB and C/EBPβ may represent the region in the IL-6 promoter that is inhibited by the presence of 17β-oestradiol.[51] Other investigators have found that peripheral blood mononuclear cells taken from women with osteoporosis release high levels of IL-1; this could be suppressed to control values with oestrogens or progestogen therapy.[52] Studies of osteoporotic bone biopsies have confirmed that levels of mRNA's coding for IL-1α, IL-1β, TNFα and IL-6 are higher in comparison to that in normal bone specimens from women taking HRT.[53] Additional research has confirmed that physiological concentrations of oestrogens inhibit the release of IL-1 from stimulated peripheral human monocytes.[54]

Other local humoral factors that affect bone metabolism include prostaglandins, particularly PGE_2 which in low concentrations stimulates bone formation. In higher concentrations, PGE_2 promotes osteoblast-mediated bone resorption. Experimental work on rats has shown that cyclo-oxygenase inhibitors, such as indomethacin, causes a decrease in bone loss.[55]

Whether oestrogens affect prostaglandin release at this level in humans is not known, although there is some evidence that they reduce prostaglandin release from cultured bone tissue of oophorectomized rats.[56]

Systemic indirect action

Evidence about the effects of oestradiol on calcitonin secretion is conflicting. Some researchers report a decrease in calcitonin after the menopause[57–59] and a rise in calcitonin levels with HRT administration in postmenopausal women.[60–63] Others have observed no change in calcitonin levels in osteoporotic women[64–66] and no effect of HRT on calcitonin levels in ovariectomized women.[67] In vitro studies[68] have shown that 17β-oestradiol can stimulate thyroid C-cells to cause an increase in calcitonin release.

NON-RESPONDERS TO OESTROGEN REPLACEMENT THERAPY

As described above there is a small proportion of women whose bone density does not increase with the administration of standard dosages of oral HRT. In such women there may be a better response if the oestrogen dose is increased. Whether non-responders to oral HRT will benefit from this therapeutic strategy remains to be determined, as does the theoretical option of androgen addition in the hope that its anabolic effects may reverse or retard bone loss. Equally, whether addition of bisphosphonate drugs to HRT regimens is of benefit to oestrogen 'non-responders' is not known, although there are some data to suggest that etidronate disodium and HRT exert a greater bone-conserving effect than HRT alone when given to early postmenopausal women without established osteoporosis.[69]

ANTI-OESTROGENS FOR THE TREATMENT OF OSTEOPOROSIS

The first drug of this kind – clomiphene – was developed in 1960 and was originally found to act as a postcoital contraceptive agent in rats. In later years this compound has, paradoxically, been used as an adjunct in the treatment of anovulatory infertility. Tamoxifen, a related anti-oestrogen, was also described as a postcoital contraceptive agent but was found to possess potent anti-oestrogenic properties. Experimental studies on rats with carcinogen-induced mammary tumours showed that tamoxifen blocked the binding of oestradiol to tumour cells. Further work in humans has clearly demonstrated the advantages of tamoxifen as an adjuvant treatment for pre- and postmenopausal women with oestrogen receptor-positive disease.[70,71] There was initial concern that long-term anti-oestrogen therapy may have a deleterious effect on bone density and lipids, but tamoxifen and clomiphene act as partial agonists with a resultant beneficial action. Recently, newer, purer anti-oestrogens have been developed and their chemical structures are shown in Figure 7.1.

Types of anti-oestrogens

Tamoxifen
Tamoxifen is a non-steroidal synthetic drug that is widely used in the treatment of breast

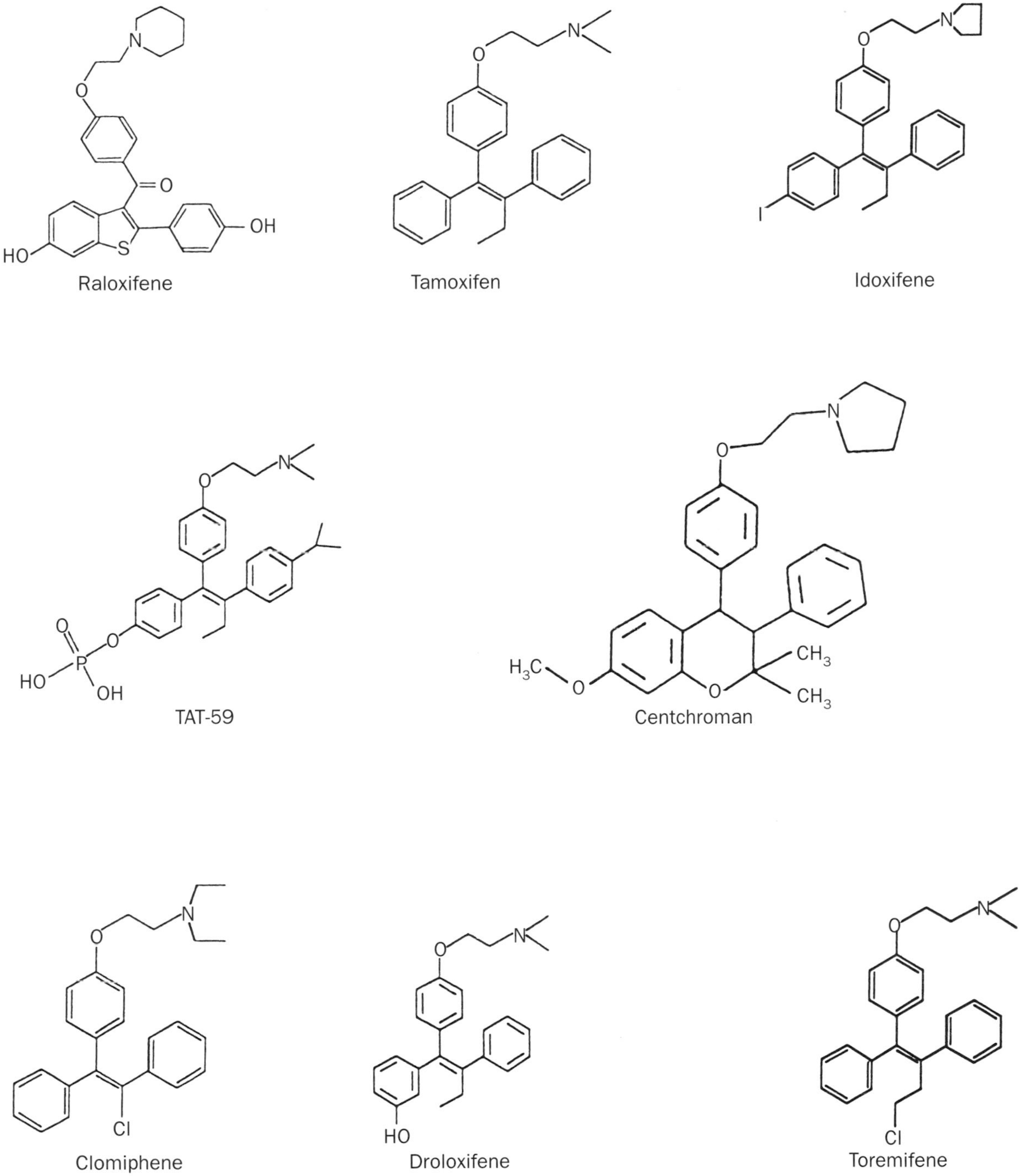

Figure 7.1 Chemical structures of newer, purer anti-oestrogens.

cancer and is taken up passively by oestrogen target tissues. In the cell tamoxifen competes with oestrogen for the nuclear oestrogen receptor. Recent work suggests that tamoxifen exerts antagonistic activity by promoting specific transactivation domains – TAF2 – and agonist activity is mediated through another region – TAF1.[72]

The effects of tamoxifen on bone vary according to the species of animal and the type of tissue[73,74] studied, but in humans there are several studies that have clearly demonstrated tamoxifen's bone-sparing effects in post-menopausal women.[75–84] One large, prospective, placebo-controlled study of 140 postmenopausal women with breast cancer showed that lumbar spine bone density increased by 0.6% over a 2-year period.[85] Other studies have shown increases in lumbar spine bone density ranging from 2.4% over 12 months[72] to 1.17% annually.[86] Premenopausal women receiving tamoxifen appear not to conserve bone in the hip, spine[84,86] and radius,[87] and this effect is consistent with experimental work on rats with intact ovarian function.[88] This suggests that the net effect of tamoxifen in the presence of endogenous ovarian steroid hormones is bone resorption. Whether this process is reversible when tamoxifen is stopped is, at the moment, unknown.

As yet there are no fracture data for tamoxifen, but one retrospective study has demonstrated a small increase in femoral neck bone density with long-term (>5 years) tamoxifen usage.[89]

Raloxifene

Raloxifene (previously known as keoxifene) is a non-steroidal compound derived from a benzothiophene series of anti-oestrogens; it competitively inhibits the actions of oestrogen in the breast and particularly the uterus.[90] It also acts as an oestrogen agonist on bone and lipid metabolism. Raloxifene differs from tamoxifen in these respects and has been classified as a selective oestrogen receptor modulator (SERM). Laboratory studies in ovariectomized rats have confirmed that raloxifene acts as a bone conserver, has no uterotrophic effects and lowers cholesterol levels.[91,92] Compared with 17β-oestradiol, raloxifene has a similar bone-conserving capacity when comparisons are made in ovariectomized rats using dual energy X-ray absorptiometry (DEXA) methods to assess bone mineral density.[93] The precise mechanism of raloxifene's action on bone is, as with oestrogen, not entirely understood but TGFβ3 may be involved. This is produced by both osteoclasts and osteoblastic cells, and surgically castrated rats express reduced TGFβ3 in bone. Both raloxifene and oestradiol can transcriptionally up-regulate TGFβ3 expression in bone which inhibits osteoclastic differentiation and reduces bone loss.[94]

There has, so far, been only one short-term study of the effects of raloxifene in postmenopausal women on bone and lipid metabolism.[95] This randomized, double-blind, placebo-controlled trial examined the effects of raloxifene, placebo or conjugated equine oestrogens on aspects of bone metabolism, endometrial histology and lipids in 251 postmenopausal women over an 8-week period. Raloxifene was found to reduce cholesterol by 5–10% and to have no stimulatory effect on the endometrium after 8 weeks of therapy. Bone turnover markers (serum osteocalcin, alkaline phosphatase, urinary pyridinoline cross-links) were reduced in both the oestrogen- and raloxifene-treated groups which implies a potential beneficial effect on the skeleton. Classic symptoms of anti-oestrogens, such as hot flushes, were experienced by 12–20% of women in the raloxifene group and this seemed to be dose dependent. Interestingly, 11% of the placebo group of women also experienced hot flushes. As would be expected, mastalgia was more common in the oestrogen-treated group. Raloxifene may be an important drug which will be used in the future to conserve bone, and large clinical trials are under way to help determine its long-term effects on this and other important metabolic processes. One main potential disadvantage of raloxifene and other anti-oestrogens is the exacerbation of menopausal symptoms and future trials should include symptomatic postmenopausal women so that side effects can be accurately assessed.

Droloxifene

This anti-oestrogen has an affinity for the oestrogen receptor which is at least 10 times that of tamoxifen; it also possesses lower oestrogenic/higher anti-oestrogenic activity on the uterus than tamoxifen.[96] In addition droloxifene has a shorter half-life than tamoxifen ($t_{\frac{1}{2}}$ of droloxifene is 24 hours compared with 7 days for tamoxifen). In breast tissue, droloxifene has an anti-oestrogenic effect and thus has been used with good effect in the treatment of advanced breast cancer in postmenopausal women.[97] Laboratory studies in ovariectomized rats have shown that droloxifene has beneficial effects on the skeleton (lumbar vertebral trabecular bone, femora and proximal tibiae), reduces cholesterol and has no effect on uterine weight.[98–100] In addition, these studies suggest that droloxifene is as efficacious as 17β-oestradiol in maintaining bone density. There have been no published studies in humans on the bone-conserving effects of droloxifene to date.

Clomiphene citrate

Experimental work in laboratory animals and in vitro studies have shown that clomiphene acts as a bone conserver,[101–104] but there have been no studies in humans examining its effects on bone mineral density.

Centchroman

This anti-oestrogen, used as a contraceptive agent in some parts of the world, has been found to inhibit osteoclastic bone resorption when studied in vitro.[105] To date it has also been used in the treatment of advanced breast cancer.[106] There are no data on this drug's effect on bone density in vivo.

Idoxifene, toremifene and TAT 59

Idoxifene is a weaker anti-oestrogen than its parent molecule (tamoxifen) and has been used in the treatment of metastatic breast cancer.[107] Toremifene is produced by chlorination of the side chain of tamoxifen and this also has reduced anti-oestrogenicity, although only theoretically less hepatic toxicity. Toremifene has also been used for advanced breast cancer.[108] TAT 59 is another tamoxifen analogue and is currently undergoing clinical trials. None of these drugs has been investigated to determine their effects on bone in either humans or animal models.

CONCLUSIONS

Hormone replacement therapy appears to be an effective option for the treatment of osteopenia and established osteoporosis in post-menopausal women. The long-term safety of other antiresorptive agents such as the bisphosphonates has not been fully elucidated. Additional advantages of HRT include cardiovascular protection which makes HRT the therapeutic drug of choice when treating women with low bone density.

The development of specific anti-oestrogens or oestrogen-like molecules is an exciting development because, in theory, these compounds have an antagonistic effect on the breast and uterus, and an agonistic effect on bone and lipid metabolism. This group of agents has obvious potential advantages in health care but their place has yet to be established in the treatment of osteopenia and osteoporosis. One main disadvantage of these drugs is their potential to exacerbate menopausal symptoms and this may restrict their use to relatively asymptomatic women.

REFERENCES

1. Cooper C, Campion G, Melton LJ III. Hip fractures in the elderly: a world-wide projection. *Osteoporosis Int* 1992; **2**: 285–9.
2. Nilas L, Christiansen C. The pathophysiology of peri- and postmenopausal bone loss. *Br J Obstet Gynaecol* 1989; **96**: 580–7.
3. Henderson BE, Ross RK, Paginini-Hill A et al. Estrogen use and cardiovascular disease. *Am J Obstet Gynecol* 1986; **154**: 1181–6.
4. Stampfer MJ, Willett WC, Colditz GA et al. A prospective study of postmenopausal estrogen therapy and coronary heart disease. *N Engl J Med* 1985; **313**: 1044–9.
5. Rymer J, Chapman MG, Fogelman I. Effect of

tibolone on postmenopausal bone loss. *Osteoporosis Int* 1994; **4:** 314–19.

6. Geusens P, Dequeker J, Gielen et al. Non-linear increase in vertebral density induced by a synthetic steroid (Org OD 14) in women with established osteoporosis. *Maturitas* 1991; **13:** 155–62.

7. Lindsay R, Hart DM, Krasewski A. A prospective double-blind trial of synthetic steroid (Org OD 14) for preventing postmenopausal osteoporosis. *BMJ* 1980; **ii:** 1207–9.

8. Felson DT, Zhang Y, Hannan MT et al. The effect of postmenopausal estrogen therapy on bone density in elderly women. *N Engl J Med* 1993; **329:** 1141–6.

9. Kiel DP, Felson DT, Anderson JJ et al. Hip fracture and the use of estrogens in postmenopausal women – the Framingham Study. *N Engl J Med* 1987; **317:** 1169–74.

10. Lafferty FW, Fiske ME. Postmenopausal estrogen replacement: a long-term cohort study. *Am J Med* 1994; **97:** 66–77.

11. Weiss NS, Ure CL, Ballard JH et al. Decreased risk of fractures of the hip and lower forearm with postmenopausal use of estrogen. *N Engl J Med* 1980; **303:** 1195–8.

12. Cauley JA, Seeley DG, Ensrud K et al. Estrogen replacement therapy and fractures in older women. *Ann Intern Med* 1995; **122:** 9–16.

13. Paganini-Hill A, Ross RK, Gerkins VR et al. Menopausal estrogen therapy and hip fractures. *Ann Intern Med* 1982; **95:** 28–31.

14. Ettinger B, Genant HK, Cann CE. Long-term estrogen replacement therapy prevents bone loss and fractures. *Ann Intern Med* 1985; **102:** 319–24.

15. Hutchinson TA, Polansky SM, Feinstein AR. Postmenopausal oestrogens protect against fractures of hip and distal radius. *Lancet* 1979; **ii:** 705–9.

16. Hillard TC, Whitcroft SJ, Marsh MS et al. Long-term effects of transdermal and oral hormone replacement therapy on postmenopausal bone loss. *Osteoporosis Int* 1994; **4:** 341–8.

17. Lindsay R, Tohme JF. Estrogen treatment of patients with established postmenopausal osteoporosis. *Obstet Gynecol* 1990; **76:** 290–5.

18. Prince RL, Smith M, Dick IM et al. Prevention of postmenopausal osteoporosis – a comparative study of exercise, calcium supplementation, and hormone replacement therapy. *N Engl J Med* 1991; **325:** 1189–95.

19. Lindsay R, Hart DM, Aitken JM et al. Long-term prevention of postmenopausal osteoporosis by oestrogen: evidence for increased bone mass after onset of oestrogen treatment. *Lancet* 1976; **i:** 1038–41.

20. Nachtigall LE, Nachtigall RH, Nachtigall RD et al. Estrogen replacement therapy. I. A 10 year prospective study in relationship to osteoporosis. *Obstet Gynecol* 1979; **53:** 277–81.

21. Lufkin EG, Wahner HW, O'Fallon WM et al. Treatment of postmenopausal osteoporosis with transdermal estrogen. *Ann Intern Med* 1992; **117:** 1–9.

22. DeCherney A. Bone-sparing properties of the oral contraceptives. *Am J Obstet Gynecol* 1996; **174:** 15–20.

23. Rozenberg S, Gevers R, Peretz A et al. Decrease of bone density during estrogen substitution therapy. *Maturitas* 1993; **17:** 205–10.

24. Hassager C, Jensen SB, Christiansen C. Non-responders to hormone replacement therapy for the prevention of postmenopausal bone loss: do they exist? *Osteoporosis Int* 1994; **4:** 36–41.

25. Stevenson JC. Postmenopausal bone loss and osteoporosis. In: *The Climacteric and Beyond* (Zichella L, Whitehead MI, van Keep PA, eds). Carnforth: Parthenon Publishing, 1988: 125–35.

26. Holland EFN, Leather AT, Studd JWW. The effect of a new sequential oestradiol valerate and levonorgestrel preparation on the bone density of postmenopausal women. *Br J Obstet Gynaecol* 1993; **100:** 966–7.

27. Lees B, Pugh M, Siddle N et al. Changes in bone density in women starting hormone replacement therapy compared with those in women already established on hormone replacement therapy. *Osteoporosis Int* 1995; **5:** 344–8.

28. Riis BJ, Thomsen K, Strøm V et al. The effect of percutaneous estradiol and natural progesterone on postmenopausal bone loss. *Am J Obstet Gynecol* 1987; **156:** 61–5.

29. Stevenson JC, Cust MP, Ganger KF et al. Effects of transdermal versus oral hormone replacement therapy on bone density in spine and proximal femur in postmenopausal women. *Lancet* 1990; **335:** 265–9.

30. Studd JWW, Holland EFN, Leather AT et al. The dose–response of percutaneous oestradiol implants on the skeletons of postmenopausal women. *Br J Obstet Gynecol* 1994; **101:** 787–91.

31. Ryde SJS, Bowen-Simpkins K, Bowen-Simpkins P et al. The effect of oestradiol implants on regional and total bone mass: a three year longitudinal study. *Clin Endocrinol* 1994; **40:** 33–8.

32. Naessén T, Persson I, Thor L et al. Maintained bone density at advanced ages after long-term treatment with low dose oestradiol implants. *Br J Obstet Gynaecol* 1993; **100**: 454–9.

33. Grey AB, Cundy TF, Reid IR. Continuous combined oestrogen/progestin therapy is well tolerated and increases bone density at the hip and spine in postmenopausal osteoporosis. *Clin Endocrinol* 1994; **40**: 671–7.

34. Fuleihan GE-H, Brown EM, Curtis K et al. Effect of sequential and daily continuous hormone replacement therapy on indexes of bone mineral metabolism. *Arch Intern Med* 1992; **152**: 1904–9.

35. Christiansen C, Riis BJ. 17β-estradiol and continuous norethisterone: a unique treatment for established osteoporosis in elderly women. *J Clin Endocrinol Metab* 1990; **71**: 836–41.

36. Nielsen SP, Bärenholdt O, Hermansen F et al. Magnitude and pattern of skeletal response to long term continuous and cyclical sequential oestrogen/progestin treatment. *Br J Obstet Gynaecol* 1994; **101**: 319–24.

37. Need AG, Horowitz M, Bridges A et al. Effects of nandrolone decanoate and antiresorptive therapy on vertebral density in postmenopausal women. *Arch Intern Med* 1989; **149**: 57–60.

38. Savvas M, Studd JWW, Fogelman I et al. Skeletal effects of oral oestrogen compared with subcutaneous oestrogen and testosterone in postmenopausal women. *BMJ* 1988; **297**: 331–3.

39. Davis SR, McCloud P, Strauss BYG et al. Testosterone enhances oestradiol's effects on postmenopausal bone density and sexuality. *Maturitas* 1995; **21**: 227–36.

40. Garnett T, Studd J, Watson N et al. The effects of plasma estradiol levels on increases in vertebral and femoral bone density following therapy with estradiol and estradiol with testosterone implants. *Obstet Gynecol* 1992; **79**: 968–72.

41. Eriksen EF, Colvard DS, Berg NJ et al. Evidence of estrogen receptors in human osteoblast-like cells. *Science* 1988; **241**: 84–6.

42. Komm BS, Terpening CM, Benz DJ et al. Estrogen binding, receptor mRNA and biologic response in osteoblast-like osteosarcoma cells. *Science* 1988; **241**: 81–3.

43. Pensler JM, Radosevich JA, Higbee R et al. Osteoclasts isolated from membranous bone in children exhibit nuclear estrogen and progesterone receptors. *J Bone Miner Res* 1990; **5**: 797–802.

44. Oursler MJ, Osdoby P, Pyfferoen J et al. Avian osteoclasts as estrogen target cells. *Proc Natl Acad Sci USA* 1991; **88**: 6613–17.

45. Ernst M, Schmid C, Foresch ER. Enhanced osteoblast proliferation and collagen gene expression by estradiol. *Proc Natl Acad Sci USA* 1988; **85**: 2307–10.

46. Ernst M, Heath JK, Rodan GA. Estradiol effects on proliferation, messenger ribonucleic acid for collagen and insulin-like growth factor-1, and parathyroid hormone-stimulated adenylate cyclase activity in osteoblastic cells from calvariae and long bones. *Endocrinology* 1989; **125**: 825–33.

47. Gray TK. Estrogens and the skeleton: cellular and molecular mechanisms. *J Steroid Biochem* 1989; **34**: 285–7.

48. Ralston SH, Russell RGG, Gowen M. Estrogen inhibits release of tumor necrosis factor from peripheral blood mononuclear cells in postmenopausal women. *J Bone Miner Res* 1990; **5**: 983–8.

49. Cantatore FP, Loverro G, Ingrosso AM et al. Effect of oestrogen replacement on bone metabolism and cytokines in surgical menopause. *Clin Rheumatol* 1995; **14**: 157–60.

50. Girasole GRL, Jilka G, Passeri S et al. 17β oestradiol inhibits interleukin-6 production by bone marrow-derived stromal cells and osteoblasts in vitro: a potential mechanism for the antiosteoporotic effect of estrogens. *J Clin Invest* 1992; **89**: 883–91.

51. Stein B, Yang MX. Repression of the interleukin-6 promoter by estrogen receptor is mediated by NF-κB and C/EBPβ. *Mol Cell Biol* 1995; **15**: 4971–9.

52. Pacifici R, Rifas L, Teitelbaum S et al. Spontaneous release of interleukin 1 from human blood monocytes reflects bone formation in idiopathic osteoporosis. *Proc Natl Acad Sci USA* 1987; **84**: 4616–20.

53. Ralston SH. Analysis of gene expression in human bone biopsies by polymerase chain reaction: evidence for enhanced cytokine expression in postmenopausal osteoporosis. *J Bone Miner Res* 1994; **9**: 883–90.

54. Polan ML, Daniele A, Kuo A. Gonadal steroids modulate human monocyte interleukin-1 (IL-1) activity. *Fertil Steril* 1988; **49**: 964–8.

55. Schoutens A, Verhas M, Dourov N et al. Bone loss and bone blood flow in paraplegic rats treated with calcitonin. *Calcif Tissue Int* 1988; **42**: 136–43.

56. Feyen JHM, Raisz LG. Prostaglandin produc-

tion by calvariae from sham operated and oophorectomised rats: effect of 17 beta oestradiol in vivo. *Endocrinology* 1987; **121**: 819–21.

57. Chestnut CH, Baylink DJ, Sisom K et al. Basal plasma immunoreactive calcitonin in postmenopausal osteoporosis. *Metab Clin Exp* 1980; **29**: 559–62.

58. Whitehead MI, Lance B, Morsman J et al. Effect of castration on calcium regulating hormones. In: *Osteoporosis* (Christiansen C, Arnaud CD, Nordin BEC, Parfitt AM, Peck WA, Riggs BL, eds). Department of Clinical Chemistry, Glostrup Hospital, Denmark,1984: 331–2.

59. Reginster JY, Deroisy R, Albert A et al. Relationship between whole plasma calcitonin levels, calcitonin secretory capacity, and plasma levels of estrone in healthy women and postmenopausal osteoporotics. *J Clin Invest* 1989; **83**: 1073–7.

60. Gennari C, Agnusdei D. Calcitonin, estrogen and the bone. *J Steroid Biochem Mol Biol* 1990; **37**: 451–5.

61. Stevenson JC, Abeyasekera G, Hillyard CJ et al. Calcitonin and the calcium-regulating hormones in postmenopausal women: effect of oestrogens. *Lancet* 1981; **i**: 693–5.

62. Stevenson JC, Abeyasekera G, Hillyard CJ et al. Regulations of calcium-regulating hormones by exogenous sex steroids in early postmenopause. *Eur J Clin Invest* 1983; **13**: 481–7.

63. Reginster JY, Deroisy R, Fontaine MA et al. Influence of estrogen replacement therapy on endogenous calcitonin production rates. *Gynecol Endocrinol* 1992; **6**: 65–71.

64. Leggate J, Farish E, Fletcher CD et al. Calcitonin and postmenopausal osteoporosis. *Clin Endocrinol* 1982; **20**: 85–92.

65. Tiegs RD, Body JJ, Wahner HW et al. Calcitonin secretion in postmenopausal osteoporosis. *N Engl J Med* 1985; **312**: 1097–100.

66. Prince RL, Dick IM, Price RI. Plasma calcitonin levels are not lower than normal in osteoporotic women. *J Clin Endocrinol Metab* 1989; **68**: 684–7.

67. Lobo RA, Roy S, Shoupe D et al. Estrogen and progestin effects on urinary calcium and calciotropic hormones in surgically induced postmenopausal women. *Horm Metab Res* 1985; **17**: 370–3.

68. Greenberg C, Kukreja SC, Bowser EN et al. Effects of estradiol and progesterone on calcitonin secretion. *Endocrinology* 1986; **118**: 2594–8.

69. Wimalawansa SJ. Combined therapy with estrogen and etidronate has an additive effect on bone mineral density in the hip and vertebrae: four-year randomised study. *Am J Med* 1995; **99**: 36–42.

70. Breast Cancer Trials Committee. Scottish Cancer Trials Office: adjuvant tamoxifen in the management of operable breast cancer: the Scottish trial. *Lancet* 1987; **ii**: 171–5.

71. Early Breast Cancer Trialists' Collaborative Group. Systemic treatment of early breast cancer by hormonal, cytotoxic or immune therapy. 133 randomised trials involving 31,000 recurrences and 24,000 deaths among 75,000 women. *Lancet* 1992; **339**: 71–85.

72. Tzukerman MT, Esty A, Santiso-Mere D et al. Human estrogen receptor transactivational capacity is determined by both cellular and promoter context and mediated by functionally distinct intramolecular regions. *Mol Endocrinol* 1994; **8**: 21–30.

73. Broulik PD. Tamoxifen prevents bone loss in ovariectomised mice. *Endocr Regul* 1991; **25**: 217–19.

74. Turner RT, Wakeley GK, Hannon KS et al. Tamoxifen inhibits osteoclast-mediated resorption of trabecular bone in ovarian hormone-deficient rats. *Endocrinology* 1988; **122**: 1146–50.

75. Love RR, Mazess RB, Barden HS et al. Effects of tamoxifen on bone mineral density in postmenopausal women with breast cancer. *N Engl J Med* 1992; **326**: 852–6.

76. Grey AB, Stapleton JP, Evans MC et al. The effect of the antiestrogen tamoxifen on bone mineral density in normal late postmenopausal women. *JAMA* 1995; **99**: 636–41.

77. Turken S, Siris E, Seldin D et al. Effects of tamoxifen on spinal bone density in women with breast cancer. *J Natl Cancer Inst* 1989; **81**: 1086–8.

78. Fornander T, Rutqvist LE, Sjöberg HE et al. Long-term adjuvant tamoxifen in early breast cancer: effect on bone mineral density in postmenopausal women. *J Clin Oncol* 1990; **8**: 1019–24.

79. Ward RL, Morgan G, Dalley D et al. Tamoxifen reduces bone turnover and prevents lumbar spine and proximal femoral bone loss in early postmenopausal women. *Bone Miner* 1993; **22**: 87–94.

80. Kristensen B, Ejlertsen B, Dalgaard P et al. Tamoxifen and bone metabolism in postmenopausal low-risk breast cancer patients: a randomised study. *J Clin Oncol* 1994; **12**: 992–7.

81. Leslie WD, Cowden EA, Maclean JP. Oestrogen

and bone density: a comparison of tamoxifen and hypo-oestrogenaemia. *Nucl Med Commun* 1995; **16:** 698–702.

82. Ryan WG, Wolter J, Bagdade GD. Apparent beneficial effects of tamoxifen on bone mineral content in patients with breast cancer: preliminary study. *Osteoporosis Int* 1991; **2:** 39–41.

83. Wright CD, Mansell RE, Gazet JC et al. Effect of long-term tamoxifen treatment on bone turnover in women with breast cancer. *BMJ* 1993; **306:** 429–30.

84. Fentiman IS, Caleffi M, Rodin A et al. Bone mineral content of women receiving tamoxifen for mastalgia. *Br J Cancer* 1989; **60:** 262–4.

85. Love RR, Barden HS, Mazess RB et al. Effect of tamoxifen on lumbar spine bone mineral density in postmenopausal women after 5 years. *Arch Intern Med* 1994; **154:** 2585–8.

86. Powles TJ, Hickish T, Kanis JA et al. Effect of tamoxifen on bone mineral density measured by dual-energy X-ray absorptiometry in healthy premonpausal and postmenopausal women. *J Clin Oncol* 1996; **14:** 78–84.

87. Gotfredsen A, Christiansen C, Palshof T. The effect of tamoxifen on bone mineral content in premenopausal women with breast cancer. *Cancer* 1984; **53:** 853–7.

88. Feldman S, Minne HW, Parvizi S. Antioestrogen and antiandrogen administration reduce bone mass in the rat. *Bone Miner* 1989; **7:** 245–54.

89. Neal AJ, Evans K, Hoskin PJ. Does long-term administration of tamoxifen affect bone mineral density? *Eur J Cancer* 1993; **29A:** 1971–3.

90. Black LJ, Jones CD, Falcone JF. Antagonism of estrogen action with a new benzothiophene derived antiestrogen. *Life Sci* 1983; **32:** 1031–6.

91. Black LJ, Sato M, Rowley ER et al. Raloxifene (LY 139481 HCL) prevents bone loss without causing uterine hypertrophy in ovariectomized rats. *J Clin Invest* 1994; **93:** 63–9.

92. Evans G, Bryant HU, Magee D et al. The effects of raloxifene on tibia histomorphometry in ovariectomized rats. *Endocrinology* 1994; **134:** 2283–8.

93. Sato M, McClintock C, Kim J et al. Dual-energy X-ray absorptiometry of raloxifene effects on the lumbar vertebrae and femora of ovariectomized rats. *J Bone Miner Res* 1994; **9:** 715–24.

94. Yang NN, Bryant HU, Hardikar S et al. Estrogen and raloxifene stimulate transforming growth factor-β3 gene expression in rat bone: a potential mechanism for estrogen- or ralox-

ifene-mediated bone maintenance. *Endocrinology* 1996; **137:** 2075–84.

95. Draper MW, Flowers DE, Huster WJ et al. A controlled trial of raloxifene (LY 139481) HCL: impact on bone turnover and serum lipid profile in healthy postmenopausal women. *J Bone Miner Res* 1996; **11:** 835–42.

96. Effenberger U, Wosikowski K, Kung W. Pharmacologic and biological properties of droloxifene, a new antiestrogen. *Am J Clin Oncol* 1991; **14**(suppl 2): S5–14.

97. Bruning PF. Droloxifene, a new antioestrogen in postmenopausal advanced breast cancer: preliminary results of a double-blind dose-finding phase II trial. *Eur J Cancer* 1992; **28A:** 1404–7.

98. Ke HZ, Simmons HA, Pirie CM et al. Droloxifene, a new estrogen antagonist/agonist, prevents bone loss in ovariectomized rats. *Endocrinology* 1995; **136:** 2435–41.

99. Chen HK, Ke HK, Jee WSS et al. Droloxifene prevents ovariectomy-induced bone loss in tibiae and femora of aged female rats: a dual-energy X-ray absorptiometric and histomorphometric study. *J Bone Miner Res* 1995; **10:** 1256–62.

100. Ke HZ, Chen HK, Qi H et al. Effects of droloxifene on prevention of cancellous bone loss and bone turnover in the axial skeleton of aged, ovariectomized rats. *Bone* 1995; **17:** 491–6.

101. Stewart PJ, Stern PH. Effects of the antiestrogens tamoxifen and clomiphene on bone resorption in vitro. *Endocrinology* 1986; **118:** 125–31.

102. Beall PT, Misra LK, Young RL et al. Clomiphene protects against osteoporosis in the mature ovariectomized rat. *Calcif Tissues Int* 1984; **36:** 123–5.

103. Chakraborty PK, Brown JL, Ruff CB et al. Effects of long-term treatment with estradiol or clomiphene citrate on bone maintenance, and pituitary and uterine weights in ovariectomized rats. *J Steroid Biochem Mol Biol* 1991; **40:** 725–9.

104. Goulding A, Fisher L. Preventive effects of clomiphene citrate on estrogen-deficiency osteopenia elicited by LHRH agonist administration in the rat. *J Bone Miner Res* 1991; **6:** 1177–81.

105. Hall TJ, Nyugen M, Schaueblin M et al. The bone-specific estrogen centchroman inhibits osteoclastic bone resorption in vitro. *Biochem Biophys Res Commun* 1995; **216:** 662–8.

106. Misra NC, Nigam PK, Gupta R et al. Centchroman – a non-steroidal anti-cancer

agent for advanced breast cancer: phase II study. *Int J Cancer* 1989; **43:** 781–3.

107. Coombes RC, Haynes BP, Dowsett M et al. Idoxifene: report of a phase I study in patients with metastatic breast cancer. *Cancer Res* 1995; **55:** 1070–4.

108. Pyrhönen S. Phase III studies of toremifene in metastatic breast cancer. *Breast Cancer Res Treat* 1990; **16:** 41–46.

8

Bisphosphonates for the treatment of osteoporosis

J-Y L Reginster, C Gosset and G Fraikin

CONTENTS • Etidronate • Clodronate • Amino-bisphosphonates • Cyclical bisphosphonates

The historical background of bisphosphonates, previously called diphosphonates, is closely linked to the history of inorganic pyrophosphates. Inorganic pyrophosphate is the simplest polyphosphate, a family of compounds characterized by the existence of at least one phosphorus–oxygen–phosphorus (POP) bridge. Polyphosphates prevent precipitation of calcium carbonate in solution, which is the main reason for their long-lasting marketing as additives that prevent calcium carbonate scaling in salt water.[1] Noticing the interest of the physicochemical properties of pyrophosphates, Russell and Fleisch, since 1970, searched for the development of analogues that were stable in vivo and resisted enzymatic hydrolysis: bisphosphonates in which a stable phosphorus–carbon–phosphorus (PCP) bridge was replacing the former POP bridge.[2] Bisphosphonates in vitro prevent the precipitation of calcium and phosphorus in solution, block transformation of amorphous calcium phosphates in hydroxyapatite and inhibit aggregation of hydroxyapatite crystals.[3]

Bisphosphonates are extremely potent inhibitors of bone resorption.[4] They interfere with several stages of the osteoresorption process. Different mechanisms of action, acting simultaneously and synergistically, are likely to be involved, including an acute phenomenon that is mainly physicochemical, and a cellular and/or biochemical effect, which has a longer latency.[5] The relative contribution of each of them depends on the nature of the respective bisphosphonate. The antiresorptive action of bisphosphonates has been widely used in human patients. Several bisphosphonates were tested in various clinical situations related to an increase of osteoclastic resorption, including Paget's disease of bone, tumour- and non-tumour-induced hypercalcaemia, primary hyperthyroidism, osteoporosis of hypodynamism, glucocorticoid-induced osteoporosis, juvenile idiopathic osteoporosis or primary involutional osteoporosis.[6]

Postmenopausal osteoporosis is a disorder characterized by an increase in bone resorption relative to bone formation, consistently linked to an increased rate of bone turnover.[7] Therefore, it was rather logical to consider bisphosphonates, which are selective inhibitors of osteoclastic bone resorption, as a potential preventive and therapeutic approach to postmenopausal osteoporosis[8] (Table 8.1).

ETIDRONATE

Etidronate has been widely investigated as a monotherapy for postmenopausal osteoporosis given either continuously[9] or intermittently.[10] This bisphosphonate has already been used in

Table 8.1 Bisphosphonates currently developed/marketed for prevention and/or treatment of osteoporosis

Generic name	Chemical names	Developers
Etidronate	(1-Hydroxyethylidene)bisphosphonate	Procter & Gamble
Clodronate	(Dichloromethylene)bisphosphonate	Boehringer Ingelheim/Leiras
Pamidronate	(3-Amino-1-hydroxypropylidene)-bisphosphonate	Ciba Geigy
Neridronate	(6-Amino-hydroxyhexylidene)bisphosphonate	Shire
Alendronate	(4-Amino-hydroxybutylidene)bisphosphonate	Merck
Mildronate	[3-(Dimethylamino)-1-hydroxypropylidene]-bisphosphonate	Gador
Ibandronate (BM 21.0955)	[1-Hydroxy-3-(methylpentyl-amino)-propylidene]-bisphosphonate	Boehringer Mannheim
Tiludronate	{[(4-Chlorophenyl)thio]-methylene}-bisphosphonate	Sanofi
EB-1053	[1-Hydroxy-3-(1-pyrrolidinyl)-propylidene]-bisphosphonate	Pharmacia/Leo
Cimadronate (YM 175)	[(Cycloheptylamino)-methylene]-bisphosphonate	Yamanouchi
Risedronate	[1-Hydroxy-2-(3-pyridinyl)-ethylidene]-bisphosphonate	Procter & Gamble
Zolendronate CGP 42,446	[1-Hydroxy-2-(1-imidazol-1-yl)-ethylidene]-bisphosphonate	Ciba-Geigy

several protocols based on the concept of a 'coherence therapy' of osteoporosis.[11,12] Discrepant outcomes resulted from the various therapeutic regimens.[9,12,13]

Storm and colleagues,[10] when giving etidronate (400 mg/day for 14 days every 4 months over 3 years) intermittently to osteoporotic women observed a significant increase (1.8% per year) in bone mineral density at the spine, with no concomitant loss of cortical bone. Notwithstanding, the rate of new vertebral fractures observed in the treated group during the 3 years of the trial was not significantly different from the one observed in the control group (treated with the placebo). A separate analysis of the second and third years (excluding the first year) of treatment was the only way to show a significant ($p = 0.023$) reduction of the fracture incidence in the group treated with etidronate. In a multicentre North American trial,[11] during which etidronate was administered after a similar regimen (400 mg/day for 14 days every 3 months for 2 years), although in half of the patients this was after the administration over 3 days of phosphorus 1 g/day, patients who received etidonate had a significant increase in spinal bone density (2.6–2.1% per year for etidronate/phosphorus and etidronate/placebo) with no cortical loss.

The incidence of new fractures was identical in the four groups involved in the trial (etidronate/phosphorus, etidronate/placebo, phosphorus/placebo, placebo/placebo) but, when pooling patients treated with etidronate independently of the former intake of phosphorus, the authors reported a slightly significant reduction in the incidence of vertebral fractures ($p = 0.043$) compared with the two other therapeutic groups. The follow-up of this trial for another year revealed an increase in the rate of vertebral fractures in the group treated with etidronate so that, at the end of the global period of 3 years, there was no more significant difference in the overall population, between patients treated with placebo and those treated with etidronate. A post-hoc analysis revealed, however, that patients, whose spinal bone mineral density (BMD) was below the 50th percentile of the distribution of BMD in osteoporotic patients and who, concomitantly, had more than two prevalent fractures at the start of the trial (17% of the population), experienced a significant reduction in the rate of vertebral fractures when treated with etidronate compared with those treated with the placebo. These results suggested a plausible role for etidronate in the treatment of severe osteoporosis.[14] Intermittent administration of etidronate, at the previously mentioned doses, for 2–3 years, appears to be related to an increased prevalence of histological abnormalities, characterized by histological osteomalacia and mineralization impairments,[15,16] but these abnormalities have not been shown to have clinical significance. [15–17] The absence of a relationship between these histological changes and the clinical pattern of patients treated with cyclical etidronate is in accordance with further results which show normal histological features and an absence of an increase in incidence of vertebral fractures when cyclical administration of etidronate was prolonged for 4 or 5 years.[18,19]

More recently, in a subset of osteoporotic women treated for up to 7 years with cyclical etidronate, results from transiliac crest bone biopsy samples suggested that, after 3 years of treatment, bone turnover returned towards baseline levels whereas bone mineralization remained within normal limits by histological and histomorphometric assessment.[20]

CLODRONATE

Clodronate has been exhaustively investigated and prescribed in several disorders characterized by enhanced bone resorption.[21] However, limited data are available concerning the use of this bisphosphonate in osteoporosis. Administration of intermittent oral clodronate (200–600 mg/day for 3 months followed by a similar washout period) to a small cohort of patients with osteoporosis yielded a significant increase in total body calcium (8%) after 20 months.[22] Oral clodronate (400 mg daily for 30 days every 3 months), with or without concomitant calcitriol, was also associated with a significant increase in lumbar bone density (3.88% and 3.2%, without and with calcitriol, respectively) after 12 months, whereas untreated patients lose 2.34% of their spinal bone during the same period.[23] Monthly intravenous infusion of 200 mg clodronate to women with low lumbar BMD, for 2 years, prevented further bone loss to a similar extent to transdermal 17β-oestradiol (50 µg/24 hour).[24] In a long-term study, evaluating the effects of intravenous infusion of 200 mg clodronate every 3 weeks for 6 years to osteoporotic patients (t-score < -2.5 for spinal BMD), lumbar BMD increased significantly and the upward trend persisted for all 6 years of therapy (5.69%) versus controls (-1.47%).[25] In a subset of patients monitored for 3 years, clodronate was reported to reduce, with borderline significance ($p = 0.067$), the number of patients experiencing new vertebral fractures, whereas the total number of vertebral fractures was significantly reduced ($p = 0.0013$).[26] However, studies evaluating the effect of clodronate in osteoporosis have been conducted either with too few patients or with inadequate methodology to demonstrate convincingly the efficacy of this bisphosphonate in postmenopausal osteoporosis.

AMINO-BISPHOSPHONATES

Amino-bisphosphonates currently developed and/or marketed for osteoporosis management include mainly pamidronate, alendronate, neridronate and ibandronate.

Pamidronate

Administration of pamidronate 150 mg/day for 2 weeks was reported to normalize calcium balance whereas such treatment given for up to 6.2 years (mean 3.7 years) was associated with a significant and sustained 3% annual increase in lumbar BMD.[27] However, this study had major methodological flaws which precluded the drawing of any significant conclusions.

More recently, a similar regimen (150 mg/day continuously) was investigated in a prospective, double-blind, placebo-controlled study in which 48 postmenopausal women with established osteoporosis were followed for 2 years. Significant increases in BMD were observed in patients treated with pamidronate for total body (1.9%), lumbar spine (7%) and femoral trochanter (5.4%), whereas the significant decrease observed for the placebo group at the femoral neck and Ward's triangle did not occur in the pamidronate group. The vertebral fracture rate was reduced non-significantly ($p = 0.07$) in the pamidronate group.[28]

The development of the oral form of pamidronate was, however, jeopardized by the report of erosive oesophagitis, which seems to be a common feature of all amino-bisphosphonates,[29] whereas its intravenous administration yielded only transient positive results in terms of BMD.[30]

Alendronate

Exhaustive preclinical assessment of alendronate evaluated the effects of this bisphosphonate on the biomechanical properties of the skeleton.

Globally, results obtained in both rats[31] and baboons[32] concluded that alendronate significantly improves both bone mineral content and biomechanical resistance of trabecular and cortical bone. In early postmenopausal women, alendronate 2.5 or 5 mg/day prevented cortical and trabecular bone loss, over 2 years, in a similar way to conjugated equine oestrogens (0.625 mg/day) and medroxyprogesterone acetate (5 mg/day) or 17β-oestradiol (1–2 mg/day) and norethisterone acetate (0–1 mg/day). The 5 mg/day dose gave better results than the 2.5 mg/day dose at all measured sites, including the spine (3.46% vs 2.28%), total hip (1.85% vs 1.06%) and total body (0.67% vs −0.03%).[33] Dose-dependent effects of alendronate in reducing bone turnover and increasing spinal bone mass were reported in postmenopausal women with low BMD. In this population, the 10 mg/day dose, suggested to correspond to the best risk/benefit ratio for treatment of osteoporosis, induced significant increases in BMD after 2 years[34] and 3 years.[35] In the 2-year study, mean increases in BMD with alendronate 10 mg/day were 7.21% at the spine, 5.27% for total hip and 2.53% for total body, whereas biochemical markers of bone remodelling declined by about 50% after 3 months for bone resorption markers and by 6 months for bone formation markers.[34]

The 3-year study shows similar results with increases of 2.4%, 5.5% and 7.2% for lumbar spine, femoral neck and trochanter BMD, respectively.[35] The results obtained from two studies, in which three doses of alendronate were given for 3 years (5 mg/day, 10 mg/day and 20 mg/day for 2 years, followed by 5 mg/day for one year) to women with low BMD (including a 20% subset with prevalent fractures), were pooled.[36] Compared with the placebo group, a significant reduction in the proportion of female patients with new vertebral fractures (3.2% vs 6.2%; $p = 0.03$) and a decreased progression of vertebral deformities (33% vs 41%; $p = 0.028$) were observed. Significant reduction of the risk of vertebral (RR = 0.54), hip (RR = 0.49), wrist (RR = 0.56) and all clinical fractures (RR = 0.72) was also suggested from a preliminary report of a prospective study evaluating a large cohort of North American women for 2–3 years[37] (RR is relative risk).

Besides the fact that the 10 mg/day continuous daily dose was not unequivocally demonstrated to be superior to other therapeutic regimens, the major issue with alendronate that still has to be resolved is its upper gastrointestinal tolerance. Oesophageal erosion and ulcerative oesophagitis were reported in association with the use of oral alendronate.[38,39] Although particular recommendations for alendronate intake (swallowing alendronate with 180–240 ml water on arising in the morning, and remaining upright for at least 30 minutes after swallowing the tablet and until the first food of the day has been ingested) may reduce the risk of oesophagitis; these problems should not be neglected and should be taken into account in the global evaluation of the risk/benefit ratio of this compound.[38]

Other amino-bisphosphonates

Ibandonate is a new bisphosphonate that is 2, 10, 50 and 500 times more potent than risedronate, alendronate, pamidronate or clodronate, respectively, as inhibitor of the retinoid-induced bone resorption in the thyroparathyroidectomized rat model.[40] Both oral and intravenous routes of administration of ibandronate have currently been investigated in postmenopausal osteoporosis. If monthly intravenous injection of ibandronate 2 mg to postmenopausal women, leading to an increase of 6.25% and 2.36% in lumbar and hip BMD after 12 months, were to be considered an interesting alternative for women with a poor compliance or tolerance to oral medications,[41] then the continuous daily oral intake of 2.5 mg for the same duration, with a recorded BMD increase of 4.8% (spine), 2.0–3.3% (hip), 2.0% (total skeleton) and 0.9% (forearm), would not compare favourably with other bisphosphonates that have been marketed or developed for osteoporosis.[42]

Neridronate was recently shown to suppress selectively peptide-bound deoxypyridinoline excretion in postmenopausal women with low BMD.[43] Further investigations of the effects and mechanisms of action of this bisphosphonate are requested and under progress.

CYCLICAL BISPHOSPHONATES

Major phase III protocols are currently evaluating the effects of tiludronate and risedronate in the prevention and treatment of osteoporosis.

Tiludronate

Preclinical studies evaluating the effects of tiludronate on skeletal metabolism are of particular interest. They demonstrate a dose-dependent inhibition of osteoclastic resorption in several models of rodent[44] or non-rodent[45] mammals (in accordance with results obtained with other bisphosphonates) and they confirm the harmless effects of this compound on the biomechanical resistance of trabecular and cortical bone.[45] The most original features of these investigations constitute the observation of an increase in the mineralization rate and an improvement of bone mechanical properties in a callus from dogs exposed to hemi-osteotomy of the ulna.[46] These results were in agreement with previous reports of the efficacy of tiludronate in Paget's disease of the bone,[47,48] where the proportion of responders to tiludronate was twice as high as that observed with etidronate. Tiludronate, given for 6 months to healthy early postmenopausal women, prevented spinal bone loss for up to 12 months, compared with women who received the placebo for the same duration.[49] This early report was later confirmed in a multicentre trial where women treated with oral tiludronate 200 mg/day, continuously for 6 months, lost significantly ($p = 0.016$) less femoral bone after 18 months than those receiving a placebo (-1% vs -2.8%). Results at the level of the lumbar spine show a similar trend (borderline significance $p = 0.065$).[50,51]

Risedronate

In rats, subcutaneous injection of risedronate 5 μg/kg per day significantly reduced histological parameters, reflecting osteoclastic resorption without interaction with bone formation or mineralization.[52] Similarly, the biochemical properties of vertebrae and femoral neck obtained from dogs treated with risedronate for 2 years at doses from 0.2 to 2 mg/kg per day were not significantly modified. In women with breast cancer and chemotherapy-induced menopause, risedronate was given intermittently (10–30 mg/day for 2 weeks every 3 months) for 2–3 years.[53,54] These doses of risedronate prevented the bone loss observed in the control population. A dose of 5 mg risedronate, given either continuously or intermittently (2 weeks of risedronate followed by 2 weeks of placebo) for 2 years, was evaluated in early postmenopausal women with normal bone mass. At the end of the trial, a significant difference ($p < 0.0001$) appeared among the three groups in the evolution of lumbar spine bone mass. At the trochanteric level, bone mass increased (2.3%) in the group treated with the continuous regimen, was maintained (0.5%) with the intermittent regimen and decreased (−1%) in the placebo arm.[55] This effect was mediated by a decreased bone resorption, as confirmed by a drastic reduction in urinary deoxypyridinoline (−31% and −15% for contin-

uous and intermittent risedronate regimens, respectively).[55] Paired bone biopsies obtained before and after one year of treatment revealed no signs of osteomalacia.[56]

When risedronate was given to North American women with low vertebral bone mass (more than 2 standard deviations below the peak), a dose–response profile (0, 2.5 and 5 mg/day) was observed for increase in spinal and femoral bone mass, as well as for reduction of bone turnover markers.[57] In severe osteoporosis (low bone mass and prevalent fractures), risedronate (two periods of 20 mg/day for 7 days each, followed by 14 days of calcium) decreased collagen cross-link urinary excretion significantly by more than half and for up to 3 months.[58] Daily administration of risedronate 2.5 mg to osteoporotic women, with prevalent spinal fractures at baseline, resulted in a significant trend towards an increased bone mass at the spine and trochanter, and a reduction of new vertebral fractures.[59] Demonstration of the minimal effective dose of risedronate for treatment of postmenopausal osteoporosis will be obtained from long-term prospective trials.

REFERENCES

1. Fleisch H. *Bisphosphonates in Bone Disease. From the Laboratory to the Patient.* London: Parthenon Publishing, 1995.
2. Russell RGG, Fleisch H. Inorganic pyrophosphate and pyrophosphatases in calcification and calcium homeostasis. *Clin Orthop* 1970; **69:** 101–7.
3. Fleisch H. Diphosphonates: history and mechanisms of action. *Metab Bone Dis Rel Res* 1981; **3:** 279–88.
4. Treschel U, Stutrer A, Fleisch H. Hypercalcaemia induced with an arotinoid in thyroparathyroidectomized rats. New model to study bone resorption in vivo. *J Clin Invest* 1986; **80:** 1979–86.
5. Fleisch H. Experimental basis for the use of bisphosphonates in Paget's disease of bone. *Clin Orthop Rel Res* 1987; **217:** 72–8.
6. Reginster J-Y. *Ostéoporose postménopausique. Traitement prophylactique.* Paris: Masson, 1993.
7. Riggs BL, Melton LJ. Involution osteoporosis. *Am J Med* 1986; **314:** 1676–84.
8. Reginster J-YL. Les bisphosphonates constituent-ils un réel progrès thérapeutique dans l'ostéoporose? *Méd Hyg* 1996; **54:** 1497–501.
9. Heaney RP, Saville PD. Etidronate disodium in postmenopausal osteoporosis. *Clin Pharmacol Ther* 1976; **20:** 593–604.
10. Storm T, Thamsborg G, Steinich T et al. Effect of intermittent cyclical etidronate therapy on bone mass and fracture rate in women with postmenopausal osteoporosis. *N Engl J Med* 1990; **322:** 1265–71.
11. Watts NB, Harris ST, Genant HK et al. Intermittent cyclical etidronate treatment of postmenopausal osteoporosis. *N Engl J Med* 1990; **323:** 73–9.
12. Pacifici R, MacMurtry C, Vered I et al. Coherence therapy does not prevent axial bone loss in osteoporotic women: a preliminary comparative study. *J Clin Endocrinol Metab* 1988; **66:** 747–53.
13. Smith ML, Fogelman I, Hart DM, et al. Effect of

etidronate disodium on bone turnover following surgical menopause. *Calcif Tissue Int* 1989; **44:** 74–9.

14. Harris ST, Watts NB, Jackson RD et al. Four years of intermittent cyclical etidronate treatment of postmenopausal osteoporosis: Three years of blinded therapy followed by one year of open therapy. *Am J Med* 1993; **95:** 557–67.

15. Axelrod DW, Teitelbaum SL. Results of long-term cyclical etidronate therapy: Bone histomorphometry and clinical corelates. *J Bone Miner Res* 1994; **9**(suppl 1): 136S.

16. Thomas T, Lafage MH, Alexandre C. Atypical osteomalacia after 2 years etidronate intermittent cyclic administration in osteoporosis. *J Rheumatol* 1995; **22:** 11.

17. Storm T, Thamsborg G, Kollerup G et al. Five years of intermittent cyclical etidronate therapy increases bone mass and reduces vertebral fracture rates in postmenopausal osteoporosis. *Bone Miner* 1992; **17**(suppl 1): 24S.

18. Jackson RD, Harris ST, Genant HK et al. Cyclical etidronate treatment of postmenopausal osteoporosis: 4-year experience. *Bone Miner* 1992; **17**(suppl 1): 154S.

19. Miller P, Huffer W, MacIntyre D et al. Bone histomorphometry after long-term treatment with cyclical phosphorus and etidronate. *Bone Miner* 1992; **17**(suppl 1): S23.

20. Storm T, Sorensen HA, Thamsborg G et al. Bone histomorphometric changes after up to seven years of cyclical etidronate treatment. *J Bone Miner Res* 1996; **11**(suppl 1): S151.

21. Plosker GL, Goa KL. Clodronate. A review of its pharmacological properties and therapeutic efficacy in resorptive bone disease. *Drugs* 1994; **47:** 945–82.

22. Chesnut CH. Synthetic calcitonin, diphosphonates and anabolic steroids in the treatment of postmenopausal osteoporosis. In: *Osteoporosis* (Christiansen C, Arnaud CD, Nordin BEC et al, eds). Copenhagen: Osteopress, 1984: 594–655.

23. Giannini S, D'Angelo A, Malvasi L et al. Effects of one-year cyclical treatment with clodronate on postmenopausal bone loss. *Bone* 1993; **14:** 137–41.

24. Filipponi P, Pedetti M, Fedell L et al. Cyclical clodronate is effective in preventing postmenopausal bone loss: a comparative study with transcutaneous hormone replacement therapy. *J Bone Miner Res* 1995; **10:** 697–703.

25. Filipponi P, Cristallini S, Rizzello E et al. Cyclical intravenous clodronate in postmenopausal osteoporosis: Results of a long-term clinical trial.

Bone 1996; **18:** 179–84.

26. Filipponi P, Cristallini S, Rizzello E et al. 6-year cyclical intravenous clodronate in postmenopausal osteoporosis effect on bone mass and vertebral fractures. *Osteoporosis Int* 1996; **6**(suppl 1): 260.

27. Valkema R, Vismans FJE, Papapoulos SE et al. Maintained improvement in calcium balance and bone mineral content in patients with osteoporosis treated with bisphosphonate APD. *Bone Miner* 1989; **5:** 183–92.

28. Reid IR, Wattie DJ, Evans MC et al. Continuous therapy with pamidronate, a potent bisphosphonate, in postmenopausal osteoporosis. *J Clin Endocrinol Metab* 1994; **79:** 1595–9.

29. Lufkin EG, Argueta R, Whitaker MD et al. Pamidronate: an unrecognized problem in gastrointestinal tolerability. *Osteoporosis Int* 1994; **4:** 320–2.

30. Devogelaer JP, Esselinckx W, Nagant de Deuxchaisnes CA. A randomized, controlled trial of APD (disodium pamidronate) given intravenously with and without sodium fluoride in involutional osteoporosis. *J Bone Miner Res* 1992; **5**(suppl 2): 252S.

31. Toolan BC, Shea M, Myers ER et al. Effects of 4-amino-1-hydroxybutylidene bisphosphonate on bone biomechanisms in rats. *J Bone Miner Res* 1992; **7:** 1399–406.

32. Balena R, Toolan BC, Shea M et al. The effects of 2-year treatment with the aminobisphosphonate alendronate on bone metabolism, bone histomorphometry, and bone strength in ovariectomized nonhuman primates. *J Clin Invest* 1993; **92:** 2577–86.

33. Hosking DJ, McClung MR, Ravn P et al. Alendronate in the prevention of osteoporosis: EPIC study two-year results. *J Bone Miner Res* 1996; **11**(suppl 1): S133.

34. Chesnut CH, McClung MR, Ensrud KE et al. Alendronate treatment of the postmenopausal osteoporotic woman: effect of multiple dosages on bone mass and bone remodeling. *Am J Med* 1995; **99:** 144–52.

35. Devogelaer JP, Broll H, Correa-Rotter R et al. Oral alendronte induces progressive increases in bone mass of the spine, hip, and total body over 3 years in postmenopausal women with osteoporosis. *Bone* 1996; **18:** 141–50.

36. Liberman U, Weiss SR, Broll J et al. Effect of oral alendronate on bone mineral density and the incidence of fractures in postmenopausal osteoporosis. *N Engl J Med* 1995; **333:** 1437–43.

37. Black DM, Cummings SR, Thompson D. Alendronate reduces the risk of vertebral and clinical fractures in women with existing vertebral fractures results of the fracture intervention trial. *Lancet* 1996; **348**: 1535–41.

38. De Groen PC, Lubbe DF, Hirsch LJ et al. Esophagitis associated with the use of alendronate. *N Engl J Med* 1996; **335**: 1016–21.

39. Maconi G, Porro GB. Multiple ulcerative esophagitis caused by alendronate. *Am J Gastroenterol* 1995; **90**: 1889–90.

40. Muhlbauer RC, Bauss F, Schenk R et al. Ibandronate, a potent new bisphosphonate to inhibit bone resorption. *J Bone Miner Res* 1991; **6**: 1003–11.

41. Schurch MA, Rizzoli R, Slosman D et al. Protein supplements increase serum IGF-1 and prevent proximal femur bone loss in elderly with a recent hip fracture. *Osteoporosis Int* 1996; **6**(suppl 1): 94.

42. Ravn P, Clemmesen B, Riis J et al. The effect on bone mass and bone markers of different doses of ibandronate – a new bisphosphonate for prevention and treatment of postmenopausal osteoporosis. A 1-year, randomized, double-blind, placebo-controlled dose-finding study. *Osteoporosis Int* 1996; **6**(suppl 1): 301.

43. Tobias JH, Laversuch CV, Wilson N et al. Neridronate preferentially suppresses the urinary excretion of peptide-bound deoxypyridinoline in postmenopausal women. *Calcif Tissue Int* 1996; **59**: 407–9.

44. Ammann P, Rizzoli R, Caverzasio J et al. Effects of the bisphosphonate tiludronate on bone resorption, calcium balance, and bone mineral density. *J Bone Miner Res* 1993; **8**: 1491–8.

45. Geusens P, Nijs J, Van der Perre G et al. Longitudinal effect of tiludronate on bone mineral density, resonant frequency, and strength in monkeys. *J Bone Miner Res* 1992; **7**: 599–609.

46. Chastagnier D, Barbier A, de Vernejoul MC et al. Effects of two bisphosphonates (tiludronate and etidronate) on bone healing. *J Bone Miner Res* 1993; **8**(suppl 1): 236S.

47. Reginster JY, Colson F, Morlock G et al. Evaluation of the efficacy and safety of oral tiludronate in Paget's disease of bone. A double-blind, multiple-dosage, placebo-controlled study. *Arthritis Rheum* 1992; **35**: 967–74.

48. Roux C, Gennari C, Farrerons J et al. Comparative, prospective, double-blind, multi-center study of the efficacy of tiludronate and etidronate in Paget's disease of bone. *Arthritis Rheum* 1995; **38**: 851–8.

49. Reginster JY, Lecart MP, Deroisy R et al. Prevention of postmenopausal bone loss by tiludronate. *Lancet* 1989; **ii**: 1469–71.

50. Roux C, Deroisy R, Basse-Cathalinat B et al. Prevention of early postmenopausal bone loss with oral tiludronate. *Osteoporosis Int* 1996; **6**(suppl 1): 249.

51. Chappard D, Minaire P, Privat C et al. Effects of tiludronate on bone loss in paraplegic patients. *J Bone Miner Res* 1995; **10**: 112–8.

52. Wronski TJ, Yen CF, Scott KS. Estrogen and bisphosphonate treatment provide long-term protection against osteopenia in ovariectomized rats. *J Bone Miner Res* 1991; **6**: 387–94.

53. Ettinger B, Genant H, Bekker P et al. A pilot three-year of risedronate in women with breast cancer and chemotherapy-induced menopause. *J Bone Miner Res* 1995; **10**(suppl 1): S198

54. Delmas PD, Hardouin C, Confavreux E et al. Intermittent risedronate prevents bone loss in women with artificial menopause induced by chemotherapy of breast cancer. *J Bone Miner Res* 1995; **10**(suppl 1): S200.

55. Mortensen L, Bekker P, Ouweland FVD et al. Prevention of early postmenopausal bone loss by risedronate: a two-year study. *J Bone Miner Res* 1995; **10**(suppl 1): S140.

56. Langdahl B, Eriksen EF, Mortensen L et al. Histomorphometry from a three-year risedronate bone loss prevention study. *J Bone Miner Res* 1995; **10**(suppl 1): S199.

57. McClung M, Bensen W, Bolognese M et al. Risedronate treatment of postmenopausal women with low bone mass: Preliminary data. *Osteoporosis Int* 1996; **6**(suppl 1): 257.

58. Zegels B, Balena R, Eastell R et al. Effect of risedronate on collagen cross links in postmenopausal osteoporosis. *J Bone Miner Res* 1995; **10**(suppl 1): S455.

59. Taquet AN, Clemmensen B, Zegels B et al. A three-year double-blind placebo controlled study of risedronate in postmenopausal osteoporosis. *Osteoporosis Int* 1996; **6**(suppl 1): 262.

9

Stimulators of bone formation for the treatment of osteoporosis

JD Ringe

CONTENTS • **Fluoride salts** • **Parathyroid hormone** • **Strontium** • **Further compounds**

The decrease in bone mass seen in osteoporosis is caused by an imbalance between bone resorption and bone formation during bone remodelling. Accordingly, treatment can try to stop excessive bone resorption, increase bone formation or do both consecutively or even simultaneously.[1]

Therapeutic agents for osteoporosis are correspondingly classified as substances primarily decreasing bone resorption ('antiresorber') and agents that appear capable of restoring bone mass previously lost ('positive bone formers' or 'osteoanabolic substances').

From a didactic point of view the distinction of these two groups is generally accepted, but pharmacologically there is a considerable overlap between the two. Some antiresorbers also have mild stimulatory effects on osteoblasts (e.g. calcitonins) and an osteoanabolic treatment to some extent may also inhibit bone resorption (e.g. fluorides, strontium). For other substances there is even still some controversy about whether they are more inhibitors of osteoclasts or stimulators of osteoblasts (e.g. anabolic steroids, alfacalcidol, calcitriol).[2]

The ideal therapeutic agent for osteoporosis should increase bone mass above the fracture threshold.[3] As in general there is only a moderate and timely limited gain in bone mass with a pure antiresorptive therapy, this goal can only be reached by an antiresorber if patients are in an early stage of osteoporosis, i.e. no severe deficit of bone substance (Figure 9.1).

Theoretically, formation-stimulating drugs should be able to increase bone mass above the critical threshold in all stages of osteoporosis (Table 9.1). It must, however, be taken into consideration that the lower the initial bone mass the more advanced the deterioration of spongy bone architecture within the bone. If an osteoanabolic treatment is able only to increase the diameter of the remaining trabeculae, this treatment should also start as early as possible and would be of limited value in very advanced cases of osteoporosis.[4] Drugs and hormones that are regarded as primarily stimulating agents of osteoblasts are shown in Table 9.2.

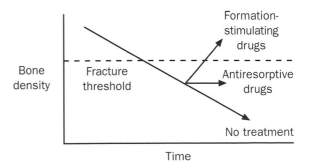

Figure 9.1 Effect of different anti-osteoporotic treatments on the course of bone density values.

Table 9.1 Clinical stages of osteoporosis on the basis of lumbar spine mineral density and prevalence of vertebral fractures

Clinical stage		Criteria
0	Osteopenia (preclinical osteoporosis)	Bone mineral density ↓ (t-score: −1 to −2.5 s.d.) No vertebral fractures
1	Osteoporosis without fractures	Bone mineral density ↓ (t-score: < minus 2.5 s.d.) No vertebral fractures
2	Established osteoporosis	Bone mineral density ↓ One to three vertebral fractures (without adequate trauma)
3	Severe established osteoporosis	Bone mineral density ↓ Multiple vertebral fractures Often nonvertebral fractures

t-score = number of standard deviations in relation to peak bone mass.

Table 9.2 Drugs and hormones with osteoanabolic potency

Fluoride salts
  Sodium fluoride (NaF)
  Monofluorophosphate (MFP)

Parathyroid hormone (PTH)
  Human PTH (1–34)
  PTHrp analogues

Strontium salts
  S12911

Anabolic steroids

Growth hormone (hGH)

Prostaglandin E_2

Local growth factors

PTHrp = PTH-related peptide.

FLUORIDE SALTS

Fluoride is one of the most avid bone-seeking elements, but as a trace element it is also present in all other human tissues.

It is well known from endemic, industrial and toxic fluorosis that fluorides may lead to severe osteosclerotic changes of the skeleton.[5–7] Prompted by studies showing a lower prevalence of osteoporotic fractures in regions with moderately increased levels of fluoride in the drinking water,[8] sodium fluoride was used for the first time in 1961 to treat osteoporosis.[9] This means that fluoride has been used now for more than 35 years in the management of osteoporosis. It is still regarded as the most potent osteoanabolic substance available. Positive effects on bone mass are well documented in humans and, moreover, it is very inexpensive and can be administered orally.

Uncertainties persist, however, about the quality of the newly formed bone tissue and the effectiveness of fluoride treatment in decreasing vertebral fracture rate.[10,11]

Pharmacology

It is important to make a clear distinction between the two fluoride salts that are mainly used: sodium fluoride (NaF) and monofluorophosphate (MFP).[12,13]

As the application of plain NaF is accompanied by a high rate of mainly epigastric side effects,[14] this fluoride salt is usually given as enteric-coated or sustained-release tablets. Although intestinal resorption of NaF amounts to 95% when used as the plain compound, the different preparations reduce the bioavailability of the fluoride ions to different degrees (Table 9.3). The advantage of the delayed-release preparations lies, however, in the fewer side effects that they have.

Disodium monofluorophosphate (Na_2PO_4F), usually called MFP, has the same high intestinal absorption rate as plain NaF (95–100%), but a significantly lower rate of gastrointestinal side effects.[15] This fluoride compound dissociates in aqueous solvents into Na^+ and $(FPO_3)^{2-}$ ions. The monofluorophosphate ion is resorbed before hydrolysis, partly in the stomach but mainly in the upper small intestine.[12] It then becomes hydrolysed by alkaline phosphatases of the intestinal mucosa into fluoride and phosphate ions. The small number of epigastric side effects of MFP result from the fact that no aggressive free fluoride ions are released in the gastrointestinal tract before resorption.[15]

Another important difference between the two fluoride salts is that the bioavailability of fluoride from NaF is significantly reduced with food and in the presence of calcium, which is not the case for MFP. Therefore calcium salts, commonly given in therapeutic regimens with fluoride, must be given separately when using NaF.

As the fluoride ion is the active therapeutic principle, the fluoride content and the differences in bioavailability from both fluoride salts and the different galenic preparations of NaF must be taken into consideration. The comparison given in Table 9.3 may be helpful for interpreting existing therapeutic studies with discrepant results and for planning treatment regimens.

Recently, a sustained-release formulation was also developed for MFP.[16] This preparation decreases the bioavailability of fluoride ions, but has the advantage of avoiding high peak serum concentrations.[17]

The non-renal clearance of fluoride (about 80 ml/min) reflects mainly accretion into bone.[18] On average, about 50% of the absorbed fluoride is deposited in the skeleton, and most

Table 9.3 Fluoride content and bioavailability of sodium fluoride (NaF) and monofluorophosphate (MFP)		
	NaF	**MFP**
Range of usual dosages/day (mg)	50–80	100–200
Fluoride content per 100 mg (mg)	45.5	13.2
Mean bioavailability (%)	60[a]	95
Average resorbed fluoride from 100 mg substance (mg)	27.3	12.5
Equivalent doses needed if 15 mg fluoride ions shall be applied (mg)	55	120

[a] Average estimated bioavailability; depends on type of enteric-coated or sustained-release preparation.

of the remainder is excreted in the urine. The uptake of fluoride by the bone tissue is not homogeneous and a higher proportion is taken up by cancellous than by cortical bone. This may account for the heterogeneous response of different skeletal regions observed in clinical studies.

Mechanisms of action

With therapeutic concentrations, fluoride increases osteoblastic proliferation, i.e. it obviously has a mitogenic effect.[19] It is currently suggested that fluoride may increase the mitogenic effect of a protein kinase by a growth factor-dependent tyrosine phosphorylation pathway, enhancing osteoblastic proliferation. A recent study gave evidence that this indirect stimulatory effect of fluoride on osteoblasts is potentiated by aluminium.[20]

From a clinical point of view, this implies that patients on fluoride therapy also exposed to aluminium may show a better response to fluoride, but may also have a much higher risk of developing iatrogenic fluorosis (Figure 9.2).

In contrast to the osteoanabolic effect of antiresorbers, which is generally rather moderate and of limited duration, fluoride stimulates osteoblastic proliferation as long as it is therapeutically adopted, i.e. there is no secondary resistance or plateau phenomenon and a linear increase of mineral content can be observed over the years.[14,21,22]

Besides the main effect of fluoride, the osteoanabolic potency, there is also an indirect, moderate inhibitory effect on osteoclastic resorption. The fluoride ion is about the same size as the hydroxyl ion and therefore it can readily substitute the latter. Fluorapatite is, however, less soluble than hydroxyapatite, thereby making bone tissue more resistant to osteoclastic resorption.[23] With therapeutic doses of fluoride, the appearance of fluorapatite will increase the stability of the mineral phase, whereas the toxic quantities of fluoride, leading to a radiologically visible osteosclerosis or even fluorosis, will alter crystal morphology more profoundly towards a decreased stability. In the

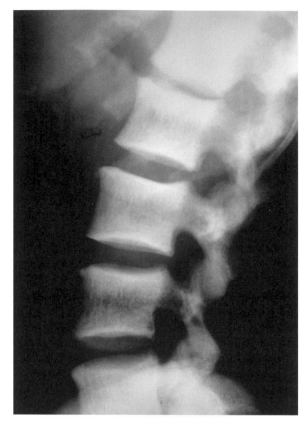

Figure 9.2 Clinical example for iatrogenic fluorosis in a 56-year-old woman: lateral radiograph of the lumbar spine after only 2 years' treatment with 80 mg enteric-coated NaF per day. There is severe osteosclerosis without extraosseous calcifications. BMD at the lumbar spine = 2.049 g/cm^2 (t-score = +7.16). (Possible explanation: no osteoporosis at onset of therapy with fluoride; co-medication with aluminium-containing antacids.)

case shown in Figure 9.2, however, fractures never occurred. Two years after withdrawal of MFP the radiograph of the spine looked quite normal, although the density for L2–L4 was still increased with 1.554 g/cm^2 (t-score = +3.00 s.d.).

It is now generally accepted that the therapeutic window of fluoride is rather small, but the existing pharmacokinetic data are not sufficient to define a clear window by plasma levels of fluoride.[24,25] There has, however, been a tendency over the last few years towards lower doses and avoidance of high peak plasma concentrations for both fluoride salts.[17,26]

Clinical results

From the 35 years of therapeutic use of fluoride for osteoporosis, there is a large body of radiological and densitometric evidence that long-term fluoride treatment increases bone mass mainly at bone sites with a high proportion of trabecular bone.[4,27,28]

Much of the earlier work is, however, methodologically unacceptable now. Another problem is that fluoride is rather cheap, so that it is difficult for industry and investigators to make the investments necessary for large long-term studies on the basis of modern recommendations.[29]

In the author's first study from 1978 with enteric-coated NaF (80 mg/day) without calcium supplementation, an increase of iliac trabecular bone volume was found but a decrease of cortical bone mass at the radius shaft was found, measured by single-photon absorptiometry.[30] This result had to be related to an increase in parathryoid hormone (PTH) secretion. In all later studies using MFP in fixed combination with calcium, it was possible to document slight increases of bone density even at cortical measuring sites.[31-33]

In the well-known study of Riggs et al[14] 75 mg/day of plain NaF were given over 4 years. The gain of bone density at the spine at the end of the study was 36% (=9% increase per annum). There was also an increase at the proximal femur but a significant loss at the radius, although 1500 mg calcium were supplemented daily. The reason is obviously the very high fluoride dose corresponding to approximately 34 mg bioavailable fluoride ions per day (compare Table 9.3).

Doubts concerning fluoride therapy were fuelled by this widely publicized study and another study with similar design and results,[21] because the rate of vertebral fractures after 4 years was not significantly lower in the fluoride plus calcium group than in the placebo–calcium group.[14]

In the meantime an extension and a new analysis of the same study were published showing a reduction of the vertebral fracture rate with lower fluoride doses,[34] i.e. it was conceded that the original dosage was too high.

Besides these initially negative and later moderately positive results from the Mayo Clinic,[14,34] several important studies have appeared since 1988 demonstrating positive effects of long-term fluoride therapy on fracture incidence in postmenopausal and idiopathic male osteoporosis.[22,32,35-37] These studies were performed with NaF or MFP at different doses, but for all the range of daily bioavailable fluoride ions was between 10 and 20 mg (see Table 9.3).

Most attention was given to the placebo-controlled randomized, 4-year trial of Pak et al[37] using 50 mg/day of a slow-release sodium fluoride at a schedule of 12 months on and 2 months off.

There was an average annual increase of lumbar bone density of 4–5% and of femoral bone density of 2.4%, and no significant change at the radius shaft. The rate of vertebral fracture-free patients was 85.4% for the fluoride group and only 56.9% for the placebo group ($p = 0.001$).[37]

In addition, two studies were published showing a highly significant increasing effect of MFP plus calcium on bone density in glucocorticoid-induced osteoporosis.[38,39] Nevertheless, the discussion about the definite clinical value of fluoride treatment is not over. Recently, negative and positive results were again reported in parallel at the same congress.

Altogether, at the present time far more positive results are documented in the literature than negative experiences. A meta-analysis is, however, difficult because of the aforementioned differences in fluoride salts, preparations and dosages.

The potential benefit of fluoride treatment is illustrated by the following case report of a patient who responded extremely well.

Case report

A 34-year-old man (height 168 cm, weight 47 kg) with established secondary osteoporosis resulting from long-term glucocorticoid therapy for colitis ulcerosa (clinical stage 3, according to Table 9.1). Six months before first consultation in the department total colectomy had been performed.

Bone mineral density:
- L2–L4   0.601 g/cm2 (t-score: −5.21 s.d.)
- Femur neck   0.692 g/cm2 (t-score: −3.15 s.d.)

Radiograph of thoracic and lumbar spine: Osteoporotic fractures of Th6,7 and L1–L4 (Figure 9.3)

Laboratory findings: Calcium, phosphorus, alkaline phosphatase, testosterone, PTH, 25-hydroxyvitamin D_3 within normal range

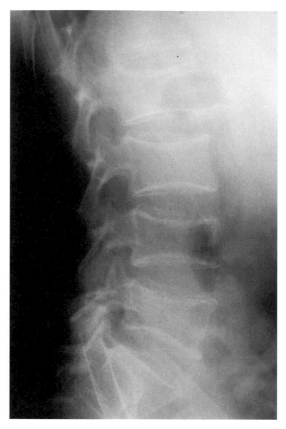

Figure 9.3 A lateral radiograph of the spine of a 34-year-old man with severe glucocorticoid-induced osteoporosis before fluoride treatment.

Table 9.4 Case report of a 34-year-old man with severe secondary osteoporosis: Bone density values before and after 3 years of therapy with MFP, calcium and vitamin D_3

Area	Month	Bone density (g/cm²)	Percentage age matched	t-score
L2–L4	0	0.601	48	−5.21
	36	1.057	93	−1.53
Femoral neck	0	0.692	72	−3.15
	36	0.703	73	−3.06
Femur–Ward	0	0.569	67	−3.01
	36	0.576	69	−2.96

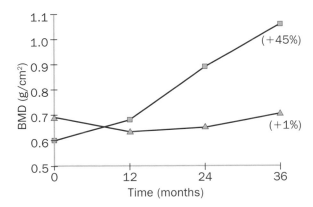

Figure 9.4 Change of bone mineral density (BMD) at the lumbar spine and the proximal femur during 3 years of treatment with MFP, calcium and vitamin D_3: ▬■▬ , L2–L4; ▬△▬ , femur neck.

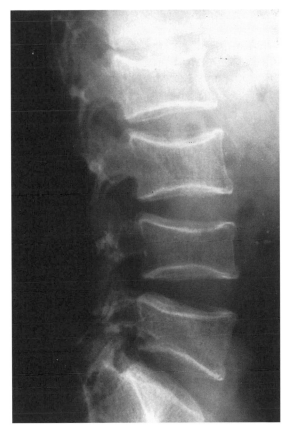

Figure 9.5 Same patient as shown in Figure 9.3: lateral radiograph of the lumbar spine 3 years after treatment with MFP, calcium and vitamin D. There was increased density of trabecular structures and endplates without further flattening of vertebrae.

Bone biopsy:
Advanced thinning of trabeculae, low bone turnover, no signs for osteomalacia

Treatment:
Three-year regimen with daily intake of:
- MFP 152 mg (=20 mg fluoride ions)
- calcium 1000 mg
- vitamin D_3 1000 IU

Results:
Continuous and rapid increase of mineral content at the lumbar spine with an average of 15% per year, no significant changes at the femoral neck and femur–Ward measuring sites (Table 9.4 and Figure 9.4). No new or progressive vertebral fractures or nonspinal fracture events during the 3 years of observation. The last radiograph of the lumbar spine shows increased bone density (Figure 9.5) in comparison with the pre-treatment picture (Figure 9.3).

Side effects

Iatrogenic fluorosis is not a drug side effect as such, but the result of incorrect therapy. In recent years two variants have been repeatedly observed. The first type very quickly (often in less than 24 months) produces a distinct sclerosed bone structure on the vertebral radiograph. In such cases, it has always been found in retrospect that the diagnosis of osteoporosis was based on a poor X-ray film, i.e. that osteo-porosis was probably not present at the start of fluoride treatment. A typical example has been shown in Figure 9.2. An individually strong response to fluoride therapy might be involved or a potentiation of the fluoride effect by aluminium, as discussed above.[20] Bone density values in these patients are greatly elevated at the lumbar spine and moderately increased in the femur and radius. The second type of iatrogenic fluorosis occurs in patients with established osteoporosis only after excessively long-term and/or high-dosage fluoride treatment, i.e. usually after 6–10 years. Densitometric measurements reveal either the same pattern as in the first type or, more frequently, greatly elevated values in the vertebrae and rather low values at peripheral sites. Although, in the first type, normally shaped vertebrae show a more or less white, ivory-like appearance (see Figure 9.2), for the second type coarsening of the previously impressed endplates and a remarkable thickening of the trabeculae are characteristic (Figure 9.6). Taking the author's own experience, it must be stressed again that iatrogenic fluorosis results either from a wrong diagnosis or from wrong treatment.

The two main adverse reactions during fluoride therapy are gastrointestinal and osteoarticular effects. As detailed above, the former occur more frequently when non-enteric-coated NaF is given. A typical example was provided by the two American double-blind studies[14,21] which used simple capsules containing plain NaF. As revealed by the third later publication, the compliance was correspondingly poor.[34] In contrast, epigastric symptoms are rarely reported with sustained-release and/or enteric-coated NaF tablets,[24] and when they did occur they were mild in nature. When MFP is used, virtually no gastric side effects are reported. The better gastric tolerance of MFP compared with NaF was also documented by a gastroscopic study.[15]

Osteoarticular symptoms, mostly affecting the ankles or the calcaneus, are referred to today as 'lower limb pain syndrome'.[42] Pronounced cases appear on the radiograph as

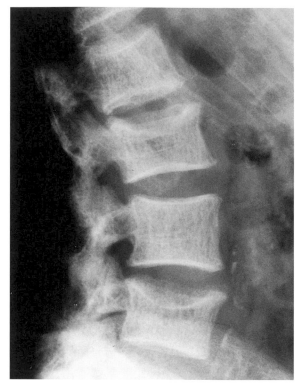

Figure 9.6 Lateral radiograph of the lumbar spine of a 67-year-old woman with postmenopausal osteoporosis: fluorosis after 6 years of therapy with MFP/calcium (BMD, L2–L4 1.709 g/cm^2 = +4.30 t-score; femur neck 0.802 g/cm^2 = −2.22 t-score).

low-contrast intraosseous coarsening and as hot spots on the scintigram (Figure 9.7). They probably correspond to mineralization defects located on the microcallus of trabecular microfractures.[43] Very rarely these microfractures or stress fracture-like lesions occur in the region of the hip or knee. Only two cases have been observed with acute pain in the hip during fluoride treatment. The case of a 70-year-old woman with severe postmenopausal osteoporosis, who complained after 2 years of fluoride treatment of acutely starting pain in the left hip, is shown in Figure 9.8.

If treatment is discontinued for 4–8 weeks,

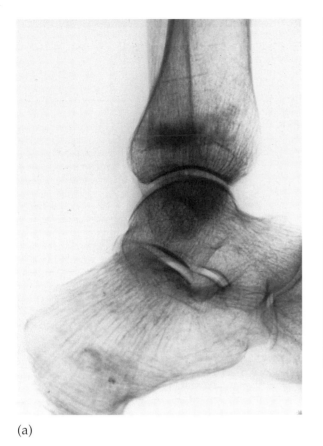

(a)

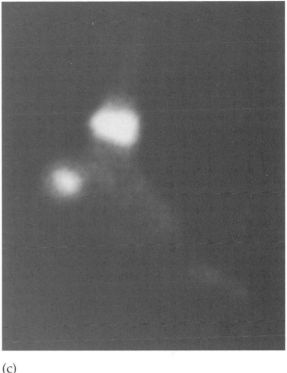

(c)

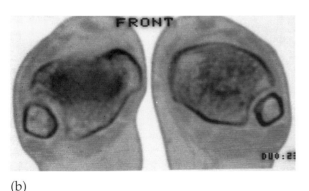

(b)

Figure 9.7 A 75-year-old woman with postmenopausal osteoporosis and acute lower limb pain syndrome after 18 months of MFP 114 mg/day. (a) The radiograph shows areas of increased density in the distal tibia and the dorsal part of the calcaneus. (b) The CT scan of the distal tibia region from the same patient proves an area of increased density (microcallus) at the right leg. (c) Bone scan from the same patient: increased uptake of the tracer at the distal tibia and dorsal calcaneus (compare (a)).

symptoms abate and radiological findings will normalize. Therapy may then be started again with an initially lower dose. Complete fractures do not occur.

No toxic or teratogenic side effects of fluoride therapy have been noted.

Early treatment and combined therapy

The classic indication for fluoride has always been established osteoporosis with at least one vertebral fracture. Most studies with fluoride were performed in manifest postmenopausal

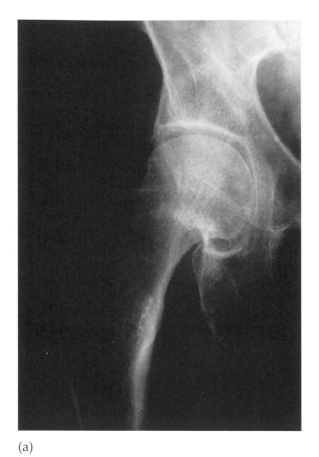

(a)

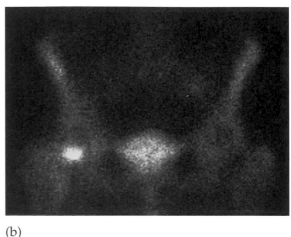

(b)

Figure 9.8 A 64-year-old woman with postmenopausal osteoporosis and acute pain in the right hip region after 2 years of MFP 114 mg/day. (a) Radiograph showing microfractures leading to a small area of increased density microcallus in the proximal–medial part of the femoral neck. (b) Bone scan from the same patient showing a 'hot spot' at the site of the microfractures.

osteoporosis with the aim to avoid *further* vertebral fractures.

Assuming, however, that fluoride will mainly build up new bone on existing intraosseous bone structures, it seems very logical to try an early treatment with the aim of bringing up bone mineral content to the normal range and avoiding the *first* vertebral fracture.

Studies with this concept were only started in recent years either for prevention of osteoporosis in healthy postmenopausal women[44] or as an early treatment in osteopenic women without fractures (stage 0, see Table 9.1).[45]

In a French double-blind study, 94 postmenopausal women were included (age range 50–70 years) with a lumbar bone density *t*-score below −2.00 s.d. and no fractures. The fluoride group received 200 mg MFP and 500 mg calcium per day; the control group received placebo and calcium.[46] Fluoride-treated patients showed a highly significant average increase of 14% at the spine over 2 years, whereas the control group showed no significant change. In both groups together, only three fracture events were recorded during the study period, which is insufficient for statistical evaluation.

With the same idea of an early fluoride therapy, the author treated 64 men with idiopathic osteoporosis. At onset spinal bone density was at a *t*-score below −2.5 s.d. and no patient had

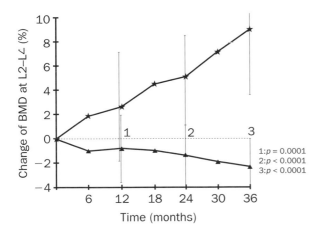

Figure 9.9 Average change of bone mineral density at the lumbar spine in men with idiopathic osteoporosis without vertebral fractures during intermittent treatment with MFP plus continuous calcium (—⋆—) or calcium alone (—▲—).

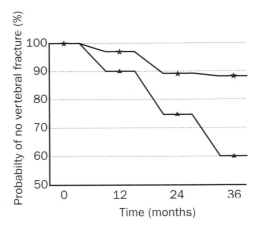

Figure 9.10 Significantly higher rate of men with no vertebral fractures after fluoride plus calcium therapy (—⋆—) than in patients treated only with calcium (—▲—).

previously had vertebral fractures. Patients were treated with either a rather low amount of MFP (114 mg/day = 15 mg fluoride ions) with an intermittent schedule of 3 months on and 1 month off plus continuous 1000 mg calcium, or with calcium alone.[41]

During the 3 years of the trial, the bone density of the fluoride group increased significantly at the lumbar spine with an average of 3% per year (Figure 9.9), and also slightly at the radius shaft and the proximal femur with an annual average of 0.4 and 0.6%, respectively. In the calcium group moderate losses of bone density were documented at all measuring sites. Despite the rather moderate increase at the spine, there was a highly significant difference in vertebral fracture events between the groups (Figure 9.10). At the end of the trial only three patients of the MFP–calcium group had established osteoporosis with, altogether, 4 vertebral fractures, whereas in the calcium group 17 fractures had occurred in 12 patients ($p = 0.008$).

One important result of this rather low-dose intermittent fluoride treatment which must be stressed again is that benefit for trabecular and cortical bone can be achieved. This was also demonstrated in a recent study from Austria using separate measurement of cortical and cancellous bone with the quantitative computed tomography (QCT) technique.[47]

The results of the aforementioned studies in postmenopausal women[44–46] and the author's own study in men[41] are encouraging for the concept of an early treatment of osteoporosis with fluoride and calcium. There is further support from corresponding intervention studies in glucocorticoid-induced osteoporosis.[38,39]

Of course, hormone replacement therapy (HRT) is still the first choice for prevention of postmenopausal osteoporosis but, in cases of significant contraindications or side effects and in men, fluoride–calcium treatment could be an alternative.

Finally, there is the option to combine osteoanabolic fluoride with antiresorptive substances. In an earlier study from the Mayo Clinic, using five different treatment groups, the one with NaF + HRT + calcium + vitamin D was the most effective in terms of reducing the vertebral fracture rate.[48] In a recent study from Italy, again with the intention of preventing osteoporosis, the combination of MFP + HRT was more effective than HRT alone in increasing bone mass.[49]

Combinations with other antiresorptive substances (calcitonin, bisphosphonates, active vitamin D metabolites) could also be very interesting and should be studied, in the future, in early stages and established cases of osteoporosis. With regard to fluoride–calcium therapy + alfacalcidol or calcitriol, it has been suggested that this combination may be of special interest in terms of ameliorating the quality of the newly formed bone and reducing the incidence of lower limb pain syndrome.[50]

PARATHYROID HORMONE

The discrepancies between bone mass and bone strength observed after fluoride treatment in some human studies[14,21] and animal trials[51,52] have been a strong promoter for research into other potentially osteoanabolic substances. One important candidate is still PTH,[53] although first indications that PTH may, in addition to the well-known resorption-inducing effect, have an anabolic action on bone tissue emerged more than 60 years ago.[54,55]

Mechanisms of action and results from animal studies

Receptors for PTH are not found in osteoclasts but are abundant in preosteoblastic cells. Increased osteoclastic resorption is therefore believed to be a consequence of secondary signalling, probably by communication of the cells lining quiescent bone surfaces with osteoclast precursors via local factors.[53]

In studies in vitro it was found that continuous application of PTH or PTH-related peptide (PTHrp) inhibited osteoblastic collagen synthesis, whereas intermittent or transient treatment had a stimulatory effect which was mediated by local production of insulin-like growth factor I (IGF-I).[56]

Parathyroid hormone may not only increase the synthesizing capacity of osteoblasts but also influence the proliferation of preosteoblasts and the programmed end of bone-forming activity of osteoblasts by apoptosis. Recent data support the concept that IGFs are also inhibitors of apoptosis,[57] i.e. PTH might have the potential to increase the number of active osteoblasts by both augmenting their rate of production and reducing their death rate.

Discontinuation of PTH treatment has been shown to cause loss of newly formed bone. Obviously the anabolic effect can only be maintained by daily administration of the hormone.[58] From a large number of animal studies, mainly performed on rats, it could be shown that PTH given by an intermittent schedule had positive effects on trabecular bone in terms of increasing volume and thickness, but not by augmenting the number of trabeculae.[53] This anabolic potency, especially on cancellous bone, can be observed rather frequently in secondary hyperparathyroidism that results from chronic renal insufficiency. A considerable augmentation of the trabecular bone mass close to the vertebral endplates is a typical radiological sign of renal osteopathy ('sandwich vertebra').

It has frequently been suggested that the pronounced osteoanabolic effect of intermittent PTH on trabecular bone mass is achieved at the expense of cortical bone, but none of the rat studies to date has shown any sign of loss of cortical bone during this therapy. There is even one study showing a positive effect on cortical bone by increasing periosteal and endosteal bone formation.[58]

As increases in bone mass may not always be in parallel with an augmentation of bone quality and hence increased biomechanical competence, measurements of bone strength were also undertaken. Again, in the rat model, it could be shown that after PTH therapy there was an increase in biomechanical stability of the vertebrae and the femoral neck.[59] However, studies are needed in a larger animal model, with intracortical remodelling comparable to the situation in humans, for further clarification of the effects of intermittent PTH therapy on cortical bone. From primary hyperparathyroidism, it is well known that continuous endogeneous PTH secretion is followed by severe cortical bone porosity.

Altogether the in vitro data and the results from animal studies were very encouraging for clinical studies in humans.

Clinical results and further perspectives

Experimental studies with parathyroid peptides in humans began 20 years ago.[60] Most studies were done with the active fragment 1–34 hPTH (human parathyroid hormone) because it was thought to be the natural cleavage product. Another fragment is currently available, the 1–38 hPTH, and also the whole molecule can easily be synthesized by recombinant technology.

The first studies with 1–34 hPTH in animals and humans were carried out using a daily dose ranging from 133 to 800 units/day given by subcutaneous injection. The units were derived from a chick hypercalcaemia-based assay. The lower doses proved to be definitely ineffective[61] and later studies were conducted in the range of 400–800 units/day. A recent study from Japan[62] reports a significant stimulation of bone formation and an increase in bone mass in patients with senile osteoporosis using only 20 units 1–34 hPTH (=6 μg). Differences in the standardization of units of hPTH may contribute to this discrepancy.

Several approaches were employed to use the anabolic effect of PTH on the spine and avoid possible negative effects on the peripheral skeleton by adding an antiresorptive drug as a second agent, e.g. calcitriol, calcitonin or oestrogen.[63,64] Some groups used a regimen with sequential application of the second agent, i.e. an 'ADFR-like' procedure (ADFR = activate–depress–free–repeat). Most of the trials were, however, of rather short-term duration and involved small numbers of patients. Nevertheless, significant and even sometimes unexpectedly high increases of lumbar bone density could be demonstrated in these studies. Antifracture efficacy studies are, however, yet to be carried out.

The very slow progress in establishing PTH as an antiosteoporotic drug during the last 20 years has several reasons:

1. Initial difficulties in manufacturing PTH fragments of adequate purity in sufficient quantity.
2. Concerns of an increase of axial bone mass at the expense of peripheral skeletal sites.
3. Lack of an effective delivery route other than parenterally, i.e. by daily injections.
4. Problems with high levels of plasma hPTH binding in some patients with the risk of reduced therapeutic efficacy as a result of antibodies.
5. The high costs of the peptide hormone in comparison to the cheap osteoanabolic fluoride.

Despite these problems there is now accumulated evidence that hPTH peptides are able to increase spinal bone mass to an extent comparable to fluoride salts or even to a greater extent. Further research should aim for strategies for the conservation of cortical bone during this treatment and for the documentation of a long-term ability to reduce vertebral and non-spinal fractures.

It is difficult to predict whether the whole PTH molecule or the rather large fragments used so far will proceed from interesting experimental drugs to developed pharmaceutical products. Modified PTH peptides and small fragments are being studied currently and may become even more interesting in the future. There is evidence that small adenylate cyclase-stimulating fragments of PTH have the potency to stimulate osteoblasts and make mechanically strong bone.[65] Furthermore a PTHrp analogue (RS-23581) has proved to be a very potent stimulator of bone in animal studies.[66]

Eventually, the intensive research into the biochemical pathways of the stimulatory effect of PTH and analogues on osteoblasts will result in the development of other potent osteoanabolic drugs with safe and easy modes of application.

STRONTIUM

It has been shown that strontium, a natural trace element, is able to increase trabecular bone volume when administered at low concentrations to normal animals.[67] On the basis of histomorphometric findings, it was suggested that this element increases bone mass by both inhibition of bone resorption and stimulation of bone formation.

In oestrogen deficiency-induced bone loss of ovariectomized rats – the classic animal model with characteristics comparable to early post-menopausal trabecular bone loss – both fluoride and PTH were shown to increase bone mass. To determine whether a strontium salt could also prevent postmenopausal bone loss, S12911, a divalent organic strontium salt (Institut de Recherches Internationales Servier, France), was used in the ovariectomized rat model.[68] The dosages of S12911 used were 77, 154 and 308 mg/kg per day and the groups of ovariectomized rats were compared with a group receiving oestradiol and a sham operated group.

Treatment with strontium prevented bone loss, measured as bone ash and restored bone mineral content against the values in placebo-treated animals. The histomorphometrically measured trabecular bone volume at the tibial metaphysis decreased by 46% after ovariectomy and was corrected by oestrogen treatment. Through treatment with S12911, it was not only corrected but increased by 30–36%. Histomorphometric indices of bone resorption and formation, and biochemical markers of bone turnover proved that, in contrast to oestrogen, which suppressed bone resorption and formation, the strontium salt decreased resorption without reducing formation. The authors concluded that the strontium compound acts as an uncoupling agent with inhibition of resorption and ongoing or even increased formation.[68]

In another recent study on rats, the osteoanabolic potency of low doses of strontium, fluoride and both substances combined were compared. The mineralized bone volume was significantly increased by 17% in the strontium-treated group, by 20% in the fluoride-treated rats and by 19% in the animals given both drugs. Furthermore, the study indicated that the treatment with low doses of strontium or fluoride increased the number of bone-forming

sites without detectable adverse effects on bone mineral chemistry or bone matrix mineralization.[69]

The data discussed, together with a large number of other preclinical studies that produced positive results, are in favour of clinical studies with this new bone-forming and antiresorptive drug. A large, prospective, placebo-controlled trial in postmenopausal osteoporosis has already been started.

FURTHER COMPOUNDS

Further compounds with osteoanabolic effects were shown in Table 9.2. Aluminium- and silicon-containing agents that are under investigation as potentially osteoanabolic substances are not listed. An additive, osteoblast-stimulating potency of aluminium salts in combination with fluoride has been mentioned above.[20] Zeolite A, a silicon-containing compound, stimulates proliferation and differentiation of cultured human osteoblast-like cells by inducing paracrine production of transforming growth factor β (TGFβ). There are also data showing an antiresorptive effect of this substance.[70]

The potentially osteoblast-stimulating effect of anabolic steroids is discussed in Chapter 10. Only growth hormone (GH), IGF-I and prostaglandin E_2 are discussed briefly here.

Growth hormone secretion reduces with ageing, resulting in decreasing amounts of circulating IGF-I. This so-called 'somatopause' is suspected of enhancing musculoskeletal changes during ageing[71] and, as GH became widely available with the advent of recombinant gene technology, interest began to increase in treating involutional osteoporosis with this hormone. This interest was fuelled by the observation that the increased prevalence of osteoporosis in patients with pituitary insufficiency might result from a lack of GH rather than from the substitution with cortisone and thyroxine.[72] Another interesting aspect was the observation, by one group of investigators, that idiopathic male osteoporosis may be related to low serum IGF-I.[73]

Both GH and IGF-I stimulate osteoblastic differentiation and enhance longitudinal bone growth, bone formation and bone mass in animals. Although most effects of GH on bone occur through induction of IGF-I, substantially different effects on bone metabolism were observed when using rhGH or rhIGF-I in children and in adults (rh = recombinant human).

Application of rhGH to healthy men stimulated bone remodelling and this effect on bone persisted after discontinuation of the hormone.[74] In children and adults with GH deficiency, rhGH and rhIGF-I proved able to increase cortical and trabecular bone density. In several small studies, GH was used to treat different forms of osteoporosis, in some trials combined with fluoride or calcitonin. Positive trends on bone histomorphometry and bone mass were reported. There are, however, also data showing an increased bone resorption and there are no trials with spinal fracture rate as a therapeutic endpoint.

Taken together, we do not currently have unequivocal evidence that GH (or IGF-I) is able to stimulate bone formation for a sustained period of time and to reduce fracture rate in patients with established osteoporosis. Therefore, neither substance can be recommended for treatment until definite positive results have been documented by properly designed trials.

Prostaglandins can modulate bone metabolism both in vitro and in vivo. In animal studies it was shown that PGE$_2$ has a profound anabolic effect on cancellous bone and, to a lesser degree, on compact bone. On the other hand, there are data that suggest that local bone resorption in periodontal disease is mediated by PGE$_2$.[75]

Recent studies support the hypothesis that PGE$_2$ stimulates the proliferation and differentiation of osteoblastic precursor cells,[76] and raise the possibility that the observed stimulation of periosteal bone formation may be mediated by increased survival of periosteal bone-forming cells, i.e. suppressed apoptosis.[77] Intensive further research is necessary to develop PGE$_2$ to a therapeutic substance for local or systemic application in bone diseases.

REFERENCES

1. Consensus Development Conference. Diagnosis, prophylaxis and treatment of osteoporosis. *Am J Med* 1993; **94**: 646–50.

2. Ringe JD. *Osteoporose. Postmenopausale Osteoporose – Senile Osteoporose – Sekundäre Osteoporose – Osteoporose des Mannes*. Stuttgart: Georg Thième Verlag, 1995.

3. Kanis JA, Melton LJ, Christiansen C et al. Perspective. The diagnosis of osteoporosis. *J Bone Miner Res* 1994; **9**: 1137–41.

4. Kleerekoper M, Mendlovic B. Sodium fluoride therapy of postmenopausal osteoporosis. *Endocrine Rev* 1993; **14**: 312–23.

5. Shortt HE, McRobert GR, Barnad TW. Endemic fluorosis in the Madras Precidency. *Ind J Med* 1937; **25**: 553–4.

6. Möller PF, Gudjonsson SV. Massive fluorosis of bones and ligaments. *Acta Radiol* 1932; **13**: 267–94.

7. Roholm K. Fluorine intoxication. *A Clinical Hygienic Study with a Review of the Literature and Some Experimental Investigations*. London: HK Lewis & Co Ltd, 1937.

8. Bernstein DS, Sadowsky N, Hegsted DM et al. Prevalence of osteoporosis in high- and low-fluoride areas in North Dakota. *JAMA* 1966; **198**: 499–504.

9. Rich C, Ensinck J. Effect of sodium fluoride on calcium metabolism of human beings. *Nature* 1961; **191**: 184–5.

10. Ringe JD. Osteoporosetherapie mit Fluoriden. State of the Art 1992. *Arzneimitteltherapie* 1992; **10**: 349–57.

11. Heaney RL. Fluoride and osteoporosis. *Ann Intern Med* 1994; **120**: 689–90.

12. Setnikar I, Ringe JD. Fluorverbindungen: Pharmakokinetik und Bioverfügbarkeit. *Arzneimitteltherapie* 1995; **13**: 73–9.

13. Delmas PD, Dupuis J, Duboeuf F et al. Treatment of vertebral osteoporosis with disodium monofluorophosphate: Comparison with sodium fluoride. *J Bone Miner Res* 1990; **5**(suppl 1): S143–7.

14. Riggs BL, Hodgson SF, O'Fallow WM et al. Effect of fluoride treatment on the fracture rate in postmenopausal women with osteoporosis. *N Engl J Med* 1990; **322:** 802–9.

15. Müller P, Schmid K, Warneke et al. Sodium fluoride-induced gastri mucosal lesions: Comparison with sodium monofluorophosphate. *Z Gastroenterol* 1992; **30:** 252–4.

16. Resch H, Libanati C, Talbot et al. Pharmakokinetic profile of a new fluoride preparation: Sustained-release monofluorophosphate. *Calcif Tissue Int* 1994; **54:** 7–11.

17. Erlacher L, Templ H, Magometschnigg D. A comparative bioavailability study on two new sustained-release formulations of disodium monofluorophosphate versus a nonsustained-release formulation in healthy volunteers. *Calcif Tissue Int* 1995; **56:** 196–200.

18. Ekstrand J, Ehrnebo M, Boreus LO. Fluoride bioavailability after intravenous and oral administration: importance of renal clearance and urine flow. *Clin Pharmacol Ther* 1978; **23:** 329–37.

19. Farley JR, Wergedal JE, Baylink DJ. Fluoride directly stimulates proliferation and alkaline phosphatase activity of bone forming cells. *Science* 1983; **222:** 330–2.

20. Caverzasio J, Imai T, Amman P et al. Aluminium potentiates the effect of fluoride on tyrosine phosphorylation and osteoblast replication in vitro and bone mass in vivo. *J Bone Miner Res* 1996; **11:** 46–55.

21. Kleerekoper M, Peterson EL, Nelson DA et al. A randomized trial of sodium fluoride as a treatment for postmenopausal osteoporosis. *Osteoporosis Int* 1991; **1:** 155–61.

22. Farley SM, Wergedal JE, Farley JR et al. Spinal fractures during fluoride therapy for osteoporosis: Relationship to spinal bone density. *Osteoporosis Int* 1992; **2:** 213–18.

23. Eriksen EF, Mosekilde L, Melsen F. Effect of sodium fluoride, calcium, phosphate, and vitamin D2 on trabecular bone balance and remodeling in osteoporosis. *Bone* 1985; **6:** 381–9.

24. Pak CYC, Sakhaee K, Gallagher C et al. Attainment of therapeutic fluoride levels in serum without major side effects using a slow-release preparation of sodium fluoride in postmenopausal osteoporosis. *J Bone Miner Res* 1986; **1:** 563–71.

25. Ringe JD, Meunier PJ. What is the future for fluoride in the treatment of osteoporosis? *Osteoporosis Int* 1995; **5:** 71–4.

26. Pak CYC, Zerwekh JE, Antich P. Anabolic effects

of fluoride on bone. *Trends Endocrinol Metab* 1995; **6:** 229–34.

27. Briancon D, Meunier PJ. Treatment of osteoporosis with fluoride, calcium and vitamin D. *Orthop Clin North Am* 1981; **12:** 629–48.

28. Eriksen EF, Hodgson SF, Riggs BL. Treatment of osteoporosis with sodium fluoride. In: *Osteoporosis: Etiology, Diagnosis and Management* (Riggs BL, Melton III LJ, eds). New York: Raven Press, 1988: 415–32.

29. Editorial (GREES). Recommendations for the registration of new chemical entities used in the prevention and treatment of osteoporosis. *Calcif Tissue Int* 1995; **57:** 247–50.

30. Ringe JD, Kruse HP, Kuhlencordt F. Long-term treatment of primary osteoporosis by sodium fluoride. In: *Fluoride and Bone* (Courvoisier B, Donath A, Baud CA, eds). Bern: Hans Huber, 1978: 228–32.

31. Ringe JD. Kombinierte Fluoridtherapie der primären Osteoporose. Ergebnisse einer zweijährigen Behandlung mit Natriummonofluorophosphat und Calcium. *Fortschr Med* 1987; **115:** 379–82.

32. Ringe JD. Monofluorophosphate prevents fractures in postmenopausal osteoporosis. In: *Current Research in Gynecology and Obstetrics* (Genazzani et al, eds). Casterton Hall: The Parthenon Publishing Group, 1991: 527–31.

33. Ringe JD, Schmidt R. Low-dose intermittent monofluorophosphate calcium therapy in idiopathic male osteoporosis. *Bone* 1995; **16**(suppl): 161S.

34. Riggs BL, O'Fallon WM, Lane A et al. Clinical trial of fluoride therapy in postmenopausal osteoporotic women: Extended observations and additional analysis. *J Bone Miner Res* 1994; **9:** 265–75.

35. Mamelle N, Dusan R, Martin JL et al. Risk–benefit ratio of sodium fluoride treatment in primary vertebral osteoporosis. *Lancet* 1988; **ii:** 361–5.

36. Pak CYC, Sakhaee K, Piziak V et al. Slow-release sodium fluoride in the management of postmenopausal osteoporosis. A randomized controlled trial. *Ann Intern Med* 1994; **120:** 625–32.

37. Pak CYC, Sakhaee K, Adams-Huet B et al. Treatment of postmenopausal osteoporosis with slow-release sodium fluoride. Final report of a randomized controlled trial. *Ann Intern Med* 1995; **123:** 401–8.

38. Meys E, Terraux-Duvert F, Beaume-Six T et al. Bone loss after cardiac transplantation: effects of

calcium, calcidiol and monofluorophosphate. *Osteoporosis Int* 1993; **3:** 1–8.

39. Rizzoli R, Chevalley Th, Slosman DO et al. Sodium monofluorophosphate increases vertebral bone mineral density in patients with corticoid-induced osteoporosis. *Osteoporosis Int* 1995; **5:** 39–46.

40. Meunier PJ. Bone forming agents. *Osteoporosis Int* 1996; **6**(suppl 1): 94.

41. Ringe JD, Kipshoven C, Rovati L et al. Therapy of idiopathic male osteoporosis: A three year study with calcium and low dose intermittent monofluorophosphate. *Osteoporosis Int* 1996; **6**(suppl 1): 96.

42. O'Duffy JD, Wahner HW, O'Fallon WM et al. Mechanism of acute lower extremity pain syndrome in fluoride-treated osteoporotic patients. *Am J Med* 1986; **80:** 561–6.

43. Boivin G, Grousson B, Meunier PJ. X-ray microanalysis of fluoride distribution in microfracture calluses in cancellous iliac bone from osteoporotic patients treated with fluoride and untreated. *J Bone Miner Res* 1991; **11:** 1183 90.

44. Affinito P, Di Carlo C, Primizia M et al. A new fluoride preparation for the prevention of postmenopausal osteoporosis: calcium monofluorophosphate. *Gynecol Endocrinol* 1993; **7:** 201–5.

45. Pouilles JM, Tremollieres F, Causse E et al. Fluoride therapy in postmenopausal osteopenic women: Effect on vertebral and femoral bone density and prediction of bone response. *Osteoporosis Int* 1991; **1:** 103–9.

46. Sebert JL, Richard P, Mennecier I et al. Monofluorophosphate increases lumbar bone density in patients with low bone mass but no vertebral fractures. A double-blind randomized study. *Osteoporosis Int* 1995; **5:** 108–14.

47. Peichl P, Zamani O, Kumpan W et al. Antiosteoporotic therapy with monofluorophosphate and calcium increases cortical and trabecular vertebral bone density. *Osteologie* 1995; **4:** 87–98.

48. Riggs BL, Seeman E, Hodgson SF et al. Effect of the fluoride/calcium regimen on vertebral fracture occurrence in postmenopausal osteoporosis. *N Engl J Med* 1982; **306:** 446–50.

49. Gambacciani M, Spinetti A, Cappagli B et al. Effects of low-dose monofluorophosphate and transdermal oestradiol on postmenopausal vertebral bone loss. *Eur Menopause J* 1995; **2:** 16–20.

50. Lundy MW, Stauffer M, Wergedal et al. Histomorphometric analysis of iliac crest bone biopsies in placebo-treated versus fluoride-treated subjects. *Osteoporosis Int* **5:** 115–29.

51. Mosekilde L, Kragstrup J, Richards A. Compressive strength, ash weight, and volume of vertebral trabecular bone in experimental fluorosis in pigs. *Calcif Tissue Int* 1987; **39:** 69–73.

52. Sogaard CH, Mosekilde I, Schwartz et al. Effects of fluoride treatment on rat vertebral body biomechanical competence and bone mass. *Bone* 1995; **16:** 163–9.

53. Dempster DW, Cosman F, Parisien M et al. Anabolic actions of parathyroid hormone on bone. *Endocrinol Rev* 1993; **14:** 690–709.

54. Seyle H. On the stimulation of new bone-formation with parathyroid extract and irradiated ergosterol. *J Endocrinol* 1932; **16:** 547–58.

55. Burrows R. Variations produced in bones of growing rats by parathyroid extracts. *Am J Anat* 1938; **62:** 237–90.

56. Canalis E, McCarthy TL, Centrella M. Differential effects of continuous and transient treatment with parathyroid hormone related peptide (PTHrp) on bone collagen synthesis. *Endocrinology* 1990; **126:** 1806–12.

57. Harrington EA, Fanidi A, Evan GI. Oncogenes and cell death. *Genet Dev* 1994; **4:** 120–9.

58. Gunness-Hey M, Hock JM. Loss of the anabolic effect of parathyroid hormone on bone after discontinuation of hormone in rats. *Bone* 1989; **10:** 447–52.

59. Wronski TJ, Yen CF. Anabolic effects of parathyroid hormone on cortical bone in ovariectomized rats. *Bone* 1994; **10:** 447–52.

60. Reeve J, Tregear GW, Parsons JA. Preliminary trial of low doses of human parathyroid hormone (1–34) peptide in treatment of osteoporosis. *Calcif Tissue Res* 1976; **21**(suppl): 469–77.

61. Tellez M, Zanelli JM, Wootton et al. Dose variation in the treatment of osteoporosis with synthetic human parathyroid hormone fragment hPTH 1–34. *Clin Sci* 1981; **60:** 26.

62. Sone T, Fukunaga M, Ono S et al. A small dose of human parathyroid hormone (1–34) increased bone mass in the lumbar vertebrae in patients with senile osteoporosis. *Min Electrolyte Metab* 1995; **21:** 232–5.

63. Reeve J, Bradbeer JN, Arlot ME et al. hPTH 1–34 treatment of osteoporosis with added hormone replacement therapy: Biochemical, kinetic and histological responses. *Osteoporosis Int* 1991; **1:** 162–70.

64. Hesch RD, Busch U, Prokop M et al. Increase of vertebral density by combination therapy with pulsatile 1–38 PTH and sequential addition of

calcitonin nasal spray in osteoporotic patients. *Calcif Tissue Int* 1989; **44:** 176–80.

65. Whitfield JF, Morley P. Small bone-building fragments of parathyroid hormone: new therapeutic agents for osteoporosis. *Trends Pharmacol Sci* 1995; **16:** 382–6.

66. Hill EL, Zuber Y, Avnur Z et al. Anabolic effects of RS-23581, a PTHrp analogue, on bone in mature, osteopenic rats. *J Bone Miner Res* 1996; **11**(suppl 1): S95.

67. Marie PJ, Garba MT, Hott et al. Effect of low doses of stable strontium on bone metabolism in rats. *Miner Electrolyte Metab* 1985; **11:** 5–13.

68. Marie PJ, Hott M, Modrowski D et al. An uncoupling agent containing strontium prevents bone loss by depressing bone resorption and maintaining bone formation in estrogen-deficient rats. *J Bone Miner Res* 1993; **8:** 607–15.

69. Grynpas M, Hamilton E, Cheung R et al. Strontium increases vertebral bone volume in rats at a low dose that does not induce detectable mineralization defect. *Bone* 1996; **18:** 253–9.

70. Schuetze N, Oursler MJ, Spelsberg TC. Zeolite A inhibits osteoclast mediated bone resorption in vitro. *J Bone Miner Res* 1995; **10**(suppl 1): S386.

71. Rudman DV, Feller AG, Nagrog HS et al. Effect of human growth hormone in men over age 60. *N Engl J Med* 1990; **323:** 52–4.

72. Wüster C, Slenczka E, Ziegler R. Increased prevalence of osteoporosis and atherosclerosis in patients with conventionally substituted pituitary insufficiency: Is there a need for additional GH substitution? *Klin Wochenschr* 1991; **69:** 769–73.

73. Ljunghall S, Johansson AG, Burman P et al. Low plasma levels of IGF-I in male patients with idiopathic osteoporosis. *J Intern Med* 1992; **232:** 59–64.

74. Brixen K, Nielsen HK, Mosekilde L et al. A short course of rhGH stimulates osteoblasts and activates bone remodeling in normal human volunteers. *J Bone Miner Res* 1990; **5:** 609–18.

75. Offenbacher S, Collins JG, Arnold RR. New clinical diagnostic strategies based on pathogenesis of disease. *J Periodontal Res* 1993; **28:** 523–35.

76. Weinreb M, Suponitzki I, Keila S. Stimulation of bone marrow osteogenic precursors as a possible mechanism of the anabolic effect of systemic PGE_2 in rats. *J Bone Miner Res* 1996; **11**(suppl 1): S139.

77. Machwate M, Rodan SB, Rodan GA et al. Prostaglandin (PG) E_2 suppresses apoptosis in two rat periosteal cell lines via a cAMP-dependent pathway. *J Bone Miner Res* 1996; **11**(suppl 1): S143.

10

Other agents for treatment of osteoporosis

C Gennari and R Nuti

CONTENTS • Calcium • Vitamin D and analogues • Calcitonin • Anabolic steroids • New agents

CALCIUM

Calcium is a major component of mineralized tissue and is needed for normal growth and development of the skeleton. Two main factors were shown to influence the occurrence of osteoporosis: the optimal peak bone mass obtained in the first two to three decades of life and the rate of bone loss in later years. Adequate calcium intake is necessary to maximize peak adult bone mass, and administration of an oral calcium supplement can reduce the acceleration of bone loss which follows the menopause. On the basis of the most current information available, optimal daily calcium intake is estimated to be: 800 mg for young children (1–5 years); 800–1200 mg for older children (6–10 years); 1200–1500 mg for adolescent and young adults; 1000 mg for women and men between 25 and 50 years; 1200 mg for pregnant and lactating women; 1000 mg for postmenopausal women on oestrogen replacement therapy; and 1500 mg for postmenopausal women not on oestrogen treatment, and for men and women over 65 years of age. In adults aged 65 years and older, calcium intake of less than 600 mg/day is common. Calcium insufficiency as a result of low calcium intake and reduced intestinal absorption can translate into an accelerated rate of age-related bone loss in older individuals. Moreover, we know that dietary constituents, hormones, drugs and genetic factors may influence the amount of calcium required for optimal skeletal health. However, a high calcium intake will not substitute for oestrogen therapy in decreasing the accelerated bone loss during the climacteric period.[1]

To assess the effect of dietary calcium intake on risk of hip fracture, a 14-year prospective population study was carried out in 947 men and women aged 50–79 years: the top tertile of calcium intake (over 705 mg calcium daily) was associated with a 60% reduction in risk of hip fractures when compared with the lower two tertiles.[2] Subsequently, it was demonstrated that healthy older postmenopausal women with a daily calcium intake of less than 400 mg can significantly reduce bone loss by increasing their calcium intake to 800 mg/day.[3] A recent prospective study (the Rancho Bernardo Cohort) showed that age-adjusted mean bone mineral density (BMD) levels increased significantly with increasing tertile of calcium intake at all hip sites in women, with the most striking difference being at the femoral neck; the data indicate that low dietary calcium predicts low BMD in older women independent of other major determinants of BMD (body mass index, smoking, exercise, alcohol intake, use of oestrogen replacement therapy, number of years postmenopausal).[4]

The value of calcium supplementation in the prevention of bone loss was confirmed by further studies. In a group of normal women at least 3 years after menopause, with a mean dietary calcium intake of 750 mg/day, calcium supplementation (1000 mg/day) for 2 years significantly slowed axial and appendicular bone loss in comparison to a controlled placebo group; the rate of loss was reduced by one-third to one-half in the calcium group.[5] The beneficial effects on both axial and appendicular BMD were confirmed in a subsequent double-blind trial, in which the rate of bone loss for total body, lumbar spine, femoral neck and trochanter was reduced in the calcium group throughout the 4-year study period; moreover, although nine symptomatic fractures occurred in seven subjects in the placebo group, only two fractures were observed in two subjects receiving calcium.[6] The different role of dietary calcium and HRT on bone turnover in the postmenopausal phase has recently been underlined. In a three-arm, placebo-controlled, randomized study, an intake of 1700 mg calcium was compared with calcium augmentation with hormone replacement therapy (HRT) and placebo.[7] The use of HRT with calcium suppressed bone resorption to a greater degree than dietary calcium alone, resulting in a positive skeletal remodelling balance; however, whereas calcium augmentation lowered calcitriol levels, these levels were maintained by HRT, possibly by an increment in the effect of parathyroid hormone (PTH) on the kidneys.

With regard to the role of calcium supplementation in the treatment of osteoporosis, earlier studies had been carried out to assess the efficacy by measuring calcium balance on high calcium intake: the results were contradictory, and only in some studies was positive calcium balance found.[8] Recently, it has been reported that only in the early phase of treatment may calcium be able to induce a positive calcium balance, which later becomes negative, increasing with length of treatment.[9] From the histological point of view, a significant decrease in bone resorption was reported after high calcium intake (2–2.5 g/day);[10] on the other hand, increased bone mineralization and bone remodelling were demonstrated in elderly osteoporotic patients after daily treatment with calcium 1200 mg.[11] Therefore, only high doses (>2 g/day) of calcium supplements appear to retard bone loss in osteoporotic patients, whereas using lower dosages, e.g. 1 g/day, the effects of calcium therapy on BMD and vertebral fracture rates have been significantly less positive in comparison to other types of treatment.[12–15] Calcium supplementation could be helpful only in osteoporotic patients who have a very low calcium intake.

VITAMIN D AND ANALOGUES

Low vitamin D status in elderly patients can become apparent either as muscle weakness, which may lead to falls and subsequent fractures, or as a secondary hyperparathyroidism.[16,17] With regard to the preventive activity of vitamin D in old age, vitamin D_3 (800 IU) and tricalcium phosphate (1.2 g/day) were administered to 1634 healthy elderly women for 18 months: BMD of the proximal femur increased by 2.7% in the vitamin D_3 calcium group and decreased by 4.6% in the placebo group; the numbers of hip and nonvertebral fractures were 43% and 32%, respectively – lower in the vitamin D_3–calcium group in comparison with the placebo group.[18] However, these results have not been entirely confirmed; in a prospective double-blind trial carried out in 2178 people, the incidence of hip fractures and other peripheral fractures did not decrease after vitamin D_3 supplementation (400 IU/day) together with a daily calcium intake of at least 800–1000 mg/day.[19]

The vitamin D–endocrine system has been taken into account in the pathogenesis of involutional osteoporosis.[20] Postmenopausal osteoporosis (type 1) is mainly related to factors triggered by oestrogen deficiency which lead to excessive and accelerated bone loss. Impaired calcium absorption has been demonstrated consistently[21] and is associated with normal or low levels of serum 1,25-dihydroxyvitamin D_3 [$1,25(OH)_2$-D_3][22] and with slightly low values for serum PTH. Age-related osteoporosis (type 2) is associated with an age-related decrease in calcium absorption, secondary hyperparathyroidism and two types of abnormalities in the vitamin D–endocrine system:[20] an earlier resistance to vitamin D action associated with a decrease in intestinal vitamin D receptor concentration and, later in life, a primary defect in 25-hydroxyvitamin D 1α-hydroxylase activity which is a sign of an ageing kidney with reduced levels of $1,25(OH)_2$-D_3. Recently, it has been reported that vitamin D receptor genotypes are predictive for differences in bone mass in the twin model.[23]

Treatment with vitamin D_2 or D_3 compounds has not been successful in reversing malabsorption of calcium in physiological doses.[24] On the other hand, it has been largely demonstrated that physiological doses of $1,25(OH)_2$-D_3 may restore intestinal calcium absorption.[24,25] 1,25-Dihydroxyvitamin D_3 (calcitriol) and its analogue, 1α-hydroxyvitamin D_3, have been shown to have beneficial effects on bone mass in women with involutional osteoporosis. In a double-blind, randomized, clinical trial of 24 months' duration, calcitriol (mean dose 0.8 µg/day) induced positive slopes for total body calcium, radium and spine BMD, and for the bone radiographic absorptiometry of the middle phalanges.[26] Similar results were observed in another double-blind, 2-year, randomized study carried out in postmenopausal women with vertebral fractures: total body calcium and spine BMD increased (0.21% and 1.94%, respectively) in the calcitriol group (0.75–1.0 µg/day) and decreased (−1.85% and −3.92%, respectively) in placebo-treated women.[27] No adverse effects on renal function were seen in both studies during calcitriol administration. In an open-label retrospective study, calcitriol (1 µg/day without calcium supplementation) restored intestinal calcium transport and total body BMD increased (1.20% and 1.58% after 12 and 24 months, respectively).[25] With regard to antifracture efficacy, a significant reduction in the rate of new vertebral fractures in women with postmenopausal fractures was reported after 3 years of calcitriol therapy (0.25 µg twice daily): 4.2 vs 31.0 fractures per 100 patient-years in calcitriol-treated women and the control group, respectively.[15]

In other studies, beneficial effects of $1,25(OH)_2$-D_3 on bone mass or fracture rate were not demonstrated.[28,29] The most likely explanation for these negative results could be an ineffective dose:[24] indeed, re-analysis of the data of one trial did show increases in bone mass in patients receiving higher doses of calcitriol.[30] The beneficial effect of $1,25(OH)_2$-D_3 for restoring calcium balance and preventing or reversing bone loss is mainly the result of the increase in intestinal calcium absorption. Recent clinical studies reported significant increase in serum osteocalcin after calcitriol administration:[31] an effect of stimulating osteoblast activity has been hypothesized.

1α-Hydroxyvitamin D_3 (1αOHD$_3$) (alfacalcidol) is a pro-drug of $1,25(OH)_2$-D_3 which has to be metabolized first in the liver before the parent compound, $1,25(OH)_2$-D, is formed. In a double-blind placebo-controlled study, 1 µg 1αOHD$_3$ daily or inactive placebo was administered for one year to osteoporotic women.[32] All patients were given 300 mg elemental calcium daily. Lumbar BMD increased by 0.65% with 1αOHD$_3$ and decreased by 1.14% with placebo; the vertebral fracture rate in the treated group was significantly less (75/1000 patient-years) than in the control group (277/1000 patient-years). No significant changes in serum creatinine were reported.

Both calcitriol and 1α derivatives may produce hypercalcaemia or hypercalciuria if given in large doses. On the other hand, the antiosteoporosis effects of these drugs appear to be improved by increasing the dose. Unfortunately, the incidence of toxic side effects also increases, indicating that these compounds may be limited in their therapeutic usefulness by their potential toxicity; toxicity can, however, be minimized by restricting calcium intake to about 500 mg/day. As a low calcium intake is not uncommon in elderly people, who represent the main target of these drugs, toxicity may be restricted to that group of patients who habitually consume a high calcium diet.[33]

CALCITONIN

Calcitonin is a 32 amino acid polypeptide hormone synthesized in the C-cells of the thyroid.

The principal role in humans is thought to be short-term fine tuning of calcium homoeostasis, and protection of the skeleton during growth, pregnancy, lactation and, briefly but repeatedly, after meals.[34] Calcitonin was known to bind to high-affinity receptors on osteoclasts, with pronounced inhibition of activity. This action appears to be related to alteration of the internal structure of osteoclasts, and probably to a decrease in the rate of osteoclast formation by blocking the fusion of mononuclear marrow cells.[35] Recently, both in vitro and in vivo data have given support to the hypothesis that calcitonin might have a direct or indirect effect on osteoblast activity. It has been postulated that oestrogen deficiency in postmenopausal women resulted in a reduction in circulating calcitonin levels.[36] However, the calcitonin deficiency theory of postmenopausal osteoporosis has been contradicted by several studies.[37] In the three decades since its identification and synthesis, calcitonin has established a place in the treatment of Paget's disease of the bone, hypercalcaemia of malignancy and algoneurodystrophy, and in the management of osteoporosis. Four species of calcitonin – salmon, human, eel and an analogue of eel calcitonin – are currently available for therapeutic administration. The hormone may be administered by intramuscular and subcutaneous injection or, less often, by intravenous injection; a relatively new route of administration is a nasal spray formulation.

As it concerns the use of calcitonin in the prevention and treatment of involutional osteoporosis, in an early study a significant increase in total body calcium, measured by neutron activation analysis, was reported in 24 postmenopausal osteoporotic women treated with 100 IU salmon calcitonin for 18 months, whereas a progressive bone loss was shown in the control group.[38] Similar positive effects of salmon calcitonin were demonstrated either at the distal radius or at the spine and femoral neck:[39,40] in the latter study, after one year of treatment, the increase in lumbar spine BMD was 8.5% in elderly osteoporotic women receiving 100 IU/day and 4% in patients receiving 100 IU every second day. Using quantitative computed tomography (QCT) to measure spinal BMD, a 2-year randomized study confirmed these data:[41] synthetic human calcitonin, administered in doses of 0.1 mg (20 IU) three times weekly, reduced vertebral bone loss in patients with established postmenopausal osteoporosis. Calcitonin treatment was demonstrated to be especially effective in osteoporotic patients with a high bone turnover: a net gain of BMD in the axial skeleton (7%) and a slowing of bone loss in the appendicular bones were reported.[42] Surgical menopause may also lead to the development of osteoporosis: salmon calcitonin 50–100 IU (given intramuscularly every other day) has been found to prevent rapid bone loss in these patients.[43]

Safety is an outstanding feature of calcitonin. Transient facial flushing and nausea, rare vomiting and diarrhoea, and mild inflammation or itching at the injection site represent the main adverse effects; very rarely they necessitate drug discontinuation.[44] To increase patient acceptability and decrease side effects, the nasal preparation of calcitonin was developed. In the first report, nasal salmon calcitonin 50 IU/day for 5 days a week plus calcium 500 mg/day were followed by an increase (1.38%) in lumbar BMD in early postmenopausal women, whereas in the control group (500 mg/day) BMD decreased significantly (−3.16%).[45] This preventive effect of nasal salmon calcitonin was subsequently confirmed with higher doses (100 IU/day, 200 IU every other day), in the case of trabecular bone;[67,68] the positive changes in lumbar BMD were associated with a progressive and significant reduction of parameters of bone turnover.[46] Conflicting results have been published regarding the optimal dosage for preventing postmenopausal bone loss. A daily dose of 200 IU nasal salmon calcitonin was demonstrated to prevent bone loss, whereas intermittent administration of 200 IU three times a week was unsuccessful.[47] Likewise, a lower dose of 100 IU/day, with no calcium supplementation, significantly reduced trabecular bone loss.[48] Recently, in a double-blind, placebo-controlled, dose-finding trial, salmon calcitonin 50 IU/day, administered nasally and intermittently, appears to prevent lumbar bone loss in early postmenopausal women.[49] In the authors' opinion the effectiveness of different dosages is strictly related to bone turnover: nasal 200 IU every other day may be adequate to stop the fast bone loss in women with high bone turnover rates. On the other hand, in established involutional osteoporosis, the recommended dose of nasal salmon calcitonin may be considered to be 200 IU/day. The treatment should be administered discontinuously.[50] In any case the increase of BMD is typically transient: after 18–24 months of treatment a stabilization of bone mass is generally found.[38,40] This potential decrease in therapeutic effectiveness with prolonged treatment presumably results from the development of neutralizing antibodies, down-regulation at receptor sites or a counter-regulatory mechanism.[38,51]

The antifracture activity of calcitonin was demonstrated in an epidemiological survey: the protective effect on hip fracture increased significantly with increase in duration of exposure, and calcitonin was equally effective in older and younger women.[52] In a 2-year retrospective study, a significant reduction in new vertebral fracture rates (−60%) was reported in osteoporotic women given intramuscular salmon calcitonin 100 IU for 10 days/month compared with the incidence observed in a control group (35%).[53] A similar effect was also observed in a 2-year prospective study carried out in elderly women with low forearm BMD: nasal salmon calcitonin reduced the rates of fractures by 66% compared with calcium alone.[46] Regarding a new route of administration, an interesting preventive approach against trabecular postmenopausal bone loss was reported using rectal calcitonin;[54] however, suppositories for long-term treatment appear unlikely to be acceptable.

The analgesic action of calcitonin has been extensively described. A significant decrease in bone pain was observed by the treatment group (nasal salmon calcitonin 200 IU/day) after only 7 days, and the pain intensity continued to decrease over the 30-day period.[55] First, this effect was associated with an improvement of bone lesions; however, many studies suggested that this property could be unrelated to the effect on bone. Several hypotheses have been proposed, concerning the local synthesis of a humoral factor that generates pain, a direct effect on the central mechanism regulating pain and the involvement of an endogenous opioid system. In conclusion, calcitonin appears to be an antiresorbing agent that is effective in preventing bone loss and reducing pathological fractures; its use is recommended by the US Food and Drug Administration for treating postmenopausal osteoporotic patients.

ANABOLIC STEROIDS

Early studies carried out in osteoporotic patients showed a markedly positive skeletal balance induced by testosterone treatment. However, the masculinizing effect of androgens in women made these agents unacceptable as a treatment for postmenopausal osteoporosis. Anabolic steroids have been developed from androgens to decrease the virilizing effect and retain the anabolic action. In the past few years, they have received attention as therapeutic agents for osteoporosis. Effects of anabolic steroids on bone result from a combined direct action on osteoblast bone formation associated with indirect effects mediated by mechanical forces caused by muscle strength improvement.[56]

Nandrolone (19-nortestosterone) is an anabolic steroid that avoids the metabolic complications of orally administered compounds, because it is given by injection and so does not pass through the liver during its assimilation.[56] In two studies carried out in postmenopausal women, nandrolone was administered at the dosage of 50 mg every 2–3 weeks and compared with antiresorptive agents (calcium, calcitriol 0.25 μg and ethinyloestradiol): in the first study nandrolone produced a significant gain in forearm BMD;[57] in the second, after a treatment period of 14 months a mean increase of 20% in spinal BMD in the nandrolone group was reported, whereas no significant changes were observed with other agents.[58] A significant rise in intestinal radioactive calcium absorption after nandrolone administration was also demonstrated.[59]

A histomorphometric study carried out in osteoporotic women treated with nandrolone 50 mg i.m. every 3 weeks for one year showed a significant increase in trabecular bone volume and active osteoid surface area.[60] Virilization effects, hoarsening and sodium retention are considered to be the main adverse effects of nandrolone;[56] they are in any case dose related and reversible. As 17α-alkylated preparations, these agents can be expected to produce liver function test abnormalities and changes in lipid high-density lipoprotein levels.

Using stanozolol, combined with a daily 1000 mg calcium intake, a substantial improvement in total bone mass (TBC-NAA) in 21 postmenopausal osteoporotic women over 29 months was reported.[61] In 23 osteoporotic women, stanozolol 5 mg/day for one year promoted, together with a decrease in the urinary calcium excretion, an increase in bone turnover and the bone formation rate; however, no significant changes in bone volume or wall thickness were observed after treatment.[62]

NEW AGENTS

Parathyroid hormone

Parathyroid hormone (PTH) is a single chain polypeptide of 84 amino acids. The hormone stimulates release of calcium and phosphate from bone, stimulates reabsorption of calcium and inhibits reabsorption of phosphate from the glomerular filtrate, and stimulates the renal synthesis of $1,25(OH)_2D$. Several studies over the past three decades have established that intermittent injections of PTH can increase trabecular bone mass in rats, dogs and sheep.[63,64] Recent studies have also demonstrated that PTH increases appendicular cortical bone mass as well as total body calcium in rats.[65] The anabolic effect of intermittent PTH administration has been achieved mainly through stimulation of osteoblast number, with a resultant marked increase in total tissue bone formation rates at trabecular, periosteal and endosteal bone surfaces; no changes in osteoclast number and bone resorption rates were reported.[66] The pat-

tern of response was found to depend on both the dose of PTH and the duration of therapy.[67]

The effects in humans of hPTH (human PTH) administration resulted in an increase in cancellous bone, with a considerable apparent variability of response regarding cortical bone mass. In early studies in patients with involutional osteoporosis, 1–34 hPTH was given alone as a daily injection (100 μg s.c.) over a period of 6–24 months, with nutritional calcium supplements when necessary and a normal intake of vitamin D;[68] the hormone promoted increased trabecular bone resorption and formation rate, together with increased cancellous bone volume, with no changes in intestinal calcium absorption, plasma calcitriol levels and cortical bone density. Histomorphometric studies carried out in the early phase of hPTH treatment indicate that the previous resorption is not essential for the anabolic response to PTH.[66] The co-administration of 1–34 hPTH 400 IU/day and calcitriol 0.25 μg twice a day to osteoporotic women in two different regimens, concomitantly every day or on alternate days (6 weeks of PTH followed by 6 weeks of calcitriol), promoted significant increases in spinal bone mass, 12% and 32% after 1 and 2 years, respectively;[69] however, after 2 years of hPTH administration, forearm BMD decreased significantly (−5.2%) in comparison to controls (−1.5%). In an open study 1–34 hPTH (500 IU daily subcutaneous injections for one year) was administered to 12 osteoporotic patients in combination with antiresorptive agents (oestrogen or nandrolone), and the results were compared with those from a group treated with sodium fluoride.[70] The patients receiving the peptide showed a substantial increase in vertebral spongiosa, with no significant changes in spinal cortical or radial BMD; a relative similar increase in cancellous and cortical bone was achieved over the same period in the fluoride group. Subsequently, in a following paper it was demonstrated that the response in iliac trabecular bone was largely preserved and was very similar, in relative terms, to the response in vertebral body cancellous bone;[71] through lack of a long-term increment in whole-body bone resorption, these authors underlined the uncertainty of whether 1–34 hPTH provided sufficient additional benefit when added to long-term HRT. However, in 11 patients (five active, six control), it was observed that bone mass increments induced by treatment with 1–34 hPTH 25 µg/day for 3 years can be maintained by oestrogens.[72] In fact, new data are arising about analogues of PTH or PTHrp (PTH-related peptide) and very recently a novel PTH receptor, the PTH2 receptor, has been described.[73,74]

Anti-oestrogens

Tamoxifen is the most commonly prescribed synthetic anti-oestrogen for the treatment of patients with breast cancer. Studies in vitro and in animals have shown that tamoxifen is characterized by an oestrogen agonist effect on skeleton and it produces antiresorptive effects in bone.[75] In postmenopausal women with breast cancer, it was demonstrated that tamoxifen preserved spinal bone mass;[76] however, this effect was not confirmed universally.[77] More recently, in a randomized, double-blind, placebo-controlled trial, tamoxifen was administered at the dosage of 20 mg/day for 2 years;[78] in the women given tamoxifen, the mean BMD of the lumbar spine increased significantly in comparison to the women given placebo. Total body BMD declined in both groups, but less so in the tamoxifen-treated patients, whereas no differences were observed in the proximal femur BMD. Regarding bone turnover, tamoxifen promoted a significant decrease of markers of bone resorption and bone formation; this effect was also observed in women over 70 years of age.[79] Adverse effects are mainly represented by vaginal discharge and vasomotor flushes. These results suggest that tamoxifen produces a transient remodelling effect, suppressing bone turnover to allow filling in the remodelling space, and may exert a small protective effect on bone mass in postmenopausal osteoporosis.

Raloxifen is a selective oestrogen receptor modulator with mixed oestrogen agonist–antagonist properties; animal models show raloxifen to have an effect, indistinguishable from that of oestrogen, of inhibiting bone resorption as a result of oestrogen deficiency. Recent reports underline that raloxifen mimics oestrogen in human bone remodelling kinetics, and it appears to inhibit bone resorption together with a decrease in total and low-density lipoprotein cholesterol in postmenopausal women.[80]

Growth hormone and insulin-like growth factors

Growth hormone (GH) promotes both direct and indirect actions on bone. On the one hand, GH improves both muscle mass and strength, and may lead to increased physical activity, with the resultant beneficial effects on bone mass; on the other, the hormone also potentiates the gonadal secretion of the sex steroids.[81] The presence of reduced BMD in patients with adult-onset GH deficiency,[82] and the evidence for skeletal growth factor deficiency in elderly people,[83] raised the possibility that human GH (hGH) may have a role in the treatment of involutional osteoporosis. Indeed, patients with osteoporosis have a lower peak GH response to insulin-induced hypoglycaemia compared with patients with osteoarthritis.[84] Densitometric studies failed to demonstrate any appreciable improvements in osteoporotic women, despite increases in total body calcium. In normal human volunteers, it was demonstrated that a short course of recombinant hGH (0.1 µg/kg twice daily for 7 days) stimulates osteoblastic cell lineage and activates bone remodelling.[85] Sustained elevations of bone turnover markers were also observed during the 12 months of a randomized placebo-controlled intervention trial of hGH in healthy elderly women; however, no significant changes were observed in BMD at either the lumbar spine or proximal femur.[86] In a treatment regimen employing cyclic administration of GH and calcitonin as an inhibitor of bone resorption, bone mass assessed by neutron activated analysis increased whereas BMD measured by dual photon absorptiometry did not change.[87] In postmenopausal women with osteopenia, short-term GH therapy in ADFR (activate–depress–free–repeat) treatment promoted a stimulation in bone formation and bone resorption.[88] Concerning body composition, GH treatment increases lean tissue mass and decreases fat mass; however, functional ability is not enhanced, even though muscular mass is increased.[89]

The most common side effect of GH therapy is fluid retention; data on long-term adverse side effects of hGH therapy are not yet available. Additional studies are needed to assess the therapeutic potential of hGH in attenuating or reversing bone loss in elderly people.

Insulin-like growth factors (IGFs) present in the skeletal matrix may be derived from the systemic circulation as synthesized by a variety of cells present in bone.[90] These factors are known to be potentially important local regulators of bone cell activity. IGF-I levels have generally been found to be decreased in patients with osteoporosis.[91] The presence of IGF-I receptors on isolated osteoblasts supports a role for IGF-I in enhancing preosteoblastic cell differentiation and increasing matrix of apposition rate.[92] In a man with idiopathic osteoporosis and low serum IGF-I, giving IGF-I at a dosage of 160 µg/kg per day for 7 days promoted an increase in biochemical bone markers.[93] Significant increases in bone turnover markers have been confirmed after short-term IGF-I administration, also in healthy young volunteers:[94] in combination with GH,

IGF-I administration (60 µg/kg twice daily) for 28 days promoted an activation of remodelling osteons in elderly women.[95] No data concerning BMD changes are available. At present, the role of IGF-I therapy in osteoporosis remains to be established.

Diuretic agents

Thiazide diuretic agents are known to lower the urinary excretion of calcium and improve calcium balance. Early data demonstrated that thiazide users had significantly more BMD at radius, ulna and os calcis than non-users.[96] A subsequent prospective study reported that, in older men and women, the use of thiazide was associated with a reduction of about one-third in the risk of hip fracture.[97] In a non-sectional study (9704 ambulatory women who were 65 years or older), thiazide users for more than 10 years had significantly higher bone mass than women who had never used thiazide diuretics; however, the incidence of falls and the risk for non-spinal and osteoporotic fractures were similar in both groups. Only a trend towards a lower risk for hip and wrist fractures was observed in thiazide users.[98] More recently, in a double-masked prospective study carried out in 113 postmenopausal women, chlorthalidone used at a dosage of 12.5–25 mg daily was associated with bone gain at the calcaneus and the distal radius, with significantly reduced bone loss at the proximal radius.[99]

REFERENCES

1. NIH Consensus Conference. Optimal calcium intake. *JAMA* 1994; **272:** 1942–8.
2. Holbrook TL, Barret-Connor E, Wingard DL. Dietary calcium and risk of hip fracture. 14-year prospective population study. *Lancet* 1988; **ii:** 1046–9.
3. Dawson-Hughes B, Dallal GE, Krall EA et al. A controlled trial of the effect of calcium supplementation on bone density in postmenopausal women. *N Engl J Med* 1990; **323:** 878–83.
4. Holbrook TL, Barret-Connor E. An 18-year prospective study of dietary calcium and bone mineral density in the hip. *Calcif Tissue Int* 1995; **56:** 364–7.
5. Reid IR, Ames RW, Evans MC et al. Effect of calcium supplementation on bone loss in postmenopausal women. *N Engl J Med* 1993; **328:** 460–4.
6. Reid IR, Ames RW, Evans MC et al. Long-term effects of calcium supplementation on bone loss and fractures in postmenopausal women: a randomized controlled trial. *Am J Med* 1995; **98:** 331–5.
7. Aloia JF, Vaswani A, Yeh JK, Russo L.

Differential effects of dietary calcium augmentation and hormone replacement therapy on bone turnover and serum levels of calciotrophic hormones. *Osteoporosis Int* 1996; **6:** 55–62.

8. Schwartz E, Chokas WV, Panariello VA. Metabolic balance studies of high calcium intake in osteoporosis. *Am J Med* 1964; **36:** 233–49.

9. Stamp T, Katakity M, Golstein AJ et al. Metabolic balance study of mineral supplementation in osteoporosis. *Clin Sci* 1991; **81:** 799–802.

10. Riggs BL, Jowsey J, Goldsmith RS et al. Short- and long-term effect of estrogen and synthetic anabolic hormone in postmenopausal osteoporosis. *J Clin Invest* 1972; **51:** 1659–63.

11. Orwoll ES, McClung MR, Oviatt SK et al. Histomorphometric effects of calcium or calcium plus 25-hydroxyvitamin D_3 therapy in osteoporosis. *J Bone Miner Res* 1989; **4:** 81–8.

12. Riggs BL, Hodgson SF, O'Fallon WM et al. Effect of fluoride treatment on the fracture rate in postmenopausal women with osteoporosis. *N Engl J Med* 1990; **322:** 802–9.

13. Riis B, Thomsen K, Christiansen C. Does calcium supplementation prevent postmenopausal bone loss? *N Engl J Med* 1987; **316:** 173–7.

14. Reid IR, Ames RW, Evans MC et al. Effect of calcium supplementation on bone loss in postmenopausal women. *N Engl J Med* 1993; **328:** 460–4.

15. Tilyard MW, Spears GF, Thomson J et al. Treatment of postmenopausal osteoporosis with calcitriol or calcium. *N Engl J Med* 1992; **326:** 357–62.

16. Fraser DR. Vitamin D. *Lancet* 1995; **345:** 104–7.

17. Freaney R, McBrinn Y, McKenna MJ. Secondary hyperparathyroidism in elderly people: combined effect of renal insufficiency and vitamin D deficiency. *Am J Clin Nutr* 1993; **58:** 187–91.

18. Chapuy MC, Arlot ME, Duboeuf F et al. Vitamin D_3 in calcium to prevent hip fractures in elderly women. *N Engl J Med* 1992; **327:** 1637–42.

19. Lips P, Graafmans WC, Ooms ME, Bezemer D, Bouter L. Vitamin D supplementation and fracture incidence in elderly persons. *Ann Intern Med* 1996; **124:** 400–6.

20. Riggs BL, Melton LJ III. Evidence for two distinct syndromes involutional osteoporosis. *Am J Med* 1983; **27:** 861–82.

21. Caniggia A, Gennari C, Bianchi V et al. Intestinal absorption of ^{45}Ca in senile osteoporosis. *Acta Med Scand* 1963; **173:** 613–17.

22. Lorè F, Nuti R, Vattimo A et al. Vitamin D metabolites in postmenopausal osteoporosis. *Horm Metab Res* 1984; **16:** 56–7.

23. Morrison NA, Qi JC, Tokita A et al. Prediction of bone density from vitamin D receptor alleles. *Nature* 1994; **367:** 284–7.

24. Gallagher JC. Treatment of osteoporosis with vitamin D, vitamin D metabolites or vitamin D analogues. In: *Proceedings of Fourth International Symposium on Osteoporosis* (Christiansen C, Riis B, eds). Aalborg, Denmark: Handelstrykkeriet Aalborg ApS, 1993: 538–40.

25. Caniggia A, Nuti R, Lorè F et al. Long-term treatment with calcitriol in postmenopausal osteoporosis. *Metabolism* 1990; **39**(suppl 1): 43–9.

26. Aloia JF, Vaswani A, Yeh JK et al. Calcitriol in the treatment of postmenopausal osteoporosis. *Am J Med* 1988; **84:** 401–8.

27. Gallagher JC, Goldgar D. Treatment of postmenopausal osteoporosis with high doses of synthetic calcitriol. *Ann Intern Med* 1990; **113:** 649–55.

28. Falch JA, Odegaard OR, Finnanger AM et al. Postmenopausal osteoporosis: no effect of three years treatment with 1,25-dihydroxycholecalciferol. *Acta Med Scand* 1987; **221:** 199–204.

29. Ott SM, Chesnut CH. Calcitriol treatment is not effective in postmenopausal osteoporosis. *Ann Intern Med* 1989; **110:** 267–74.

30. Ott SM, Chesnut CH. Tolerance dose of calcitriol is associated with improved bone density in women with postmenopausal osteoporosis. *J Bone Miner Res* 1990; **5**(suppl 1): 186.

31. Geusens P, Vanderschueren D, Verstraeten A, Dequeker J, Devos P, Bouillon R. Short term course of $1,25(OH)_2D_3$ stimulates osteoblasts but not osteoclasts in osteoporosis and osteoarthritis. *Calcif Tissue Int* 1991; **49:** 168–73.

32. Orimo H, Shiraki M, Hayashi Y et al. Effects of 1α-hydroxyvitamin D_3 on lumbar bone mineral density and vertebral fractures in patients with postmenopausal osteoporosis. *Calcif Tissue Int* 1994; **54:** 370–6.

33. Gallagher JC. Prevention of bone loss in postmenopausal and senile osteoporosis with vitamin D_3 analogues. *Osteoporosis Int* 1993; suppl 1: S172–5.

34. Azria M, Copp DH, Zanelli JM. 25 years of salmon calcitonin: from synthesis to therapeutic use. *Calcif Tissue Int* 1995; **57:** 405–8.

35. Nicholson GC, Moseley JM, Sexton PM et al. Abundant calcitonin receptors in isolated rate osteoclasts. Biochemical and autoradiographic characterization. *J Clin Invest* 1986; **78:** 355–70.

36. Stevenson JC, Whitehead MI. Postmenopausal osteoporosis. *BMJ* 1982; **285:** 585.

37. Prince RL, Dick IM, Price RI. Plasma calcitonin levels are not lower than normal in osteoporotic women. *J Clin Endocrinol Metab* 1989; **68:** 684–7.

38. Gruber HE, Ivey JL, Baylink DJ et al. Long-term calcitonin therapy in postmenopausal osteoporosis. *Metabolism* 1984; **33:** 295–303.

39. Mazzuoli GF, Passeri M, Gennari C et al. Effects of salmon calcitonin in osteoporosis: a controlled double-blind study. *Calcif Tissue Int* 1986; **38:** 3–8.

40. Gennari C, Chierichetti SM, Bigazzi S et al. Comparative effects on bone mineral content of calcium and calcium plus salmon calcitonin given in two different regimen in postmenopausal osteoporosis. *Curr Therap Res* 1985; **38:** 455–64.

41. McIntyre I, Whitehead MI, Banks LM et al. Calcitonin for prevention of postmenopausal osteoporosis. *Lancet* 1988; **i:** 900–2.

42. Civitelli R, Gonnelli S, Zacchei F et al. Bone turnover in postmenopausal osteoporosis: effects of calcitonin treatment. *J Clin Invest* 1988; **82:** 1268–74.

43. Mazzuoli GF, Tabolli S, Bigi F et al. Effects of salmon calcitonin on the bone loss induced by ovariectomy. *Calcif Tissue Int* 1990; **47:** 209–14.

44. Wimalawansa SJ. Long- and short-term side effects and safety of calcitonin in man: a prospective study. *Calcif Tissue Int* 1993; **52:** 90–3.

45. Reginster JY, Albert A, Lecart MP et al. 1-year controlled randomized trial of prevention of early postmenopausal bone loss by intransal calcitonin. *Lancet* 1987; **ii:** 1481–3.

46. Gennari C, Agnusdei D, Camporeale A. Effect of salmon calcitonin nasal spray on bone mass in patients with high turnover osteoporosis. *Osteoporosis Int* 1993; suppl 1: 208–10.

47. Stevenson JC, Lees B, Ellerington MC et al. Postmenopausal osteoporosis: a double-blind placebo-controlled study. *J Bone Miner Res* 1992; **7**(suppl 1): 325.

48. Meunier PJ, Gozzo I, Chaumet R et al. Dose–effect on bone density and parathyroid function of intranasal salmon calcitonin when administered without calcium in postmenopausal women. *J Bone Miner Res* 1992; **7**(suppl 1): 325.

49. Reginster JY, Deroisy R, Lecart MP et al. A double-blind, placebo-controlled, dose-finding trial of intermittent nasal salmon calcitonin for prevention of postmenopausal osteoporosis. *Am J Med* 1995; **98:** 452–8.

50. Overgard K. Effect of intranasal salmon calcitonin therapy on bone mass and bone turnover in early postmenopausal women: a dose–response study. *Calcif Tissue Int* 1994; **55:** 82–6.

51. Muff R, Dambacher MA, Fisher JA. Formation of neutralizing antibodies during intranasal synthetic salmon calcitonin treatment of postmenopausal osteoporosis. *Osteoporosis Int* 1991; **1:** 72–5.

52. Kanis JA, Johnell O, Gullberg B et al. Evidence for efficacy of drugs affecting bone metabolism in preventing hip fracture. *BMJ* 1992; **305:** 1124–8.

53. Rico H, Hernandez ER, Revilla M et al. Salmon calcitonin reduces vertebral fracture rate in postmenopausal crush fracture syndrome. *Bone Miner* 1992; **16:** 131–8.

54. Reginster JY, Jupsin I, Deroisy R et al. Prevention of postmenopausal bone loss by rectal calcitonin. *Calcif Tissue Int* 1995; **56:** 539–42.

55. Gennari C, Agnusdei D, Camporeale A. Use of calcitonin in the treatment of bone pain associated with osteoporosis. *Calcif Tissue Int* 1991; **49**(suppl 1): 9–13.

56. Dequeker J, Geusens P. Anabolic steroids, muscle function and bone. In: *Update on Osteoporosis, 69–76* (Duursma SA, Raymakers JA, Scheven BAA, eds). Utrecht: Stichting Education Permanente, 1990.

57. Need AG, Horowitz M, Walker CJ et al. Crossover study of fat-corrected forearm mineral content during nandrolone decanoate therapy for osteoporosis. *Bone* 1989; **10:** 3–6.

58. Need AG, Horowitz M, Bridges A et al. Effects of nandrolone decanoate and antiresorptive therapy on vertebral density in osteoporotic postmenopausal women. *Arch Intern Med* 1989; **149:** 57–60.

59. Gennari C, Agnusdei D, Gonnelli S et al. Effects of nandrolone decanoate therapy on bone mass and calcium metabolism in women with established osteoporosis: a double-blind placebo-controlled study. *Maturitas* 1989; **11:** 187–9.

60. Need AG, Durbridge TC, Nordin BEC. Clinical experience with nandrolone decanoate therapy in established osteoporosis. In: *Proceedings of Fourth International Symposium on Osteoporosis* (Christiansen C, Riis B, eds). Aalborg, Denmark: Handelstrykkeriet Aalborg Aps, 1993: 311–14.

61. Chesnut CH, Ivey JL, Gruber HE et al. Stanozolol in postmenopausal osteoporosis: therapeutic efficacy and possible mechanism of action. *Metabolism* 1983; **32:** 571–80.

62. Beneton MNC, Yates AJP, Rogers S et al. Stanozolol stimulate remodelling of trabecular

bone and net formation of bone and endocortical surface. *Clin Sci* 1991; **81**: 543–9.

63. Dempster DW, Cosman F, Parisien M et al. Anabolic actions of parathyroid hormone on bone. *Endocrinol Rev* 1993; **14**: 690–709.

64. Podbesek R, Edouard C, Meunier PJ et al. Effects of two treatment regimes with synthetic human parathyroid hormone fragment on bone formation and the tissue balance of trabecular bone in greyhounds. *Endocrinology* 1983; **112**: 1000–6.

65. Ejersted C, Andreassen TT, Nilsson MH et al. Human parathyroid hormone (1–34) increases bone formation and strength of cortical bone in aged rats. *Eur J Endocrinol* 1994; **130**: 201–7.

66. Hock JM, Gera I. Effects of continuous and intermittent administration and inhibition of resorption on the anabolic response of bone to parathyroid hormone. *J Bone Miner Res* 1992; **7**: 65–72.

67. Mitlak BH, Burdette-Miller P, Shozneeld D et al. Segmential effects of chronic human PTH (1–134) frammint of estrogen-deficiency osteopenia in the rats. *J Bone Miner Res* 1996; **11**: 430–9.

68. Reeve J, Meunier PJ, Parsons JA et al. The anabolic effect of human parathyroid hormone fragment (hPTH) 1–34 therapy on trabecular bone in involutional osteoporosis: report of a multicentre trial. *BMJ* 1980; 1340–4.

69. Neer R, Slovik D, Daly M et al. Treatment of postmenopausal osteoporosis with daily parathyroid hormone plus calcitriol. In: *Osteoporosis* (Christiansen C, Overgaard K, eds). Copenhagen: Osteopress, 1990: 1314–17.

70. Reeve J, Davies UM, Hesp R et al. Treatment of osteoporosis with human parathyroid peptide and observations on effect of sodium fluoride. *BMJ* 1990; **301**: 314–18.

71. Reeve J, Bradbeer N, Arlot M et al. hPTH 1–34 treatment of osteoporosis with added hormone replacement therapy: biochemical, kinetic and histological response. *Osteoporosis Int* 1991; **1**: 162–70.

72. Lindsay R, Cosman F, Shen V et al. Bone mass increments induced by PTH treatment can be maintained by estrogen. *J Bone Miner Res* 1995; **10**(suppl 1): S200.

73. Weir EC, Terwilliger G, Sartori L et al. Synthetic parathyroid hormone-like protein (1–74) is anabolic for bone in vivo. *Calcif Tissue Int* 1992; **51**: 30–4.

74. Usdin TB, Gruber C, Bonner TJ. Identification and functional expression of a receptor selectively recognizing parathyroid hormone, the PTH2 receptor. *J Biol Chem* 1995; **270**: 15455–8.

75. Turner RT, Wakley GK, Hannon KS et al. Tamoxifen inhibits osteoclast-mediated resorption of trabecular bone in ovarian hormone-deficient rats. *Endocrinology* 1988; **122**: 1146–50.

76. Ryan WG, Wolter J, Bagdade JD. Apparent beneficial effect of tamoxifen on bone mineral contents in patients with breast cancer: a preliminary study. *Osteoporosis Int* 1991; **2**: 39–41.

77. Neal AJ, Evans K, Hoskin PJ. Does long-term administration of tamoxifen affect bone mineral density? *Eur J Cancer* 1993; **29A**: 1971–3.

78. Grey AB, Stapleton JB, Evans MC et al. The effect of the antiestrogen tamoxifen on bone mineral density in normal late postmenopausal women. *Am J Med* 1995; **99**: 636–41.

79. Kenny AM, Prestwood KM, Pilbeam CC et al. The short-term effects of tamoxifen on bone turnover in older women. *J Clin Endocrinol Metab* 1995; **80**: 3287–91.

80. Draper MW, David EF, Huster WJ et al. A controlled trial of raloxifene (LY139481) HC1: impact on bone turnover and serum lipid profile in healthy postmenopausal women. *J Bone Miner Res* 1996; **11**: 835–42.

81. Inzucchi SE, Robbins RJ. Clinical Review 61. Effects of growth hormone on human bone biology. *J Clin Endocrinol Metab* 1994; **79**: 691–4.

82. Holmes SJ, Economou G, Whitehouse RW et al. Reduced bone mineral density in patients with adult onset growth hormone deficiency. *J Clin Endocrinol Metab* 1994; **78**: 669–74.

83. Boonen S, Aerssens J, Broos P et al. Age-related bone loss and senile osteoporosis: evidence for both secondary hyperparathyroidism and skeletal growth factor deficiency in the elderly. *Aging Clin Exp Res* 1996; **7**: 414–22.

84. Dequeker J, Burssens A, Bouillon R. Dynamics of growth hormone secretion in patients with osteoporosis and in patients with osteoarthrosis. *Horm Res* 1982; **16**: 353–6.

85. Brixen K, Nielsen HK, Mosekilde L et al. A short course of recombinant human growth hormone treatment stimulates osteoblasts and acitvates bone remodeling in normal human volunteers. *J Bone Miner Res* 1990; **5**: 609–18.

86. Marcus R, Holloway L, Butterfield G. Clinical use of growth hormone in older people. *J Reprod Fert* 1993; **46**: 115–18.

87. Aloia JF, Vaswani A, Meunier PJ et al. Coherence treatment of postmenopausal osteoporosis with growth hormone and calcitonin. *Calcif Tissue Int* 1987; **40**: 253–9.

88. Brixen K, Kassem M, Nielsen HK et al. Short term treatment with growth hormone stimulates osteoblastic and osteoclastic activity in osteopenic postmenopausal women: a dose response study. *J Bone Miner Res* 1995; **10:** 1865–74.

89. Papadakis MA, Grady D, Black D et al. Growth hormone replacement in healthy older men improves body composition but not functional ability. *Ann Intern Med* 1996; **124:** 708–16.

90. Canalis E. Growth factors and their potential clinical value. *J Clin Endocrinol Metab* 1992; **75:** 1–4.

91. Wuster C, Blum W, Schlemilch S et al. Decreased insulin-like growth factors and IGF binding protein in osteoporosis. *J Intern Med* 1993; **234:** 249–55.

92. Canalis E. Skeletal growth factors and aging. *J Clin Endocrinol Metab* 1994; **78:** 1009–10.

93. Johansson AG, Lindh E, Ljunghall S. Insulin-like growth factor stimulates bone turnover in osteoporosis. *Lancet* 1992; **339:** 1619.

94. Mauras N, Doi SQ, Shapiro JR. Recombinant human insulin-like growth factor I, recombinant human growth hormone, and sex steroids: effects on markers of bone turnover in humans. *J Clin Endocrinol Metab* 1996; **81:** 2222–6.

95. Ghiron LJ, Thompson JL, Holloway L et al. Effects of recombinant insulin-like growth factor I and growth hormone on bone turnover in elderly women. *J Bone Miner Res* 1995; **10:** 1844–52.

96. Wasnich RD, Benfante RJ, Yano K et al. Thiazide effect on the mineral content of bone. *N Engl J Med* 1983; **309:** 344–7.

97. LaCroix AZ, Wienpahl J, White LR et al. Thiazide diuretics agents and the incidence of hip fracture. *N Engl J Med* 1990; **322:** 286–90.

98. Cauley JA, Cummings SR, Seeley DG et al. Effects of thiazide diuretic therapy on bone mass, fractures and falls. *Ann Intern Med* 1993; **118:** 666–73.

99. Wasnich RD, Davis JW, He YF et al. A randomized, double-masked, placebo-controlled trial of chlortalidone and bone loss in elderly women. *Osteoporosis Int* 1995; **5:** 247–51.

11

Non-pharmacologic prevention of osteoporosis: nutrition and exercise

RP Heaney

Osteoporosis is recognized to be a multifactorial disorder. In this sense it is similar to most of the chronic disorders that increase in prevalence with age. Fractures represent structural failure of the skeleton and, in individuals past middle life, most skeletal fractures occur as a result of low-energy trauma (i.e. falls from standing height or less). The incidence of fractures increases with age for many reasons: the bony structure becomes intrinsically more fragile; falls occur more frequently; protective postural reflexes slow with age; and there is decreased soft tissue protection over bony prominences, especially in fragile elderly people. Each of these factors has its own set of causes. Intrinsic bone strength may be reduced not solely for the obvious reason that bone mass may be low, but because of severed cross-bracing trabecular connections, and because of an increased burden of unrepaired fatigue damage. Finally, bone mass may be reduced because of hormonal deficiency, a sedentary lifestyle or immobilization, or nutritional deficiency.

This galaxy of causal factors is arranged in a hierarchy in Figure 11.1. The pharmacologic and nutritional measures currently available for prevention and treatment focus mainly on preservation or restoration of bone mass. Figure 11.1 helps us to see that, however effective these modalities may be, on their own they will never be a sufficient solution to osteoporosis,

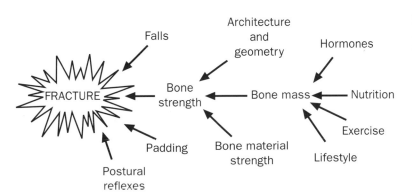

Figure 11.1 Hierarchical arrangement of factors contributing to osteoporotic fracture. (© Robert P Heaney, 1995. Reproduced with permission.)

simply because they have bearing on only one part of the fracture problem. A comprehensive approach to prevention or treatment will ultimately need to be as multifaceted as the condition itself is multifactorial.

In this chapter the focus is primarily on nutrition and exercise, and more specifically on how they protect bone mass. It must be noted, however, that both play extraskeletal protective roles as well: in the maintenance of total body health; in the preservation of muscle strength and coordination; in protection against falls; and in the provision of adequate soft tissue mass (which incidentally serves as padding over bony prominences).

NUTRITION: CALCIUM

The primitive function of the skeleton is to serve as a source and a sink for calcium and phosphorus, i.e. as a reserve to offset shortages and as a place for safely storing surpluses. This reserve feature of skeletal function is expressed, for example, in laboratory animals such as cats, rats and dogs, which, when placed on low calcium intakes, will reduce bone mass as needed to maintain near constancy of calcium levels in the extracellular fluid.[1] This activity is mediated by parathyroid hormone (PTH)[2] and involves actual bone destruction, not leaching of calcium from bone.

In the course of evolution, bone in the higher vertebrates acquired a second role, namely internal stiffening and rigidity. This structural role has become, for contemporary humans, the most apparent feature of the skeleton. Calcium and phosphorus are the only nutrients with a reserve that possesses such a secondary function. Now reserves, by their very nature, are designed to tide the organism over external shortages. When intake is inadequate, the reserve is mobilized. With most nutrients this has no detectable impact on the health or functioning of the organism. Only after the reserve is exhausted and the metabolic pool begins to be depleted, does clinical disease express itself. For some nutrients (e.g. vitamin A), the reserve can be quite large, and the latent period may last many months. For others (e.g. the water-soluble vitamins), however, the reserve may be very small and detectable dysfunction develops quickly when intake drops.

With calcium, by contrast, the reserve is vast relative to the cellular and extracellular metabolic pools of calcium. As a result, dietary insufficiency virtually never impairs those cellular metabolic functions that depend upon calcium, at least in ways that are now recognized. However, as bone strength is a function of bone mass, it follows inexorably that any decrease whatsoever in the size of the calcium reserve – any decrease in bone mass – will produce a corresponding decrease in bone strength. We literally walk about on our calcium reserve. It is this unique feature of calcium nutrition that is the basis for the linkage of calcium intake and osteoporosis.

The primitive calcium intake

Calcium was abundant in the environment in which hominids evolved. Edible foliage, tubers, nuts and other plant foods available to herbivorous and omnivorous mammals have a relatively high calcium content. Omnivorous animals, in addition to the calcium from plants, had access to the calcium in bones of animal prey, calcium in the chitinous exoskeletons of insects, and calcium in insect larvae and grubs.

Analysis of the foods consumed on a year-round basis by chimpanzees, our closest primate relatives, indicates that their diets had a calcium nutrient density of 80–100 mg Ca/100 kcal (19–24 mg Ca/100 kJ).[3] The !Kung people of South Africa have been found to have diets almost as high in calcium (70–80 mg Ca/100 kcal (17–19 mg Ca/100 kJ)). Studies of other hunter–gatherer people indicate that their diets also have calcium nutrient densities in the range of those of the high primates. Scaling the energy expenditure of a hunter–gatherer or chimpanzee up to the body size of contemporary peoples in industrialized nations allows translation of these nutrient density figures to what would be, for us today, a total calcium intake in the range of 2100–3000 mg/day. This is entirely from plant sources. Riverine people, with bony fish in their diets, had even higher calcium intakes. By way of contrast with these pre-technological kinds of intakes, the diet calcium density of urbanized or industrialized nations is commonly under 25 mg/100 kcal (6 mg Ca/100 kJ).[4]

The reason for the difference between primitive and contemporary diets is found in the shift to cereal-based diets at the time of the agricultural revolution. Farming exploited natural hybrid forms of cereal grasses which required humans for their propagation (mainly because the excess starch of the seed kernels made them too heavy for efficient dispersal by the wind). Nevertheless, the extra starch of the hybrid cereals made it possible to feed a great many more people. The hunter–gatherer lifestyle makes very inefficient use of the land, and population pressures were probably a major reason for the shift to farming.

With this development calcium intake fell. Cereals typically have calcium densities under 10 mg/100 kcal (2.4 mg Ca/100 kJ). Nevertheless, it is likely that the actual calcium intake of the agriculturists was higher than this low nutrient density would suggest, because of the adventitious entry of calcium into the food supply in the process of flour milling. Grain was typically dehulled in limestone mortars, and the dehulled kernels then ground to flour in limestone querns.[5] Limestone is, of course, a calcium carbonate mineral; it is relatively soft and workable, and it probably added a great deal of calcium to the flour produced for bread-making. Hence, it is likely that only with the development of a more advanced technology, which allowed large-scale milling, and the construction of mill stones from harder minerals (silicon-based rather than calcium-based), that the calcium intake of technologically advanced urban peoples fell to the present levels.

The calcium requirement

As far as the bony reserves are concerned, calcium functions as a 'threshold' or 'plateau' nutrient. This means that, below some critical value, bone mass will be limited by available calcium supplies, whereas, above that value, i.e. the threshold or plateau, no further benefit will accrue from additional increases in intake. This biphasic relationship is illustrated in Figure 11.2, in which the intake – effect relationship is depicted first schematically, and then as exemplified by data derived from a growing animal model. The requirement for calcium can be defined as the intake at which the plateau is reached. In Figure 11.2b the effect of the nutrient is expressed directly as the amount of bone calcium that an animal is able to accumulate from any given intake. However, if 'effect' is broadened to mean 'any change whatsoever', then the diagram fits mature adults as well, and the best representation of the requirement at all ages is the intake value just at or above the effect threshold of Figure 11.2.

There has been much uncertainty and confusion in recent years about what that intake may be for various ages and physiological states. With the 1994 Consensus Development Conference on Optimal Calcium Intake,[7] the bulk of that confusion has been resolved. The evidence for the intakes recommended by the consensus panel is summarized both in the Conference report and in recent reviews of the relationship of nutrition and osteoporosis,[8] and only the highlights will be mentioned in the remainder of the section.

Briefly, the Consensus panel of the National Institutes of Health (NIH) recommended increases in calcium intake for almost all age groups: specifically, for adolescents, 1200–1500 mg/day; for adults up to age 65, 1000 mg/day; for postmenopausal women not receiving estrogen, 1500 mg/day; and for everyone above age 65, 1500 mg/day. The most persuasive of the evidence leading to these recommendations came in the form of several randomized controlled trials showing both reduction in age-related bone loss and reduction in fractures after augmentation of prevailing calcium intakes.[9–16] As a result of the bone remodeling transient induced by any change in calcium intake,[17] randomized controlled trials are not, by their nature, well suited to dose ranging. For this reason, these recommendations, although expressed in quantitative terms,

(a)

(b)

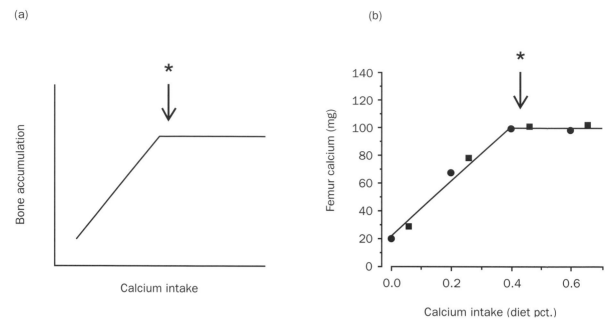

Figure 11.2 Threshold behavior of calcium intake: (a) theoretical relationship of bone accumulation to intake. Below a certain value – the threshold or plateau – bone accumulation is a linear function of intake (the ascending line); in other words, the amount of bone that can be accumulated is limited by the amount of calcium ingested. Above the threshold (the horizontal line), bone accumulation is limited by other factors, and is no longer related to changes in calcium intake. (b) Actual data from two experiments in growing rats, showing how bone accumulation does, in fact, exhibit a threshold pattern. *Minimum requirement. (Redrawn from data in Forbes et al.[6] with permission. © Robert P Heaney, 1992.)

are basically qualitative: contemporary calcium intakes by both men and women are too low for optimal bone health.

Factors that influence the requirement

There are several nutritional factors that influence or have been proposed to influence the calcium requirement. The principal interacting nutrients are sodium, protein, caffeine and fiber. Fiber and caffeine influence calcium absorption[18–21] and typically exert relatively minor effects, whereas sodium and protein influence urinary excretion of calcium,[20,22] and can be of much greater significance for the calcium economy. By contrast, the effects of dietary phosphorus and fat in humans are minor to non-existent.

The impact of protein and sodium intakes, in particular, can be profound. A nutritionally adequate diet low in protein and sodium may be incompatible with a calcium intake as low as 500 mg/day, whereas a diet high in sodium and protein may elevate the calcium requirement to as much as 2000 mg/day.

The acquisition of genetically programmed bone mass

The human skeleton contains, at birth, about 25–30 g calcium and, at maturity in women, 900–1200 g. All of this difference must come in by way of the diet. Further, unlike other structural nutrients such as protein, the amount of calcium retained is always substantially less than the amount ingested. This is both because absorption efficiency is relatively low even during growth and because calcium is lost daily through shed skin, nails, hair and sweat, as well as in urine and non-reabsorbed digestive secretions. Only about 4–8% of ingested calcium is actually retained. This inefficient retention is not so much because ability to build bone is limited, but because the primitive calcium intake to which our physiologies are adapted was high. An absorptive barrier is a protection against calcium surfeit, and inefficient retention reflects primitive environmental abundance.

When ingested calcium is less than optimal, the balance between formation and resorption, normally positive during growth, falls towards zero. This occurs because parathyroid hormone (PTH) augments bone resorption at the endosteal–trabecular surface in order to sustain the level of ionized calcium in the extracellular fluid. When the demands of mineralization at the periosteum and growth plates exceed the amount of calcium absorbed from the diet and released from growth-related bone modeling, more PTH is secreted, and resorption increases still further, until the balance becomes zero or even negative. Growth in bone size continues, however, and a limited quantity of mineral now has to be distributed over an ever larger volume. The animals receiving calcium intakes below the threshold in Figure 11.2b had bones of normal *size*; they simply contained less bony *material*.

Net bone accumulation will be greater as calcium intake increases above these inadequate levels, but only to the point where endosteal–trabecular resorption results solely from the genetic program governing growth, and is no longer being driven by bodily needs for calcium. Above that level, as seen in Figure 11.2, further increases in calcium intake will produce no further bony accumulation. The intake required to achieve the full genetic program, and thus to assure peak bone mass, is the intake that corresponds to the beginning of the plateau region in Figure 11.2. This value will be different for different stages of growth, partly because growth rates are not constant and

partly because, as body size increases, obligatory calcium losses through skin and excreta increase as well.

In a meta-analysis of published balance studies during growth, Matkovic and Heaney[23] estimated these threshold intakes as 1090 mg/day for infants, 1390 mg/day for children, 1480 mg/day for adolescents, and the low 957 mg/day for young adults. These values, based on a retrospective analysis of balance data, are buttressed by three randomized controlled trials of calcium supplementation in children and adolescents,[12,13,24] and by a longitudinal observational study in young adults.[25] The controlled trials demonstrated that bone gain during growth was greater when intake was elevated above the RDA. This suggests that the current RDAs lie on the ascending portion of the threshold curves of Figure 11.2 rather than on the plateau, as they should. However, it must be noted that some of the increase in bone mass observed in these trials was the result of a bone remodeling transient,[17] and was hence lost when treatment was withdrawn. How large the residual effect may be is still unknown.

The longitudinal study of young adults[25] showed prospectively that bone augmentation continues into the third decade. Bone mass gains in this study ranged from 0.5% per year for the forearm to 1.25% per year for total body bone mineral. The single most important correlate of the rate of bone accumulation in the subjects of this study was calcium intake. The rate of bone accumulation was inversely proportional to age, with the best estimate of the age at which the rate reached zero being about 29–30 years. Thus, the window of opportunity for achieving the full genetic program appears to remain at least partly open until about age 30.

The conservation of acquired bone mass

Studies of calcium requirement in mature, but still premenopausal, women have, in general, yielded results compatible with the NIH recommendations. Welten et al,[26] in a meta-analysis of studies in this age group, concluded that calcium intake was positively associated with bone mass. Heaney et al,[27] in a study of estrogen-replete women ingesting their habitual calcium intakes, found a mean intake for zero balance of slightly under 1000 mg/day, and Nordin et al[28] a figure closer to 600 mg/day. Recker et al,[29] in a prospective study of bone mass in premenopausal women, found no detectable bone loss over a 2-year period on an estimated mean daily calcium intake of 651 mg.

Menopause

Estrogen seems to adjust the bending setpoint of the mechanical feedback loop that regulates bone mass (see below). Accordingly, whenever women lose ovarian hormones, whether naturally at menopause or earlier as a result of anorexia nervosa or athletic amenorrhea, the skeleton appears to sense that it has more bone than it needs, and hence allows resorption to carry away more bone than formation replaces. (Precisely the same change occurs when men lose testosterone for any reason.) This is equivalent to raising the setpoint of the feedback loop which functions to maintain the degree of bone bending within safe limits. Although varying somewhat from site to site across the skeleton, the downward adjustment in bone mass caused by lack of gonadal hormones amounts to about 15% of the bone a woman had before menopause.[30]

The importance of this phenomenon in a discussion of nutrient effects is to distinguish menopausal bone loss from nutrient deficiency loss, and to stress that menopausal loss, which results mainly from absence of gonadal hormones (not to nutrient deficiency), cannot be substantially influenced by diet. Almost all of the published studies of calcium supplementation within 5 years of the menopause failed to prevent bone loss. Even Elders et al,[31] who employed a calcium intake in excess of 3100 mg/day, succeeded only in slowing menopausal bone loss, not in preventing it. Both Aloia et al[16] and Riis et al[32] showed evidence for a benefit of a high calcium intake at this life stage, but estrogen produced a significantly greater effect. Thus, it may be that, in

any group of early menopausal women, there are some whose calcium intake is so inadequate that they are losing bone for two reasons: estrogen lack *plus* calcium insufficiency.

Important as menopausal bone loss is, it is only a one-time downward adjustment and, if nutrition is adequate, the loss continues for only a few years, after which the skeleton comes into a new steady state (although at about 15% lower bone mass). It is in this context that the importance of achieving a high peak skeletal mass during growth becomes apparent. One standard deviation for lumbar spine bone mineral content in normal women is about 15% of the young adult mean and, for total body bone mineral, about 12%. Hence a woman at least one standard deviation above the mean can sustain the 15% menopausal loss and still end up with about as much bone as the average women has before menopause. By contrast, a woman at or under one standard deviation below the young adult mean premenopausally drops to 2 standard deviations below the mean as she crosses menopause and is therefore, by WHO criteria,[33] already osteopenic and verging on frankly osteoporotic.

As noted, the menopausal bone mass adjustment theoretically stops with a loss of about 15%, but this is true only so long as calcium intake is adequate. In this regard, it is important to note that estrogen has non-skeletal effects on the calcium economy as well, i.e. it improves intestinal calcium absorption and renal calcium conservation.[30,34,35] As a result, an estrogen-deficient woman has a higher calcium requirement and, unless she raises her calcium intake after menopause, she will continue to lose bone after the estrogen-dependent quantum has been lost, even if the same diet would have been adequate to maintain her skeleton before menopause. In other words, early in the menopausal period, her bone loss is mainly (or entirely) because of estrogen withdrawal, whereas later it will be because of inadequate calcium intake.

Figure 11.3 integrates the set of factors contributing to bone loss in the postmenopausal period. The figure shows both the self-limiting character of the loss resulting from estrogen deficiency and the usually slower, but continuing, loss caused by nutritional deficiency (when present). Unlike estrogen-related loss, which expresses most of its effect in the first 3–6 years after menopause, an ongoing calcium deficiency will continue to deplete the skeleton indefinitely for the remainder of a woman's life, i.e. unless calcium intake is raised to a level sufficient to stop it. Furthermore, as both absorption efficiency[34] and calcium intake[4] decline with age, the degree of calcium shortfall actually tends to worsen with age.

Thus it is important for a woman to increase her calcium intake after menopause. Both the 1984 NIH Consensus Conference on Osteoporosis,[36] and the 1994 Consensus Conference on Optimal Calcium Intake[7] recommended intakes of 1500 mg/day for estrogen-deprived postmenopausal women. It may be that the optimal intake is higher still (see below), but median intakes of women of this age in the USA and many northern European countries are in the range 500–600 mg/day[4,37] and, if the bulk of them could be raised even to 1500 mg/day, the impact on skeletal health would be considerable.

Senescence

Age-related bone loss occurs in both sexes, regardless of gonadal hormone levels, generally starting some time after the age of 50. However, such loss is obscured in the years immediately after menopause in women by the substantially larger effect of estrogen withdrawal (see Figure 11.3). It probably occurs, however, even in estrogen-treated women, at about the same rate as in men. Age-related loss involves both cortical and trabecular bone and can be brought about by several mechanisms: disuse, remodeling errors and nutritional deficiency. This rate is generally reported to be of the order of 0.5% per year during the sixth and seventh decades, but accelerates substantially with advancing age. For example, loss from the hip in the control subjects of the study by Chapuy et al,[10] at an average age of 84 and an average calcium intake of about 500 mg/day, was 3% per year.

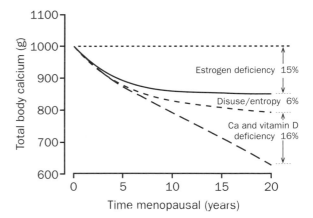

Figure 11.3 Partition of age-related bone loss in a typical postmenopausal woman with an inadequate calcium intake. (Based on a model described in detail elsewhere[29] and reproduced with permission. © Robert P Heaney, 1990.)

Although nutrient deficiency is clearly only a part of the total problem, nevertheless it is common. That the 3% loss in the control subjects of Chapuy et al[10] was related to their calcium intakes is indicated by the fact that this loss was completely obliterated in the supplemented women. Intestinal calcium absorption efficiency declines with age,[34] at the same time as nutrient intake itself generally declines;[4] the result is that the diet of aging individuals becomes more and more inadequate. McKane et al[38] have recently shown that the high PTH levels and abnormal PTH secretory dynamics typically found in elderly women are the result of calcium deficiency, and that PTH function can be entirely normalized by calcium intakes of 2400 mg/day.

It is in this age group also that the most dramatic and persuasive evidence for fracture prevention by high calcium intakes has been produced in recent years. This is partly because most fragility fractures rise in frequency with age, and hence the opportunity to see a fracture benefit (if one exists) is greater then. Chapuy et al[10] showed a reduction in hip fracture risk of about 40% by 18 months after starting supplementation with calcium plus vitamin D, and an approximately 30% reduction in other extremity fractures. Chevalley et al[14] in another study in elderly women, showed that, even when vitamin D was given to both groups, extra calcium reduced femoral bone loss *and* vertebral fracture incidence. More recently Recker et al,[39] in a 4-year, randomized controlled trial in elderly women (mean age 73), demonstrated that a calcium supplement reduced both age-related bone loss and incident vertebral fractures.

The calcium intake achieved in the Chapuy study was about 1700 mg/day, 1400 mg/day in the Chevalley study and about 1600 mg/day in the Recker study. These values are in the range of the intake found earlier by Heaney et al[27] to be the mean requirement for healthy estrogen-deprived older women (1500–1700 mg/day). All these studies are, therefore, consistent with the NIH recommendation of 1500 mg/day.[7]

An often unremarked feature of these controlled trials in already elderly individuals is the fact that bone mass was low in *both* treated and control groups at the start of the study; although a significant difference in fracture rate was produced by calcium supplementation, even the supplemented groups would have to be considered as having an unacceptably high fracture rate. What these studies do not establish is how much lower the fracture rate might have been if a high calcium intake had been provided for the preceding 20–30 years of these women's lives. The studies of Matkovic et al[40] and Holbrook et al,[41] although not randomized trials, strongly suggest that the effect may be larger than has been found with treatment started in the eighth and ninth decades of life. Both of these observational studies reported a hip fracture rate that was roughly 60% lower in elderly women whose habitual calcium intakes had been high. Although findings from observational studies such as these had not been considered persuasive in the absence of proof from controlled trials, the Chapuy, Chevalley and Recker studies have now met that need, and taken together indicate that adequate calcium intake throughout life can be counted on to reduce osteoporotic fractures by 40–60%. At the same time, it must be stressed, once again, that osteoporosis is a multifactorial condition, and

that removing one of the pathogenic factors (i.e. insuring an adequate calcium intake) cannot be expected to eradicate all osteoporotic fractures.

Calcium in treatment

Although calcium alone is insufficient to treat established osteoporosis, treatment with any of the pharmacological or hormonal modalities discussed in this book will be less than optimally effective if attention is not given to ensuring an adequate intake of calcium. Given the generally poor absorption efficiency in patients with osteoporosis, and the high prevalence of osteoporosis in calcium malabsorbers,[42] any therapy theoretically capable of favorably altering bone remodeling balance will need extra calcium if it is to realize its potential for improvement in skeletal mass. Moreover, therapies with a preferential trophic effect on the spine (e.g. fluoride, PTH) may actually deplete the peripheral skeleton to support the increase in spinal bone mass if oral calcium intake is not adequate.[43,44] Clearly, bone cannot be built without adequate provision of the raw materials from which it is constructed.

Almost no studies have addressed the questions of how much calcium may be required during treatment with bone-active pharmacologic agents. Dure-Smith et al[44] reported striking bone hunger in fluoride-treated patients, suggesting a need for as much as 2500 mg Ca/day with fluoride therapy. In this regard it should be noted that the recommendation of 1500 mg/day made by the NIH Consensus Conference is a *maintenance* recommendation, i.e. it is judged to be optimal to maintain skeletal mass. Unless there are dramatic changes in the calcium economy induced by therapy, it follows that 1500 mg/day may not be sufficient to support the full potential of the drug for bony restoration.

The bone density data of Liberman et al,[45] observed in the 3-year alendronate trial, showed continuing bone gain during years 2 and 3. Although most of the first year change would be the result of a remodeling transient, this later change indicates a positive shift in remodeling balance. What is presumably happening is that the drug is inducing resistance of osteoclasts to PTH, leading to increased PTH secretion, with a consequent improvement in calcium absorption and renal calcium conservation. In other words, the drug produced changes that allowed the patients to make better use of dietary calcium. The trial was, however, designed with a calcium supplement of only 500 mg/day, and thus it is doubtful whether the observed increase in bone density was as large as it might have been.

An example of this point is seen in a meta-analysis by Nieves et al[46] of patients treated with either estrogen or calcitonin. They found that the treatment-induced improvement in bone density was two- to fourfold greater if calcium was combined with the active agent. Davis et al[47] reported the same effect in their observational study of postmenopausal women treated with estrogen.

In summary, at least 1500 mg/day must be provided in patients receiving other treatments and, with some treatments (e.g. fluoride and PTH), at least 2500 mg/day.

NUTRITION: VITAMIN D

Vitamin D facilitates active transport of calcium across the intestinal mucosa, at least partly by inducing the formation of a calcium-binding transport protein in intestinal mucosal cells. This function is particularly important for adaptation to low calcium intakes. Calcium absorption also occurs passively, probably mainly by way of paracellular diffusion. This route is not dependent upon vitamin D, and is not as well studied. The proportion of absorption by the two mechanisms varies with intake and is not well characterized in humans; at high calcium intakes (above 2000 mg/day) absorption fraction approaches 10–15% of intake. Under these circumstances it is likely that active transport contributes relatively little to the total absorbed load. Nevertheless, it is generally considered that vitamin D status influences absorptive performance and that it thereby influences the calcium requirement.

Vitamin D status commonly deteriorates in elderly people whose plasma 25-hydroxyvitamin D levels are generally lower than in young adults.[48] This difference is partly the result of age-related decreases in solar exposure, efficiency of skin vitamin D synthesis and, in the USA and Canada, intake of milk, the principal dietary source of the vitamin in those nations. Moreover, elderly people exhibit other abnormalities of the vitamin D–endocrine system which may further impair their ability to adapt to reduce calcium intake. These include decreased responsiveness of the renal 1α-hydroxylase to PTH[49] and decreased mucosal responsiveness to calcitriol.[50]

For all these reasons there is a growing body of opinion that the requirement for vitamin D rises with age, and a body of data that strongly suggests that relative vitamin D deficiency plays a role in several components of the osteoporosis syndrome. Perhaps most persuasive of all is the finding by Heikinheimo et al,[51] in a randomized, controlled trial, of a substantial reduction in all fractures in an elderly Finnish population given a single injection of 150 000–300 000 IU vitamin D each autumn. It is also worth recalling in this connection that, in the Chapuy trial also, the subjects received 800 IU vitamin D as well as calcium.

The foregoing studies (as well as others) lead inexorably to the conclusion that vitamin D insufficiency is prevalent in middle-aged and elderly citizens of northern Europe and North America. Moreover, in virtually none of these studies was frank osteomalacia a significant feature of the problem. This former criterion for true vitamin D deficiency must today be recognized as much too insensitive to be nutritionally useful. Holick[52] has shown that it takes an intake of about 600 IU/day, from all sources, to sustain serum 25-hydroxyvitamin D levels, and the doses of vitamin D used in the studies summarized above also suggest that an intake in the range of 500–800 IU/day is required for full expression of the known effects of vitamin D in adults. This is substantially above the current recommended daily allowance (RDA) in the USA of only 200 IU for adults.[53] For comparison purposes, 800 IU/day is substantially less than daily dermal production of vitamin D in individuals working outdoors in sunny climates.

EXERCISE

It has long been recognized that, when a body region is paralyzed or immobilized, the bones involved undergo atrophy.[54,55] This is as true for bedrest and space flight in otherwise healthy individuals as it is for such conditions as paralysis, spinal cord injury and simply casting of an extremity. Clearly, therefore, usage of bone is important for its maintenance.

Mechanical control of bone mass and density

Once peak bone mass has been achieved, the principal forces acting on the skeleton are the mechanical loads imposed in ordinary, everyday usage. Skeletal structures, like all engineering structures, deform slightly under load (a dimensional change technically called 'strain'). The skeleton senses that deformation and attempts to adjust its mass (by controlling the balance between bone resorption and bone formation), so that the resulting deformation remains of the order of 0.1–0.15% in any given dimension. If a bone is loaded so heavily that it consistently bends more than that amount, then the balance between local formation and resorption is adjusted to favor formation, thereby increasing local density and making that region stiffer. Conversely, if a bony segment is used little, and its bending is less than that critical amount, the skeleton senses that it has an excess of bone in the region concerned, and adjusts the remodeling balance to remove some of the apparent surplus. If strains exceed some critical value, estimated to be about 0.3%, periosteal new bone formation is activated as well,[56] even in adults who have stopped growing. External bone size then actually increases. As stiffness of a tube increases approximately as the square of its radius, this bony change is a more efficient way of resisting excessive strain

than could be produced by addition of bone on the endosteal–trabecular envelope.

The reference level of bending is one of the fascinating physiological constants of nature. Across the vertebrates, for all species and all bones studied to date, bone mass is regulated such that any given bone deforms by about that critical 0.1–0.15% in ordinary use. This reference level of bending is termed a 'setpoint', and the bone remodeling apparatus operates to minimize local deviations from this critical value. The cellular basis for the setpoint and the precise nature of the apparatus that detects departures from it remain largely unknown; however, there is suggestive evidence that localizes this sensing apparatus to the network of osteocytes embedded in bone. For several years it has seemed likely that one of the principal determinants of the setpoint of this mass-regulating system is the level of gonadal hormones. Circumstantial evidence in support of this connection includes the recent finding that estrogen receptors in bone are concentrated in osteocytes,[57] and the facts that true bone density rises sharply at puberty[58] and declines by about the same amount as menopause (whether natural or artificial).[30] These life-phase changes are what one would expect if estrogen did affect the setpoint.

Exercise and osteoporosis prevention

Over 25 years ago, Chalmers and Ho[59] hypothesized, on the basis of international differences in hip fracture rates, that some of the age-related bone loss and the burden of bone fragility resulted from a decline in physical activity, particularly in the more technologically advanced societies with high use of labor-saving devices. Since then it has become clear that age-specific hip fracture rates have increased substantially in most industrialized nations.[60–62] As no amount of nutrition can be expected to offset an exercise-related decline in bone mass, it is clearly important to maintain or institute a pattern of exercise that optimizes bone mass in the young and that will sustain bone density in the aging.

There have been few controlled trials of fracture prevention with exercise intervention, at any life stage. However, there is strong evidence from observational studies that exercise during growth increases achieved bone mass, and that exercise slows age-related bone loss after menopause and can actually produce a modest (2–6%) increase in bone mass in elderly people.[63–70] Bone mass is a recognized factor in bone strength, and there is a scientific consensus that protection of bone mass will reduce fracture risk. The importance of starting exercise at a young age is highlighted in several studies, most notably, perhaps, that of Kannus et al,[71] who found that the effect of exercise on bone mass was two to four times greater in those who started their exercise at or before puberty.

As both mechanical loading and adequate nutrition are essential for the maintenance of bone mass, it is not surprising that studies evaluating the combined effect of increased calcium intake and increased exercise have shown more striking benefits than produced by either modality alone.[72,73]

The osteotrophic effect of exercise is seen most clearly in those forms of mechanical activity that involved impact loading,[74] and is less prominent, or absent altogether, from resistance exercises such as swimming.[75] Thus an exercise regimen that improves cardiovascular fitness and maintains joint mobility and flexibility, while advantageous for the total person, may not provide as much protection of bone as one that involves impact. Nevertheless, impact loading can itself be risky in fragile elderly people and, for them, the major benefit of exercise may reside in its non-skeletal effects.

CONCLUSION

The human organism evolved in an environment providing a high calcium intake and requiring moderate to strenuous physical exertion. The calcium economy and skeletal mechanics are adapted to these paleolithic conditions. Three forces in modern civilization work against the skeleton: a decline in physical work; a decline in the calcium density of the food supply; and a decline in total food intake associated with a decreased need for physical work. Optimal protection of bone will require individuals and societies to find suitable countermeasures for all three.

REFERENCES

1. Gershon-Cohen J, Jowsey J. The relationship of dietary calcium to osteoporosis. *Metabolism* 1964; **13:** 221–6.

2. Jowsey J, Raisz LG. Experimental osteoporosis and parathyroid activity. *Endocrinology* 1968; **82:** 384–96.

3. Eaton SB, Nelson DA. Calcium in evolutionary perspective. *Am J Clin Nutr* 1991; **54:** 281S–7S.

4. Carroll MD, Abraham S, Dresser CM. Dietary intake source data: US, 1976–80. *Vital and Health Statistics*, Serv. 11-NO. 231, DHHS. Publ. No. (PHS) 83-PHS, March 1983. Washington DC: Government Printing Office.

5. Molleson T. The eloquent bones of Abu Hureyra. *Sci Am* 1994; **271**(2): 70–5.

6. Forbes RM, Weingartner KE, Parker HM et al. Bioavailability to rats of zinc, magnesium, and calcium in casein-, egg- and soy protein-containing diets. *J Nutr* 1979; **109:** 1652–60.

7. NIH Consensus Conference. Optimal calcium intake. *JAMA* 1994; **272:** 1942–8.

8. Heaney RP. Nutritional factors in osteoporosis. *Annu Rev Nutr* 1993; **13:** 287–316.

9. Dawson-Hughes B, Dallal GE, Krall EA et al. A controlled trial of the effect of calcium supplementation on bone density in postmenopausal women. *N Engl J Med* 1990; **323:** 878–83.

10. Chapuy MC, Arlot ME, Duboeuf F et al. Vitamin D_3 and calcium to prevent hip fractures in elderly women. *N Engl J Med* 1992; **327:** 1637–42.

11. Reid IR, Ames RW, Evans MC et al. Effect of calcium supplementation on bone loss in postmenopausal women. *N Engl J Med* 1993; **328:** 460–4.

12. Johnston CC Jr, Miller JZ, Slemenda CW et al. Calcium supplementation and increases in bone mineral density in children. *N Engl J Med* 1992; **327:** 82–7.

13. Lloyd T, Andon MB, Rollings N et al. Calcium supplementation and bone mineral density in adolescent girls. *JAMA* 1993; **270**: 841–4.

14. Chevalley T, Rizzoli R, Nydegger V et al. Effects of calcium supplements on femoral bone mineral density and vertebral fracture rate in vitamin D-replete elderly patients. *Osteoporosis Int* 1994; **4**: 245–52.

15. Reid IR, Ames RW, Evans MC et al. Determinants of the rate of bone loss in normal postmenopausal women – the importance of fat mass and renal calcium handling. *Am J Med* 1995; **98**: 331–5.

16. Aloia JF, Vaswani A, Yeh JK et al. Calcium supplementation with and without hormone replacement therapy to prevent postmenopausal bone loss. *Ann Intern Med* 1994; **120**: 97–103.

17. Heaney RP. The bone remodeling transient: implications for the interpretation of clinical studies of bone mass change. *J Bone Miner Res* 1994; **9**: 1515–23.

18. Pilch SM, ed. *Physiological effects and health consequences of dietary fiber.* Prepared for the Center for Food Safety and Applied Nutrition, Food and Drug Administration under Contract No. FDA 223-84-2059 by the Life Sciences Research Office, Federation of American Societies for Experimental Biology. 1987. Available from FASEB Special Publications Office, Bethesda, MD.

19. Barger-Lux MJ, Heaney RP. Caffeine and the calcium economy revisited. *Osteoporosis Int* 1995; **5**: 97–102.

20. Heaney RP, Recker RR. Effects of nitrogen, phosphorus, and caffeine on calcium balance in women. *J Lab Clin Med* 1982; **99**: 46–55.

21. Barrett-Connor E, Chang JC, Edelstein SL. Coffee-associated osteoporosis offset by daily milk consumption. *JAMA* 1994; **271**: 280–3.

22. Nordin BEC, Need AG, Morris HA et al. The nature and significance of the relationship between urinary sodium and urinary calcium in women. *J Nutr* 1993; **123**: 1615–22.

23. Matkovic V, Heaney RP. Calcium balance during human growth. Evidence for threshold behavior. *Am J Clin Nutr* 1992; **55**: 992–6.

24. Chan GM, Hoffman K, McMurray M. Effects of dairy products on bone and body composition in pubertal girls. *J Pediatr* 1995; **126**: 551–6.

25. Recker RR, Davies KM, Hinders SM et al. Bone gain in young adult women. *JAMA* 1992; **268**: 2403–8.

26. Welten DC, Kemper HCG, Post GB et al. A meta-analysis of the effect of calcium intake on bone mass in females and males. *J Nutr* 1995; **125**: 2802–13.

27. Heaney RP, Recker RR, Saville PD. Menopausal changes in calcium balance performance. *J Lab Clin Med* 1978; **92**: 953–63.

28. Nordin BEC, Polley KJ, Need AG et al. The problem of calcium requirement. *Am J Clin Nutr* 1987; **45**: 1295–304.

29. Recker RR, Lappe JM, Davies KM et al. Change in bone mass immediately before menopause. *J Bone Miner Res* 1992; **7**: 857–62.

30. Heaney RP. Estrogen-calcium interactions in the postmenopause: a quantitative description. *Bone Miner* 1990; **11**: 67–84.

31. Elders PJM, Lips P, Netelenbos JC et al. Long-term effect of calcium supplementation on bone loss in perimenopausal women. *J Bone Miner Res* 1994; **9**: 963–70.

32. Riis B, Thomsen K, Christiansen C. Does calcium supplementation prevent postmenopausal bone loss? *N Engl J Med* 1987; **316**: 173–7.

33. Kanis JA, Melton LJ III, Christiansen et al. The diagnosis of osteoporosis. *J Bone Miner Res* 1994; **9**: 1137–41.

34. Heaney RP, Recker RR, Stegman MR et al. Calcium absorption in women: relationships to calcium intake, estrogen status, and age. *J Bone Miner Res* 1989; **4**: 469–75.

35. Nordin BEC, Need AG, Morris HA et al. Evidence for a renal calcium leak in postmenopausal women. *J Clin Endocrinol Metab* 1991; **72**: 401–7.

36. Osteoporosis. Consensus Conference. *JAMA* 1984; **252**: 799–802.

37. Alaimo K, McDowell MA, Briefel RR et al. Dietary intake of vitamins, minerals, and fiber of persons ages 2 months and over in the United States: Third National Health and Nutrition Examination Survey, Phase 1, 1988–1991. *Advance data from vital and health statistics; no. 258.* Hyattsville, MA: National Center for Health Statistics, 1994.

38. McKane WR, Khosla S, O'Fallon WM et al. Role of calcium intake in modulating age-related increases in parathyroid function and bone resorption. *J Clin Endocrinol Metab* 1996; **81**: 1699–703.

39. Recker RR, Hinders S, Davies KM. Correcting calcium nutritional deficiency prevents spine fractures in elderly women. *J Bone Miner Res* 1997, in press.

40. Matkovic V, Kostial K, Simonovic I et al. Bone

status and fracture rates in two regions of Yugoslavia. *Am J Clin Nutr* 1979; **32:** 540–9.

41. Holbrook TL, Barrett-Connor E, Wingard DL. Dietary calcium and risk of hip fracture: 14-year prospective population study. *Lancet* 1988; **ii:** 1046–9.

42. Horowitz M, Need AG, Philcox JC et al. Biochemical effects of a calcium supplement in osteoporotic postmenopausal women with normal absorption and malabsorption of calcium. *Miner Electrolyte Metab* 1987; **13:** 112–16.

43. Slovik DM, Rosenthal DI, Doppelt SH et al. Restoration of spinal bone in osteoporotic men by treatment with human parathyroid hormone (1–34) and 1,25-dihydroxyvitamin D. *J Bone Miner Res* 1986; **1:** 377–81.

44. Dure-Smith BA, Farley SM, Linkhart SG et al. Calcium deficiency in fluoride-treated osteoporotic patients despite calcium supplementation. *J Clin Endocrinol Metab* 1996; **81:** 269–75.

45. Liberman UA, Weiss SR, Bröll J et al. Effect of oral alendronate on bone mineral density and the incidence of fractures in postmenopausal osteoporosis. *N Engl J Med* 1995; **333:** 1437–43.

46. Nieves JW, Komar L, Cosman F, Lindsay R. Calcium potentiates the effect of estrogen and calcitonin on bone mass: review and analysis. *Am J Clin Nutr* 1997; in press.

47. Davis JW, Ross PD, Johnson NE et al. Estrogen and calcium supplement use among Japanese–American women: Effects upon bone loss when used singly and in combination. *Bone* 1995; **17:** 369–73.

48. Francis RM, Peacock M, Storer JH et al. Calcium malabsorption in the elderly: the effect of treatment with oral 25-hydroxyvitamin D$_3$. *Eur J Clin Invest* 1983; **13:** 391–6.

49. Slovik DM, Adams JS, Neer RM et al. Deficient production of 1,25-dihydroxyvitamin D in elderly osteoporotic patients. *N Engl J Med* 1981; **305:** 372–4.

50. Francis RM, Peacock M, Taylor GA et al. Calcium malabsorption in elderly women with vertebral fractures: evidence for resistance to the action of vitamin D metabolites on the bowel. *Clin Sci* 1984; **66:** 103–7.

51. Heikinheimo RJ, Inkovaara JA, Harju EJ et al. Annual injection of vitamin D and fractures of aged bones. *Calcif Tissue Int* 1992; **51:** 105–10.

52. Holick MF. Vitamin D – new horizons for the 21st century (McCollum Award Lecture 1994). *Am J Clin Nutr* 1994; **60:** 619–30.

53. *Recommended Dietary Allowances*, 10th edn. Washington DC: National Academic Press, 1989.

54. Whedon GD, Heaney RP. Effects of physical inactivity, paralysis, and weightlessness. In: *Bone*, Vol. 7 (Hall B, ed.). Boca Raton: CRC Press, 1991: 57–77.

55. LeBlanc A, Schneider V, Krebs J et al. Spinal bone mineral after 5 weeks of bed rest. *Calcif Tissue Int* 1987; **41:** 259–61.

56. Frost HM. The mechanostat: a proposed pathogenic mechanism of osteoporosis and the bone mass effects of mechanical and nonmechanical agents. *Bone Miner* 1987; **2:** 73–85.

57. Braidman IP, Davenport LK, Carter DH et al. Preliminary in situ identification of estrogen target cells in bone. *J Bone Miner Res* 1995; **10:** 74–80.

58. Gilsanz V, Gibbens DT, Roe TF et al. Vertebral bone density in children: effect of puberty. *Radiology* 1988; **166:** 847–50.

59. Chalmers J, Ho KC. Geographical variations in senile osteoporosis. The association with physical activity. *J Bone Joint Surg* 1970; **52:** 667–75.

60. Lau E, Donnan S, Barker DJP et al. Physical activity and calcium intake in fracture of the proximal femur in Hong Kong. *BMJ* 1988; **297:** 1441–3.

61. Law MR, Wald NJ, Meade T. Strategies for prevention of osteoporosis and hip fracture. *BMJ* 1991; **303:** 453–9.

62. Lüthje P. Incidence of hip fracture in Finland: A forecast for 1990. *Acta Orthop Scand* 1985; **56:** 223–5.

63. Mosekilde L. Osteoporosis and exercise. *Bone* 1995; **17:** 193–5.

64. White MK, Martin RB, Yeater RA et al. The effects of exercise on the bones of postmenopausal women. *Int Orthop* 1984; **7:** 209–14.

65. Heinonen A, Oja P, Kannus P et al. Bone mineral density in female athletes representing sports with different loading characteristics of the skeleton. *Bone* 1995; **17:** 197–203.

66. Leichter I, Simkin A, Marguilies JY et al. Gain in mass density of bone following strenuous physical activity. *J Orthop Res* 1989; **7:** 86–90.

67. Bevier WC, Wiswell RA, Pyka G et al. Relationship of body composition, muscle strength, and aerobic capacity to bone mineral density in older men and women. *J Bone Miner Res* 1989; **4:** 421–32.

68. Simkin A, Ayalon J, Leichter I. Increased trabecular bone density due to bone-loading exercises in postmenopausal osteoporotic women. *Calcif Tissue Int* 1987; **40:** 59–63.

69. Heinonen A, Oja P, Kannus P et al. Bone mineral density of female athletes in different sports. *Bone Miner* 1993; **23:** 1–14.

70. Dalsky GP, Stocke KS, Ehsani AA et al. Weight-bearing exercise training and lumbar bone mineral content in postmenopausal women. *Ann Intern Med* 1988; **108:** 824–8.

71. Kannus P, Haapasalo H, Sankelo M et al. Effect of starting age of physical activity on bone mass in the dominant arm of tennis and squash players. *Ann Intern Med* 1995; **123:** 27–31.

72. Kanders B, Dempster DW, Lindsay R. Interaction of calcium nutrition and physical activity on bone mass in young women. *J Bone Miner Res* 1988; **3:** 145–9.

73. Prince R, Devine A, Dick I et al. The effects of calcium supplementation (milk powder or tablets) and exercise on bone density in postmenopausal women. *J Bone Miner Res* 1995; **10:** 1068–75.

74. Rubin CT, Lanyon LE. Regulation of bone mass by mechanical strain magnitude. *Calcif Tissue Int* 1985; **37:** 411–17.

75. Orwoll ES, Ferar J, Oviatt SK et al. The relationship of swimming exercise to bone mass in men and women. *Arch Intern Med* 1989; **149:** 2197–200.

12

Practical management of the patient with osteoporotic vertebral fracture

R Eastell

Osteoporotic vertebral fracture is one of the most common types of referral to the physician with an interest in metabolic bone disease. Each physician will approach the diagnostic evaluation and treatment in a different way. This chapter is a personal view and is based on the experience of the author in offering a metabolic bone service with orthopaedic surgeons, rheumatologists, endocrinologists and geriatricians. Readers are encouraged to consider alternative views such as those of Kleerekoper,[1] Rapado,[2] and Riggs and Khosla.[3]

EVIDENCE OF VERTEBRAL FRACTURE

History of back pain

The back pain of vertebral fracture has some characteristic features. The pain often comes on within a day of some strain on the back, such as lifting a suitcase or a grandchild, a jolt on a bus or working in the garden. The pain soon becomes very severe and the patient may need to stay in bed for several days. The pain is usually localized to the back; it is uncommon for pain to radiate into the legs and rare for there to be symptoms of cord compression such as bladder dysfunction. The pain from the fracture is present throughout the day and night and gradually eases and goes by 4–6 months. If pain persists longer, or if there is a second peak of pain during the first 6 months, this usually indicates a second vertebral fracture. This is not an uncommon occurrence.

Patients do not always complain of back pain. Indeed, it has been estimated that at least half of vertebral fractures are asymptomatic.[4] These asymptomatic fractures appear to be particularly common in patients taking corticosteroids – episodes of back pain may have been forgotten. The patient commonly recalls a painful episode when confronted with the appearance of a fracture on the spinal radiograph. This incontrovertible evidence prompts the recall of a painful event occurring many decades previously, often in relation to heavy manual work or after pregnancy.

Loss of height

Loss of height is an effect of ageing, resulting from the change of posture caused by degenerative changes in the intervertebral discs. Patients do not report this symptom spontaneously and it needs to be sought by asking about the patient's height in early adult life (more easily recalled by men than women, possibly as a result of its importance in military service). The patient may have noticed that it is more difficult to reach high shelves. It is unusual to have sudden height loss as the presenting complaint for vertebral fracture.

Kyphosis

This may have been noticed by a relative or the patient may report being 'round-shouldered'. Clothes may no longer fit. These symptoms are not specific to vertebral fracture, and are more commonly caused by disc degeneration. In a young person, kyphosis may be caused by Scheuermann's disease.

Other symptoms of vertebral fracture

Vertebral fractures in the lumbar region result in decreased abdominal volume. This causes the abdomen to protrude. Patients with osteoporosis are commonly slender, so this appearance is new. They may also result in impingement of the costal margin on the iliac crest. This 'iliocostal friction syndrome' causes pain and a grating sensation.[5] This pain is postural, occurring on sitting.

Vertebral fractures in the thoracic spine result in decreased lung capacity. This may result in respiratory symptoms such as dyspnoea, or in delayed recovery from chest infections.

Clinical examination

Two aspects of the clinical examination are useful in the patient with suspected vertebral fracture. The first relates to the location of the pain. It is often assumed that the back pain is associated with the deformity on the radiograph. However, a careful palpation of the spinal processes by counting down from vertebra prominens (seventh cervical vertebra) often reveals that the site of the pain does not correspond to the level of the deformity on the radiograph.

It is helpful to evaluate the size of the gap between the costal margin and the iliac crest. This is normally three fingerbreadths (as measured by the patient's fingers).

Spinal radiographs

Plain radiographs are required of the thoracic and lumbar spine in the anteroposterior and lateral position. It is a common mistake to take the radiograph only of the painful area. This would miss asymptomatic fractures in other parts of the spine. Also, it is common only to take lateral radiographs. The anteroposterior radiograph is useful to identify the vertebral level of the fracture and to exclude other causes of deformity, such as a malignancy (associated with absent pedicles).

Types of deformity

Vertebral deformities may be wedge, endplate ('biconcave', when both endplates are affected) and compression (also called 'crush') (Figure 12.1). Wedge deformities are particularly common in the thoracic spine, because the normal kyphosis in the region results in the main force running anteriorly. Endplate deformities are particularly common in the lumbar spine, because the normal lordosis results in the main force running through the middle of the vertebra. There appears to be no association between the type of deformity and the severity of pain or the level of bone mineral density. The level of the deformities should be recorded to allow comparison at follow-up visits.

Deformities that mimic fractures

The most common deformity to mimic fracture is Scheuermann's disease. This is a form of epiphysitis that occurs during adolescence ('juvenile epiphysitis') and gives the appearance of wedging and elongation of the vertebral bodies. The characteristic feature is the wavy appearance of the superior and inferior borders.[6]

Malignancy may cause vertebral deformity. The isotope bone scan is particularly useful in this situation as it is unusual to have a single bone lesion.[7] Increased uptake in multiple sites

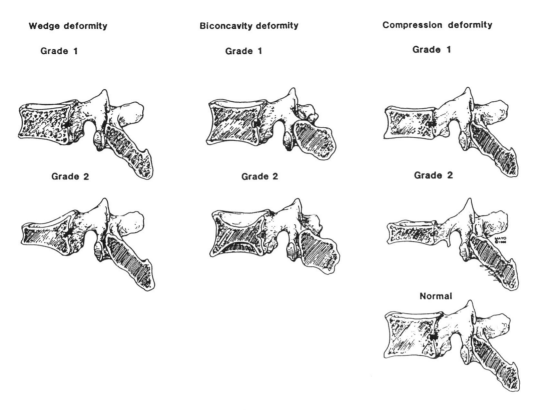

Figure 12.1 Classification of vertebral fractures.[9] The figure illustrates the types of deformity (wedge, endplate and compression) and the grade of deformity. The reference range was obtained by calculating the mean and standard deviation in normal women and the critical values are 3 s.d. below the mean.

in the skeleton is typical of malignancy and may occur in prostate cancer which affects the sacrum, lumbar spine and ribs (via Batson's venous plexus). Malignancy may cause erosion of the pedicle, an appearance not found with osteoporotic vertebral fractures.

Paget's disease of bone commonly affects the spine. The bone may appear sclerotic, but it is weak and can fracture. The bone texture has a disorganized appearance and the vertebrae may be enlarged.

Osteomalacia may result in vertebral deformities. Often adjacent vertebrae are affected and the endplates are deformed. This gives rise to a 'cod-fish' appearance. There may be other radiological clues such as the ground-glass appearance of the vertebral body bone and the presence of pseudofractures (Looser's zones) in the pelvis, long bones or ribs.

Use of vertebral morphometry in the clinic
The thoracic vertebrae normally appear a little wedged and the lumbar vertebrae often appear a little biconcave. The problem of the normal ranges for shape of vertebrae has been addressed by several authors and a consensus reached.[8] The algorithms that have been described for the definition of vertebral fractures were developed for epidemiological surveys and clinical trials. They can be useful in individual patients. For this purpose, it is advisable to keep a transparent ruler, pencil, calculator and table[9] in the clinic for borderline cases.

Isotope bone scan

This can be a useful diagnostic tool in certain cases. There is increased isotope uptake in a vertebra for at least 6 months after it has fractured[7] and typically there is uniform distribution in the vertebral body. This can be useful if the radiological appearances are borderline but the symptoms are characteristic. In patients with a suspicion of malignancy (previous breast cancer, history of weight loss), the scan is helpful in that metastases often affect many bones. Increased uptake may also be found in Paget's disease.

The scan is helpful in patients with corticosteroid-induced osteoporosis with pelvic pain. These patients commonly develop insufficiency fractures and these show up as a symmetrical appearance affecting the sacral alae and the pubic rami.[10]

Morphometric X-ray absorptiometry

Dual energy X-ray absorptiometry may be used to image the spine. The resolution of these images is inferior to the spinal radiograph, but the technique has a number of advantages over radiographs including lower radiation exposure (one-sixtieth), clearer images of vertebra covered by the diaphragm (thoracic vertebrae 10 to 12) and ease of storage. They are being introduced into the author's practice and their use compared with radiographs. They may become particularly useful during follow-up visits (see below).

Magnetic resonance imaging

This approach can be useful in identifying a recent deformity and distinguishing a fracture from a malignant deposit. It is very useful at identifying cord compression.

EVIDENCE OF OSTEOPOROSIS

The definition of osteoporosis

Vertebral fractures may occur as a result of severe trauma, particularly in young men. These patients should not be considered osteo-porotic. In clinical practice it is often difficult to decide on the level of trauma. Mild to moderate trauma is defined as a fall from standing height or less, but this is inappropriate for vertebral fracture because the stress on the spine often occurs as a result of lifting a heavy object.

An alternative way to establish the presence of osteoporosis is to measure the bone mineral density (BMD). This is usually done by dual energy X-ray absorptiometry (DXA) which is the preferred method because it is rapid, precise, accurate and has a low radiation dose. It allows measurement of the sites that commonly fracture, namely the lumbar spine and proximal femur. The World Health Organization has proposed a definition of osteoporosis that uses BMD in comparison to the young normal level[11] (Figure 12.2). Thus the average young person

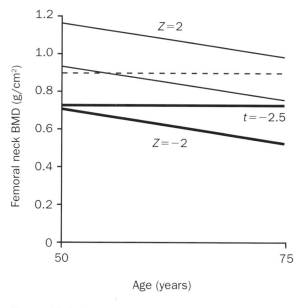

Figure 12.2 The interpretation of femoral neck BMD includes the use of the t-score and Z-score. Low bone mass is indicated by a t-score that is −1 s.d. below the mean for young women; osteoporosis is indicated by a t-score that is −2.5 s.d. below the mean for young women. The Z-score defines the BMD results adjusted for age. At any age the reference range is −2 to 2 and the average BMD Z-score is 0. A value below −2 indicates the need to investigate further for factors that accelerate bone loss.

would have a mean value of zero (the 't-score') and 95% of young people would have BMD values of between −2 and 2 standard deviation units (s.d.). The term 'low bone density' refers to those with a t-score of less than −1 s.d., the term 'osteoporosis' to those with a t-score of less than −2.5 s.d., and the term 'established osteoporosis' to those with a t-score of less than −2.5 s.d. and an osteoporosis-related fracture.

This approach has a number of problems in both practice and theory. The relationship between fracture risk and bone mineral density is affected by age. Thus, a t-score of −2.5 s.d. at age 85 results in greater fracture risk than a similar t-score at age 60.[12] Bone mineral density is not the only determinant of bone fragility, and factors such as bone geometry, architecture and turnover are also likely to be important, although they may be more difficult to measure.[13] There is no agreement on which site should be measured – if several sites are measured then it is likely that one of these may meet the criterion for osteoporosis.

Nevertheless, this type of approach is useful if applied in a flexible manner. A fracture in association with a t-score of −4 s.d. indicates severe osteoporosis and the likelihood of further fractures. A fracture in association with a t-score of 0 raises a question about the level of trauma. If the level of trauma was mild then it would raise a question about other causes for the vertebral deformity (see above).

Bone densitometry in osteoporosis

Range of values

There is a wide range of BMD values of the spine and hip in osteoporosis. The lower the bone density, the greater the risk of future fractures. The femoral neck has been found particularly useful for fracture prediction, and so more weight is put on this measurement for prognosis. The presence of a vertebral fracture increases the risk of a further vertebral fracture eightfold, regardless of the BMD level.[14] The presence of another osteoporosis-related fracture, such as a hip fracture, also increases the risk of a vertebral fracture. Presumably, the presence of these fractures indicates that some factors are present that are not captured by BMD, such as architecture and bone turnover.

Problems in its use

Bone densitometry is more difficult in the patient with a vertebral fracture than in the perimenopausal woman. The patients tend to be older and so degenerative findings are common, even though osteoarthritis tends to be protective of osteoporosis.[15] Endplate sclerosis has a particularly big effect on BMD. The fractures can occur in the lumbar spine, and so these need to be removed from the analysis. The result from fewer vertebrae will be less reliable. Patients with severe kyphosis may find the procedure uncomfortable as it is difficult for them to lie flat.

Measurement of the hip can be difficult in osteoporosis. The patients tend to be more slender than normal and in very slender patients the machine has insufficient soft tissue for its baseline measurement. This has to be addressed by placing rice bags behind the buttocks.

Occasionally patients may be so obese that DXA is unreliable. The solution here may be to measure the forearm or to use ultrasonography of the calcaneus, because the obesity tends to affect central areas more than the limbs.

Problems in interpretation

The t-score approach is appropriate for the diagnosis of osteoporosis, although there are some reservations, as noted above. However, for prognosis and identifying those patients who have had accelerated bone loss, it is better to apply the reference range for age, also called the 'Z-score' approach (see Figure 12.2).

A patient's risk of future fracture depends on the current BMD, the predicted rate of loss and the lifespan.[16] It is difficult to predict the rate of loss, although attempts have been made, using biochemical markers of bone turnover, with some success in the perimenopausal woman. The lifetime fracture risk can be predicted by assuming average bone loss and average life expectancy and using published tables.[16] A simpler approach is to use the Z-score. The lower the Z-score, the higher the risk of future fracture. Indeed, for every standard deviation decrease of BMD the risk of fracture increases two- to threefold.[17] This risk is multiplicative so that, for a patient with a Z-score of −3, the risk of fracture is 8 to 27 times higher than that of the average woman of the same age.

The reference range for age is defined as a Z-score of −2 to 2. A value below this range is likely to have resulted from accelerated bone loss. The converse is not true, i.e. a patient with normal BMD may have also had accelerated bone loss. Nevertheless, this Z-score of −2 provides a convenient level to consider that it is likely that there is some disease or drug that is accelerating bone loss and to carry out investigations accordingly.

Alternative approaches to fracture assessment

The WHO guidelines for the definition of osteoporosis have given a pre-eminent position for BMD measurements in the assessment of osteoporosis. There are other approaches to assessing fracture risk that may be less expensive and easier to apply in the community setting.

Risk factor questionnaires
The risk of fracture is increased by a number of factors that are independent of BMD. These include factors such as a maternal history of hip fractures. Such a questionnaire has been developed by the Study of Osteoporotic Fracture Group,[18] and this is useful in assessment of the individual.

Quantitative ultrasound
This approach usually measures a superficial bone such as the calcaneus, finger, tibia or patella. The velocity of sound through bone relates to its density and elasticity, and the broadband ultrasound attenuation relates to density and microarchitecture. This may prove complementary to BMD or an alternative. Once this approach has been validated by prospective studies[19] then it may prove very useful. Currently it is used only in practice by the author's group when BMD cannot be measured.

Biochemical markers of bone turnover
These may be used at the initial assessment to identify those patients with high turnover who may have increased fracture risk,[20] respond better to treatment,[21] or have an accelerating factor present (such as thyrotoxicosis). Their use in each of these settings is controversial and this has not yet become part of the author's routine evaluation. The markers can be useful in monitoring therapy when lumbar spine BMD measurements are not available (see below).

RISK FACTORS FOR OSTEOPOROSIS

A model for explaining low bone mineral density

The patient who presents with a vertebral fracture and low BMD is likely to have had one of four causes (Figure 12.3). It is impossible to know the importance of peak bone mass and the rate of bone loss in retrospect. Questions can be asked about early menopause and about the drugs and diseases known to accelerate bone loss.

Risk factors are usually assessed by administering a questionnaire before first attendance at the clinic, by carrying out a limited biochemical

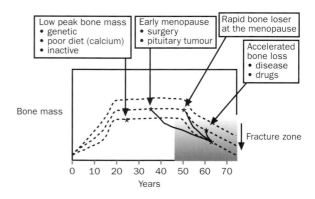

Figure 12.3 Schematic diagram of changes in bone mass across life in women. The broken lines represent the mean BMD ± 2 s.d. There are four important mechanisms which may result in low BMD in the older woman shown here.

work-up before the clinic visit, and after the clinical evaluation exploring alternative diagnoses. The limited biochemical work-up includes full blood count and erythrocyte sedimentation rate, protein electrophoresis, urinary Bence Jones protein, serum calcium, phosphate, alkaline phosphatase, albumin, creatinine, γ-glutamyl transpeptidase (GGT), thyroid-stimulating hormone, testosterone (in men), and 24-hour urinary calcium and creatinine.

Lifestyle factors

The consumption of alcohol and smoking of cigarettes are always enquired about and heavy consumption of alcohol (>24 units a week) or heavy smoking (>20 cigarettes a day) is regarded as a risk factor. Calcium intake (especially diary produce) and physical activity are also asked about. This information is useful in devising an individualized treatment plan.

Disease factors

Endocrine
Sex steroid deficiency is important to diagnose as it is reversible. In the man, a careful history is taken about fertility and secondary sex characteristics.[22] Testosterone is measured and, if low, sex hormone-binding globulin, luteinizing hormone (LH) and follicle-stimulating hormone (FSH) and prolactin are measured. Magnetic resonance imaging (MRI) of the pituitary is done if there is any abnormality suggesting pituitary disease. In women, attention is paid to age at menarche and menopause, and any periods of amenorrhoea other than for pregnancy. If the menopause occurred before age 45, LH, FSH and prolactin are measured. A number of cases of hypopituitarism and prolactinoma can be found using this approach. With hypopituitarism it is important to replace deficiencies in cortisol and thyroxine, and with prolactinoma it is important to monitor prolactin (and pituitary size by MRI) if hormone replacement therapy (HRT) is started.

Primary hyperparathyroidism is a common

condition in the postmenopausal woman and is a reversible cause of bone loss.[23] The diagnosis is made with an increase in serum calcium with a high or high–normal parathyroid hormone level. The only disorder that may be confused with these changes is familial hypercalcaemia (FBH). A careful family history should be taken and the urinary calcium measured (low or low–normal in FBH). If there is any doubt, a family study is carried out, measuring serum calcium in first-degree relatives. Thyrotoxicosis is another common condition in the postmenopausal woman and is a reversible cause of bone loss. The diagnosis is made with a decrease in TSH levels. Even suppressed TSH with thyroxine replacement therapy may contribute to the development of osteoporosis.[24]

Cushing's disease is rare but may present with osteoporosis and has been seen several times at the author's department. Usually the progress of the disease is quite rapid, with one fracture following another in quick succession. The bone loss is partially reversible when the underlying disease is cured.[25] The diagnosis is particularly difficult and includes the finding of increased urinary free cortisol and failure to suppress serum cortisol after dexamethasone. These tests are not so reliable and may be abnormal in other diseases, e.g. depression. They may need to be repeated.

Hypopituitarism results in osteoporosis and this may be aggravated if the replacement doses of thyroxine and hydrocortisone are excessive.

Rheumatological
Rheumatoid arthritis is associated with osteoporosis and is more common in postmenopausal women. The bone loss relates to disease activity and functional impairment, and to the use of corticosteroids.[26] Ankylosing spondylitis is also associated with osteoporosis.

Gastrointestinal
Primary biliary cirrhosis is associated with osteoporosis and is suspected when the findings are of raised alkaline phosphatase and GGT, and the diagnosis is supported by the finding of positive antimitochondrial antibod-

ies. There has been reluctance to use oral HRT, but transdermal oestrogen is used at the author's hospital because this preparation has been shown to be safe and effective by the Mayo Clinic Group.[27]

Malabsorption syndrome, especially coeliac disease, can be difficult to diagnose. If the urinary calcium and haemoglobin are low then the urinary calcium is rechecked and a malabsorption work-up carried out which includes serum magnesium, ferritin, red cell folate, vitamin B_{12}, and antiendomysial and antigliadin antibodies. Pernicious anaemia is another common disease in the older woman and is associated with increased fracture risk and low BMD.[28]

Alcoholism should always be suspected, especially in men. An alcohol history should be taken in a non-threatening way as well as checking the GGT and mean corpuscular volume.

Neurological

Periods of paralysis and immobilization may result in regional bone loss. Patients with epilepsy may be taking anticonvulsants that impair calcium absorption, e.g. phenytoin. If there is any difficulty in walking or bladder dysfunction[29] (see above), signs of cord compression should be sought and further investigated by MRI of the spinal column.

Haematological

Every year several cases of myeloma presenting with osteoporosis are identified. Most cases are identified by the serum protein electrophoresis and urinary Bence Jones protein. The non-secretory cases of myeloma (1%) are suspected if there are a lot of vertebral fractures and the marrow should be examined during bone biopsy examination.

The place of bone biopsy

Bone biopsy is helpful in difficult cases of osteoporosis. The author reserves it for patients with atypical features of osteoporosis, such as several fractures in a young person. It may be useful if the diagnosis of osteomalacia is suspected, because the biochemical changes are not always characteristic. Tetracycline should be adminis-

tered before biopsy to allow calculation of mineralization lag time, the most reliable indicator of osteomalacia. Biopsy is probably not so useful for assessing bone turnover because the site of the biopsy (iliac crest) is not representative of the whole skeleton and the variability of the measurement is too high.

Bone marrow aspirate may be helpful if a haematological cause is suspected, such as systemic mastocytosis (in patients with urticaria pigmentosa) or occult skeletal metastases.

Osteogenesis imperfecta

This familial condition results in fractures that are particularly common during childhood and then become frequent again after the menopause.[30] Attention should be paid during the clinical examination to blue sclerae, joint laxity, deafness and cardiac murmurs.

Osteomalacia

This may present as vertebral deformity and should be suspected in patients with malabsorption syndrome and those receiving anticonvulsant therapy. The initial investigations show an increase in alkaline phosphatase and a decrease in 24-hour urinary calcium. Further investigations show increased parathyroid hormone and decreased 25-hydroxyvitamin D. The diagnosis can be confirmed by bone biopsy, if there is doubt.

Drugs

The most important agent here is corticosteroid. Inhaled steroids are not considered a risk factor for osteoporosis by the author, but patients with asthma taking intermittent courses of oral steroids develop osteoporosis, as do patients with rheumatoid arthritis taking low doses, e.g. prednisolone 5 mg/day. Men taking high doses of corticosteroids commonly become hypogonadal and so a careful evaluation of testicular function is made.[31] Patients taking corticosteroids commonly develop vertebral fractures. The author's group found that postmenopausal women with rheumatoid arthritis on long-term prednisolone had an odds ratio of 6 for vertebral fracture.[26] These fractures are commonly painless and so spinal radiographs should be done in these patients if there is height loss or kyphosis.

Patients taking corticosteroids are prone to fractures that are not so common in other patients with vertebral fractures. Rib fractures are common and heal with abundant callus. The patients may develop insufficiency (stress) fractures of the pelvis (see above).

MANAGEMENT OF SYMPTOMS

General measures

The patient is advised to avoid heavy lifting and reaching. Information on the care of the back is provided concerning bending and performing exercises that strengthen the back muscles. These exercises should encourage extension but not flexion. The latter type of exercise has been shown to increase the risk of fracture.[32]

The patient is advised to take a diet rich in calcium, although care is needed to avoid a high-fat diet if the calcium is taken in the form of dairy produce. Regular physical activity is recommended, particularly walking. Excessive consumption of alcohol and cigarettes is not recommended.

The patient is advised to join a patient group, such as the National Osteoporosis Society (in the UK). This will provide information and support, and arranges meetings with other patients to discuss experiences.

Analgesics

Analgesics that contain morphine derivatives cause constipation and this can be a particular problem, especially as calcium supplements commonly cause constipation. It is preferable to use other analgesics such as paracetamol.

During the first few days after fracture, the pain is severe and in addition to simple analgesics calcitonin is recommended. Salmon calcitonin 50 IU is administered subcutaneously by the author at night and an antihistamine pre-scribed to prevent nausea. The analgesic effect takes about a week to start.

Other measures

Local heat may relieve pain during the acute episode. If the pain is very severe then the patient should rest in bed with the pillows arranged to relax the spine.[5] A lumbosacral support corset is recommended for those patients with fracture in the lumbar or lower thoracic spine. Patients appear to benefit most from fabric corsets in a criss-cross design. In the long-term management of pain, analgesic use can be decreased by the use of transcutaneous electrical nerve stimulation.

TREATMENT OF UNDERLYING CONDITIONS

Endocrine

Men with hypogonadism are treated using testosterone either by intramuscular injection (testosterone esters, 250 mg every 3 weeks) or transdermally. The men and their partners are warned that this treatment may result in increased libido and increased energy and muscle strength. Checks are made annually of the prostate, and the prostate-specific antigen, haemoglobin and cholesterol levels. Sex hormone replacement in men often results in increased BMD, but it needs to be given in a sufficient dose and this underlines the importance of monitoring[33] (see below).

Surgery is recommended for patients with primary hyperparathyroidism because this results in an increase in BMD towards normal. In patients unwilling to consider surgery, or in whom surgery has failed, HRT is recommended, and seems to be equally effective at restoring BMD.[23,34]

Thyrotoxicosis is treated with radioactive iodine unless a large goitre is present, and then surgery is recommended. In patients on suppressive doses of thyroxine the dose of thyroxine is reduced unless the suppression is required, as for thyroid cancer or goitre suppression. This has been shown to result in increased BMD.[24]

Treatment of Cushing's disease restores BMD towards normal.[25] Patients with hypopituitarism are often taking excessive amounts of hydrocortisone, as assessed by the 24-hour urinary free cortisol and serum cortisol profile. When the hydrocortisone dose was decreased it was found that the osteocalcin level returned towards normal.[35]

Rheumatological

It is difficult to know the relative contributions made by rheumatoid arthritis and corticosteroids towards bone loss. Indeed, there is evidence that bone loss is less in patients whose disease is controlled by a low dose of steroids (prednisolone <7.5 mg/day) than in patients not taking steroids.[36] It may be best to aim towards adequate suppression of disease severity rather than stopping steroids. Use of deflazecort is considered in younger patients requiring high doses of steroids.

Gastrointestinal

Transdermal oestrogen is used in primary biliary cirrhosis (see above). The bone loss is reversed after liver transplantation.[37] However, there is a phase of rapid bone loss in the first 6 months after transplantation, which is associated with rapid bone loss and fractures. It is preferable to prevent bone loss before transplantation. Calcium or calcitriol may be useful for preventing bone loss in the first 6 months after transplantation.

Treatment of malabsorption syndrome results in improvement of BMD. Vitamin D deficiency is suspected and calcium and vitamin D supplements are given to patients with coeliac disease.

Drugs

Corticosteroid-induced osteoporosis is treated in a similar way to postmenopausal osteoporosis.[38] In younger patients, replacement of prednisolone by deflazecort should be considered and use of calcitriol to prevent bone loss. This is at doses of 0.5–1 µg/day, taking care not to cause hypercalcaemia or renal impairment.

DRUG THERAPY FOR OSTEOPOROSIS

The drug approved for use in osteoporosis in the UK include HRT, bisphosphonates (cyclical etidronate and alendronate) calcitriol, calcitonin (by subcutaneous injection) and anabolic steroids.

Hormone replacement therapy

This is the drug therapy of first choice for osteoporosis, and it can be used up to any age because there seems to be no upper age limit on its efficacy.

Use of different types

Transdermal oestrogen (with cyclical progestin) is used in patients with a history of deep venous thrombosis, hypertension or malabsorption (or in those women who dislike tablets). Oral conjugated equine oestrogens are used in women who have had hysterectomy (15–20% in the author's practice). No-bleed HRT, such as tibolone, or continuous combined HRT is used in women over 60 years, where return of menstrual periods would have a big impact on compliance. It must be ensured that the dose of HRT is bone sparing, i.e. 0.625 mg/day for conjugated equine oestrogens, 50 µg/day for transdermal oestradiol and 2 mg/day for oestradiol valerate.[39] The dose is higher for younger women, especially if they have a large frame.

Pros and cons

The longest part of the patient consultation is taken up by talking about HRT. This discussion is supplemented with reading material and an open telephone line to an osteoporosis specialist nurse. Consideration should be given to the reduction in relative risk of fracture[40] and ischaemic heart disease,[41] and possibly to Alzheimer's disease.[42] The benefit is noted on symptoms such as hot flushes and vaginal dryness and the increased risk of breast carcinoma,[43] endometrial carcinoma[44] and deep venous thrombosis[45] is explained. A warning is also given about menstrual bleeding (or spotting with continuous combined HRT), breast

Table 12.1 The benefits and risks of taking long-term hormone replacement therapy	
Benefits	**Risks**
Relief of menopausal symptoms	Return of menstrual bleeding
Prevention of bone loss and fractures	Risk of endometrial carcinoma
Prevention of ischaemic heart disease	Breast tenderness
Prevention of dementia	Risk of breast carcinoma
	Migraine
	Risk of deep venous thrombosis

tenderness (usually limited to the first 4 months of treatment), recurrence of migraine and skin irritation with transdermal patches (Table 12.1).

Duration of therapy

Treatment is usually recommended for at least 10 years. After that the risk of breast cancer versus the benefits of ischaemic heart disease is weighed up. If the breast cancer risk is a concern or there is a first-degree relative with breast cancer an alternative, such as bisphosphonates is recommended. In patients who have had breast cancer, tamoxifen may be effective at preventing bone loss,[46] although it has long-term adverse effects such as endometrial carcinoma.

Bisphosphonates

Use of different types

Cyclical etidronate and alendronate are approved for use in the UK. The author prefers to use etidronate as the first choice because it has been used for longer and is less expensive. In patients who have particularly low BMD at the hip or who appear not to respond to etidronate, alendronate is used, although it should be avoided if there is a history of oesophagitis, oesophageal stricture or achalasia.[47]

Pros and cons

The bisphosphonates have few side effects and these are uncommon. Some patients develop skin rash a few days after starting etidronate and patients can develop diarrhoea, flatulence and constipation, the bowel effects commonly being related to the calcium supplement. Change to other calcium supplements should be considered, taking care to provide written instructions about taking the calcium at a different time to the etidronate.

One drawback to the use of bisphosphonates in elderly people is the disruption of their usual routine by the timing of tablet taking. Alendronate needs to be taken on an empty stomach half an hour before breakfast with a full glass of water and the patient is not allowed to lie down.[47] This is inconvenient for many patients. The need to take etidronate 2 hours after and 2 hours before a meal is also inconvenient, but allows more flexibility.

Duration of therapy

The author started to use etidronate shortly after the two fracture prevention trials were published in 1990.[48,49] Patients have taken the treatment for up to 7 years, which is about the same time as the longest of the clinical trials with etidronate. With the bisphosphonates the concern is that, for treatment periods longer than this, the bone may become uniformly contaminated with bisphosphonate with the result that there will be an indefinite state of low bone turnover which could cause increased risk of insufficiency fracture. For this reason the author usually avoids using bisphosphonates under the age of 50.

Calcium

Calcium supplements may benefit patients over the age of 65 when the adaptation to a low calcium diet is impaired. There is some evidence that it has a synergistic effect with HRT and bisphosphonates. Calcium on its own is never used by the author in patients with vertebral fracture. Soluble calcium salts, such as calcium citrate, are absorbed better than insoluble salts. Insoluble salts, such as calcium carbonate, should be taken with meals because fasting achlorhydria is common among elderly people, and gastric acid is required for their absorption.[50]

Vitamin D and its metabolites

Vitamin D and calcium prevent hip fracture in housebound elderly people.[51] This usual dose of vitamin D is 800 IU/day orally to most patients, but if compliance is of concern then 300 000 units of vitamin D by intramuscular injection can be given once a year. The active forms of vitamin D, calcitriol and alfacalcidol, are used by the author in younger patients with corticosteroid-induced osteoporosis and older patients who have mild to moderate renal impairment. The osteoporosis specialist nurse runs a clinic and checks serum calcium and creatinine 4 weeks after starting therapy and then every 3 months.

Other treatments

The author never uses any other treatment: anabolic steroids because their side effect profile is unfavourable, including hirsutism and fluid retention; sodium fluoride because the author is not convinced of the antifracture effect and the side effects of gastric irritation and lower extremity pain syndrome (insufficiency fracture) do not justify this marginal benefit;[52] subcutaneous calcitonin for long-term use is too expensive, too inconvenient for marginal benefit on BMD, and causes nausea, diarrhoea and metallic taste; intranasal calcitonin probably has a better analgesic effect than injectable calcitonin without these side effects, but it is not available for use in the UK.

MONITORING OF THERAPY

Concept of response

It is difficult to define a responder in the treatment of osteoporosis because it is not ethical to observe the rate of bone loss in a period before therapy. The definition needs to be based on information from clinical trials. Information from the placebo group can then be used to define a responder, for example, an increase in lumbar spine BMD that is more than 2.77 times the standard deviation above the placebo group mean would indicate a response (at $p = 0.05$). The author used the information from an alendronate trial to calculate this as 5%[53] (Figure 12.4). The least significant change for the femoral neck was 8%. These estimates of least significant change were made in a clinical trial setting, but are likely to be higher in a clinic setting where quality assurance may not be so stringent. The author's group has used a similar approach to least significant change for biochemical markers of bone turnover. Bone resorption markers were studied in postmenopausal women, giving a figure of 25% for free deoxypyridinoline by immunoassay and 55% for N-telopeptides of type I collagen by immunoassay.

These estimates of least significant change are rather high and may be too large given the current treatments available for osteoporosis which often result in a 5–10%[54,55] decrease over 3 years on BMD, and a 20–60% decrease over 3 months in bone resorption markers. Better response could be detected by making multiple measurements of BMD or markers, or by using a less stringent p value.

In practice, a p value of 0.2 is used by the author, which requires a change in BMD of 3% for the lumbar spine before a patient can be considered to be responding to treatment. In this approach the 3% is a comparison between what happened and what would have happened with

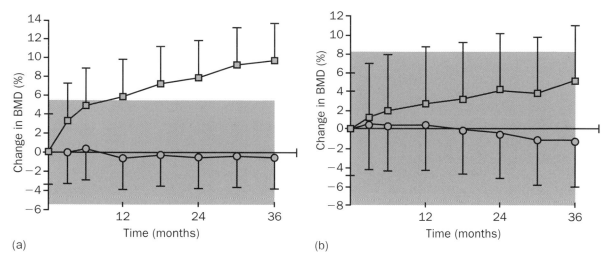

Figure 12.4 Changes in (a) lumbar spine and (b) femoral neck in response to alendronate 10 mg/day orally for 3 years in comparison to placebo. The shaded area represents the least significant change limits. The average patient will be considered a responder at the lumbar spine at 6 months, whereas he or she will never be considered a responder at the femoral neck. —○—, Placebo; —□— alendronate 10 mg/day. (Reproduced, with permission, from Eastell.[53])

no treatment. Thus, in patients with rapid bone loss, such as those just starting corticosteroids, this calculation must be taken into account.

New vertebral fractures

It is important to make accurate height measurements using a stadiometer. A decrease in height of 1 cm or more may indicate a new fracture.

Radiographs
The follow-up radiographs need be taken only in the lateral projection. Identifying a new vertebral fracture is usually straightforward and should be corroborated by the clinical examination and described in the manner given earlier. In clinical trials a decrease in vertebral height of 20% is required[55] but in the clinical setting the combination of history, examination and spinal radiographs (taking into account changes in vertebral height and changes in the endplates) usually makes the diagnosis straightforward. If

there is doubt, an isotope bone scan will show increased uptake in the case of a recent fracture.

The major difficulty with radiographs is the high radiation dose. This makes annual radiographs impractical. They should only be taken when there is a high index of suspicion of new fracture, e.g. typical back pain, height loss or change in shape of the back. The change in appearance of a vertebra on the DXA image may also indicate a fracture.

It is important to have realistic treatment goals. A new fracture does not mean treatment failure. The established treatments for osteoporosis only decrease the fracture risk by 50%.[48,49,54,55] However, several fractures over a short period would be alarming and would indicate the need to examine for secondary causes and consider a bone biopsy.

MXA
The major advantage of this technique is the low radiation dose, as noted above. This is only being used in the author's clinic as a research tool, but may prove useful in the future.

Bone mineral densitometry

This is the most useful method of monitoring treatment response. It is important to examine for treatment response to identify poor compliance, patients who do not absorb the drug or patients who do not respond for unknown reasons. Compliance can be improved by encouragement. Poor absorption of an orally administered drug might indicate malabsorption syndrome. Poor response would indicate the need to change the dose or the type of treatment.

The best bone density measurement would show a large response to treatment and have good precision. The lumbar spine measurement comes closes to this ideal with the femoral neck, total body, forearm and ultrasonic measurements all being poor. An alternative to lumbar spine measurement used by the author is the proximal femur (total hip) measurement. If this is unavailable, biochemical markers of bone turnover are used.

As mentioned above, the figure for a response at the lumbar spine (at $p = 0.2$) is 3%. This will be the response of most patients to HRT or a bisphosphonate at 2–3 years. The ideal timing for the second measurement would be 2 years if DXA is a scarce resource; most patients want to know earlier if they respond, so a compromise can be made by measuring at one-year intervals.

Lumbar spine BMD is frequently unsuitable for analysis because of fractures in the region of interest developing degenerative changes during the follow-up period. It is important to examine the image for such changes at the monitoring visit. These changes are particularly common after the age of 60, the usual age for vertebral fractures. There is a need for alternative methods of monitoring therapy.

Biochemical markers of bone turnover

These markers reflect bone formation or bone resorption.[56] The bone formation markers include osteocalcin, the bone isoform of alkaline phosphatase and the propeptides of type I collagen (PICP, PINP). These are all measured in the serum; the last three are stable and do not require immediate freezing; they all show low day-to-day variation. The response to therapy is slower than for the resorption markers and is maximum at 6 months with HRT and bisphosphonates. The mean decrease after these treatments is between 20% and 40%. The ratio of response to variation will probably result in these markers being most useful for monitoring therapy.

The bone resorption markers include deoxypyridinoline (and its related telopeptides), galactosyl hydroxylysine and hydroxyproline. These are all measured in the urine; they are stable and do not require immediate freezing, but they all show high day-to-day variation, especially hydroxyproline. The response to therapy is faster than for the formation markers and is maximal at 3 months with HRT and bisphosphonates. The mean decrease after these treatments is between 30% and 70%. The ratio of response to variation will probably result in these markers being most useful for identifying early response.

Currently, the author uses the markers only in selected cases when lumbar spine BMD cannot be used to monitor response. They will probably be used much more in the future because they are becoming more freely available and there is more experience in their use.

REFERENCES

1. Kleerekoper M. Extensive personal experience: the clinical evaluation and management of osteoporosis. *J Clin Endocrinol Metab* 1995; **80:** 757–63.
2. Rapado A, Baba H, Maezawa Y et al. General management of vertebral fractures. *Bone* 1996; **18:** 191S–6S.
3. Riggs BL, Khosla S. Practical clinical management. In: *Osteoporosis: Etiology, Diagnosis and Management* (Riggs BL, Melton LJ III, eds). Philadelphia: Lippincott-Raven, 1995: 487–502.
4. Cooper C, Atkinson EJ, O'Fallon WM III et al. Incidence of clinically diagnosed vertebral frac-

tures: A population-based study in Rochester, Minnesota, 1985–1989. *J Bone Miner Res* 1992; **7:** 221–7.

5. Sinaki M. Musculoskeletal rehabilitation. In: *Osteoporosis: Etiology, Diagnosis and Management* (Riggs BL, Melton LJ III, eds). Philadelphia: Lippincott-Raven, 1995: 435–74.

6. Lopez RA, Burke SW, Levine DB et al. Osteoporosis in Scheuemann's disease. *Spine* 1988; **13:** 1099–103.

7. Fogelman I, Collier BD, Brown ML. Bone scintigraphy: part 3, bone scanning in metabolic bone disease. *J Nucl Med* 1993; **34:** 2247–52.

8. National Osteoporosis Foundation Working Group on Vertebral Fractures. Assessing vertebral fractures. *J Bone Miner Res* 1995; **10:** 518–23.

9. Eastell R, Cedel SL, Wahner HW et al. Classification of vertebral fractures *Bone Miner Res* 1991; **6:** 207–15.

10. Cooper KL. Insufficiency stress fractures. *Curr Probl Diagn Radiol* 1994; **23:** 29–68.

11. Kanis JA, Melton LJ III, Christensen C et al. The diagnosis of osteoporosis. *J Bone Miner Res* 1994; **9:** 1137–41.

12. Eastell R, Riggs BL, Wahner HW et al. Colles' fracture and bone density of the ultradistal radius. *J Bone Miner Res* 1989; **4:** 607–13.

13. Marcus R. Clinical review 76: the nature of osteoporosis. *J Clin Endocrinol Metab* 1996; **81:** 1–5.

14. Ross PD, Davis JW, Epstein RS et al. Pre-existing fractures and bone mass predict vertebral fracture incidence in women. *Ann Intern Med* 1991; **114:** 919–23.

15. Peel NF, Barrington NA, Blumsohn A et al. Bone mineral density and bone turnover in spinal osteoarthrosis. *Ann Rheum Dis* 1995; **54:** 867–71.

16. Melton LJ III, Kan SH, Wahner HW et al. Lifetime fracture risk: an approach to hip fracture risk assessment based on bone mineral density and age. *J Clin Epidemiol* 1988; **41:** 985–94.

17. Cummings SR, Black DM, Nevitt MC et al. Bone density at various sites for prediction of hip fractures. *Lancet* 1993; **341:** 72–89.

18. Cummings SR, Nevitt MC, Browner WS et al. Risk factors for hip fracture in white women. Study of osteoporotic fractures research group. *N Engl J Med* 1995; **332:** 767–73.

19. Hans D, Dargent-Molina P, Schott AM et al. Ultrasonographic heel measurements to predict hip fracture in elderly women: the Epidos prospective study. *Lancet* 1996; **348:** 511–14.

20. Garnero P, Sornay-Rendu E, Chapuy MC et al. Increased bone turnover in late postmenopausal women is a major determinant of osteoporosis. *J Bone Miner Res* 1996; **11:** 337–49.

21. Civitelli R, Gonnelli S, Zacchei F et al. Bone turnover in postmenopausal osteoporosis. Effect of calcitonin treatment. *J Clin Invest* 1988; **82:** 1268–74.

22. Scane AC, Francis RM. Commentary – risk factors for osteoporosis in men. *Clin Endocrinol* 1993; **38:** 15–16.

23. Guo CY, Thomas WE, Al-Dehaimi AW et al. Longitudinal changes in bone mineral density and bone turnover in postmenopausal women with primary hyperparathyroidism. *J Clin Endocrinol Metab* 1996; **81:** 3487–91.

24. Guo GY, Weetman AP, Eastell R. Longitudinal changes of bone mineral density and bone turnover in postmenopausal women on thyroxine. *Clin Endocrinol* 1997; **46**(3): 301–7.

25. Hermus AR, Smals AG, Swinkels LM et al. Bone mineral density and bone turnover before and after surgical cure of Cushing's syndrome. *J Clin Endocrinol Metab* 1995; **80:** 2859–65.

26. Peel NF, Moore DJ, Barrington NA et al. Risk of vertebral fracture and relationship to bone mineral density in steroid treated rheumatoid arthritis. *Ann Rheum Dis* 1995; **54:** 801–6.

27. Crippin JS, Jorgensen RA, Dickson ER et al. Hepatic osteodystrophy in primary biliary cirrhosis: effects of medical treatment. *Am J Gastroenterol* 1994; **89:** 47–50.

28. Eastell R, Vieira NE, Yergey AL et al. Pernicious anaemia as a risk factor for osteoporosis. *Clin Sci* 1992; **82:** 681–5.

29. Baba H, Maezawa Y, Kamitani K et al. Osteoporotic vertebral collapse with late neurological complications. *Paraplegia* 1995; **33:** 281–9.

30. Paterson CR, McAllion S, Stellman JL. Osteogenesis imperfecta after the menopause. *N Engl J Med* 1984; **310:** 1694–6.

31. Reid IR, Veale AG, France JT. Glucocorticoid osteoporosis. *J Asthma* 1994; **31:** 7–18.

32. Sinaki M, Mikkelsen BA. Postmenopausal spinal osteoporosis: Flexion versus extension exercises. *Arch Phys Med Rehabil* 1984; **65:** 593–6.

33. Guo CY, Jones TH, Eastell R. Treatment of isolated hypogonadotropic hypogonadism and its effect on bone mineral density and bone turnover. *J Clin Endocrinol Metab* 1997; **82:** 658–65.

34. Grey AB, Stapleton JP, Evans MC et al. Effect of hormone replacement therapy on bone mineral density in postmenopausal women with mild primary hyperparathyroidism: a randomized, control trial. *Ann Intern Med* 1996; **125:** 360–8.

35. Peacey SR, Guo CY, Robinson AM et al. Glucocorticoid replacement therapy: are patients overtreated and does it matter? *Clin Endocrinol* 1997; **46**(3): 255–61.

36. Gough AKS, Lilley J, Eyre S. Generalised bone loss in patients with early rheumatoid arthritis. *Lancet* 1994; **344**: 23–7.

37. Eastell R, Hodgson SF, Dickson ER et al. Rates of vertebral bone loss before and after liver transplantation in women with primary biliary cirrhosis. *Clin Res* 1988; **36**: 395A.

38. Eastell R. Management of corticosteroid-induced osteoporosis. *J Intern Med* 1995; **237**: 439–47.

39. Christiansen C, Lindsay R. Estrogens, bone loss and preservation. *Osteoporosis Int* 1990; **1**: 7–13.

40. Cauley JA, Seeley DG, Ensrud K et al. Estrogen replacement therapy and fractures in older women. Study of osteoporotic fractures research group. *Ann Intern Med* 1995; **122**: 9–16.

41. Grodstein F, Stampfer MJ, Manson JE et al. Postmenopausal estrogen and progestin use and the risk of cardiovascular disease. *N Engl J Med* 1996; **335**: 453–61.

42. Tang MX, Jacobs D, Stern Y et al. Effect of oestrogen during menopause on risk and age at onset of Alzheimer's disease. *Lancet* 1996; **348**: 429–32.

43. Colditz GA, Hankinson SE, Hunter DJ et al. The use of estrogens and progestins and the risk of breast cancer in postmenopausal women. *N Engl J Med* 1995; **332**: 1589–93.

44. Beresford SAA, Weiss NS, Voigt LF et al. Risk of endometrial cancer in relation to use of oestrogen combined with cyclic progestogen therapy in postmenopausal women. *Lancet* 1997; **349**: 458–61.

45. Grodstein F, Stampfer MJ, Goldhaber SZ et al. Prospective study of exogenous hormones and risk of pulmonary embolism in women. *Lancet* 1996; **348**: 983–7.

46. Grey AB, Stapleton JP, Evans MC et al. The effect of the antiestrogen tamoxifen on bone mineral density in normal late postmenopausal women. *Am J Med* 1995; **99**: 636–41.

47. de Groen PC, Lubbe DF, Hirsch LJ et al. Esophagitis associated with the use of alendronate. *N Engl J Med* 1996; **335**: 1016–21.

48. Watts NB, Harris ST, Genant HK et al. Intermittent cyclical etidronate treatment of postmenopausal osteoporosis. *N Engl J Med* 1990; **323**: 73–9.

49. Storm T, Thamsborg G, Steiniche T et al. Effect of intermittent cyclical etidronate therapy on bone mass and fracture rate in women with postmenopausal osteoporosis. *N Engl J Med* 1990; **322**: 1265–71.

50. Recker RR. Calcium absorption and achlorhydria. *N Engl J Med* 1985; **313**: 70–3.

51. Chapuy MC, Arlot ME, Duboeuf F et al. Vitamin D_3 and calcium to prevent hip fractures in elderly women. *N Engl J Med* 1992; **327**: 1637–42.

52. Riggs BL, Hodgson SF, O'Fallon WM et al. Effect of fluoride treatment on the fracture rate in postmenopausal women with osteoporosis. *N Engl J Med* 1990; **322**: 802–9.

53. Eastell R. Assessment of bone density and bone loss. *Osteoporosis Int* 1996; **6**: S36–7.

54. Lufkin EG, Wahner HW, O'Fallon WM et al. Treatment of postmenopausal osteoporosis with transdermal estrogen. *Ann Intern Med* 1992; **117**: 1–9.

55. Liberman UA, Weiss SR, Broll J et al. Effect of oral alendronate on bone mineral density and the incidence of fractures in postmenopausal osteoporosis. *N Engl J Med* 1995; **333**: 1437–43.

56. Eastell R. Biochemical markers. *Spine: State Art Rev* 1994; **8**: 155–70.

13

Pathophysiology and prevention of hip fractures in elderly people

M-C Chapuy and PJ Meunier

CONTENTS • **Pathophysiology of hip fractures** • **Prevention of falls** • **Prevention of bone fragility** • **Conclusions**

As a result of the marked increase in life expectancy, the number of elderly people has progressively grown and this demographic change has an important health policy consequence related to the increasing number of fractures occurring in elderly people. The lifetime risk of hip fracture in a 50-year-old woman is about 18% and this risk increases exponentially after 70 years,[1] the incidence in women at all ages being about twice that in men. In addition, during the past 20 years the age incidence for hip fracture in European countries has increased[2] and the number of hip fractures in men has also progressively increased. For all these reasons, projections indicate that the number of hip fractures occurring in the world each year will rise from 1.66 million in 1990 to 6.26 million by 2050. It is well known that the fractures in elderly people represent a major cause of mortality, morbidity and cost. As an example, costs are expected to increase in the USA from US$7 billion in 1986 to US$62 billion by the year 2020.[3]

As a consequence, preventive strategies are urgently required and research for such strategies should become a priority in the field of osteoporosis. Precise and accurate non-invasive methods of bone measurements can now detect the risk of osteoporosis and hip fracture early.

The relationship between densitometric and ultrasonic parameters and the risk of subsequent osteoporotic fractures have been confirmed by several prospective studies.[4–6] Biochemically, measurement of serum calciotropic hormones can also be a useful tool for the evaluation of risk factors for fractures. The prediction of fractures on the basis of bone turnover marker values is not completely validated but recent published data are encouraging.[7]

The purposes of this chapter are to review the pathophysiological mechanisms leading to hip fractures in older people and the relative merits of the different strategies for preventing falls and cortical bone loss which are the two major determinants of these fractures (Table 13.1).

PATHOPHYSIOLOGY OF HIP FRACTURES

Falls

The vast majority of hip fractures are induced by a fall from standing height or less in men and women (90%). A minority of fractures result from specific lesions of the femur.[8] Falls are a relatively common event among elderly

---

Table 13.1 Risk factors for hip fracture

Fall

Reduced protective response
    Neuromuscular impairment
    Visual impairment
    Neurological disorders
    Decreased postural balance
    Increased in reaction time
Low energy absorption
    Low body weight

Increased bone fragility

Low bone mass
Senile secondary hyperparathyroidism

---

people; around 30% of community dwelling elderly people fall once or several times each year and, in institutionalized elderly people the proportion of those who fall is higher and reaches about 40–50% per year.[9] The percentage of elderly people who fall increases more steeply with age after 75 years: about 3–5% of falls result in a fracture but only 1% result in a hip fracture.[10] During a fall, the risk of fracture, and especially of hip fracture, depends on orientation of the defensive responses, structures surrounding the hip and bone strength.

The point of impact of a fall influences the type of fracture; old people generally fall sideways, straight down or on the hip while walking slowly, and so the risk of hip fracture is high.[11] During the fall, the effectiveness of reflex actions depends on the speed of reaction and the strength of the muscles initiating the protective movement.[12] Ageing leads to a decrease of postural balance and an increase in reaction time, which does not allow a change in orientation of the fall and a reduction in its energy. The protective response is altered by several diseases that may cause falls: neuromuscular impairment (e.g. reduction in gait speed, lower

limb dysfunction), visual impairment, and neurological disorders such as Parkinson's disease.[10,13–16] The use of psychotropic medications (hypnotics, anxiolytics antidepressive and antipsychotics) are associated with increased risk of falls.[10–13] In the EPIDOS study, however, current use of psychotropic drugs was not an independent predictor of hip fracture, possible because, in France, psychotropic drugs are prescribed less often to frail old patients than in other countries.[16] For Tinetti[10] the use of benzodiazepines, phenothiazines and antidepressants was associated with falling independently of other risk factors, including dementia and depression, the two diseases for which these drugs are most commonly prescribed in elderly people.

Other drugs such as diuretics and hypotensives may cause a propensity to fall. Vitamin D deficiency and even vitamin D insufficiency, very frequent in elderly people, could cause muscle weakness and disability of the lower extremities.[17] The risk of falling increased in a linear fashion with the number of risk factors, suggesting that the predisposition to fall may result from the accumulated effect of multiple disabilities.

Energy absorption rather than bone strength has been suggested as one of the main determinants of fractures, with insufficient soft tissue energy dissipation during the fall.[18] A lower prevalence of injury on falling occurs in people with higher body weight[14,18,19] and when the fall occurs on a not too hard surface.[19] A possible explanation for the association between fracture and body weight includes greater bone mass in heavier people, the conversion of adrenal androgens to oestrogens in adipose tissue and the protection offered by fatty tissue during a fall.[15,20] The height of the fall is actually a very important parameter. Lotz and Hayes[21] have documented that a fall from a standing height has enough potential energy to fracture even a normal hip. Even if many of these risk factors for falls cannot easily be changed, medical, rehabilitative and environmental interventions may be effective in reducing the importance of several risk factors.[22] Prevention of falls appears to be at least as important as prevention of bone loss in order to reduce the incidence of hip fractures.

Increased bone fragility

With falls, the other main determinant of hip fracture is a reduction in bone strength, which is primarily caused by the age-related bone loss. Over 70% of bone strength in the hip results from its mineral density.[23] The remainder is largely accounted for by the microarchitecture and quality of bone.

Bone mineral density

From longitudinal studies measuring bone mass and carried out on the lumbar spine, it has been claimed that the bone loss was less important after 65 years than just after the menopause. This conventional view, based on measurements performed on the lumbar spine, is wrong and we know that the real loss still carries on in a linear manner until death. In elderly people, there is no bone loss on the lumbar spine, but there is still a substantial annual bone loss on femur, radius and also os calcis. The over-estimation of the lumbar bone mass in elderly people is the result of the development of osteoarthritis. Until the development of precise and accurate non-invasive methods of measurement of femoral bone mass on peripheral sites, it was also claimed that people who fractured their hip after a fall did not have increased fragility compared with people who had fallen but did not fracture.[24] In fact, recent cross-sectional[25,26] and prospective studies[4,16,27] using dual X-ray absorptiometry (DXA) have actually shown that people who had had a hip fracture had a lower mean femoral bone mineral density (BMD) than sex- and age-matched subjects,[25,26] and that people with low femoral BMD had a greater risk of hip fracture.[10,16,27] Cummings[4] has shown that one standard-deviation (s.d.) decrease in femoral neck bone density was associated with an increase in the risk of hip fracture equivalent to a doubling of risk of fracture, which is equivalent to a 14.5-year increase in age. A recent meta-analysis by Swedish researchers showed that the relative risk (RR) for all fractures increases 1.5 for each standard deviation decrease of BMD at any skeletal site; however, femoral BMD was superior for the prediction of hip fracture: RR = 2.6.[28]

Ultrasonography of the calcaneus has emerged recently as a promising alternative technique for predicting hip fracture.[29] Indirect and in vitro experience has suggested that ultrasonography may give information not only about the bone density but also about the architecture and elasticity.[30] Through the EPIDOS study, which was the first prospective longitudinal study, Hans et al[6] have shown that quantitative ultrasonography predicts the risk of hip fracture in elderly women living at home as well as femoral BMD. The relative risk of hip fracture for 1.0 s.d. reduction was 2.0 (95% CI = 1.6–2.4) for broadband ultrasound attenuation (BUA) and 1.7 (1.4–2.1) for speed of sound, compared with 1.9 (1.6–2.4) for BMD (Table 13.2). The combination of both methods makes it possible to identify women at very high or very low risk of fracture. The strength of bone depends not only on its quantity (BMD), but also on its structure (architecture), both of which deteriorate with ageing. Histomorphometric analysis of bone of patients with trochanteric and cervical hip fractures has shown different profiles. Patients with trochanteric fractures showed a low trabecular bone volume and loss of trabecular plates with decreased trabecular thickness, similar to

Table 13.2 Relative risk (95% CI) for hip fracture corresponding to one s.d. decrease		
	Unadjusted	**Adjusted**[a]
BUA (dB/MHz)	2.1 (1.7–2.6)	2.0 (1.6–2.4)
SOS (m/s)	1.9 (1.5–2.3)	1.7 (1.4–2.1)
Femoral neck BMD (g/cm^2)	2.1 (1.7–2.5)	1.9 (1.6–2.4)

[a] Adjusted for age, weight and centre.
BUA, broadband ultrasonic attenuation; SOS, speed of sound.

changes seen in patients with vertebral fractures. In contrast, in patients with femoral neck fractures, there are minor changes in trabecular bone volume and thin cortices.[31,32] This increased femoral fragility may be the result of several additive causes: a low peak bone mass at maturity, the age-related bone loss occurring in adults of both sexes, the accelerated postmenopausal bone loss in women, and an additional cause of fragility very common in old age – senile secondary hyperparathyroidism.

Peak bone mass

During the first 20 years of life, rapid skeletal growth results in an increased age-related bone mass. The age at which the skeleton reaches its maximal BMD appears to range between 18 and 25 years. Many factors account for this bone mass, such as heredity which is the most important determinant accounting for about 80% of the variability, but also exercise and calcium intake. It is evident that the higher the peak bone mass, the lower the risk of fracture in old age.

Age-related bone loss

In 1983, Riggs and Melton[33] hypothesized that involutional osteoporosis was, in fact, heterogeneous and could be subdivided into two distinct syndromes: type I (postmenopausal) osteoporosis responsible for wrist and vertebral fractures and mainly caused by oestrogen deficiency, and type II (age-related) osteoporosis.[33] Type II osteoporosis occurs in both sexes, becomes increasingly more prevalent with ageing, and is associated with hip fracture and also with proximal humerus, tibia and pelvis fractures.

The two most important factors causing age-related osteoporosis in elderly people are impaired bone formation at the cellular level, and increased bone turnover caused by either oestrogen deficiency or secondary hyperparathyroidism.[34] Histomorphometric data have demonstrated that there was a decreased bone formation at the tissue level with ageing, most probably caused by a decrease in the number of osteoblasts or their decreased responsiveness to growth factors and cytokines,

by a depletion of other cells necessary for the continuous supply of osteoblasts for normal formation or by combinations of all these abnormalities.[34] In women, postmenopausal bone loss is an additional factor of hip fracture and prolonged oestrogen replacement therapy has been shown to be capable of decreasing bone turnover[35] and hip fracture incidence.[36,37]

Senile secondary hyperparathyroidism (Figure 13.1)

Many studies reviewed in a recent paper[24] have shown an increase in parathyroid hormone (PTH) concentrations with ageing, in elderly people living either at home or in an institution. This senile hyperparathyroidism, which has been mentioned by Riggs and Melton[33] as a potential pathophysiological factor of type II or senile osteoporosis, is secondary to the combination of decreased calcium absorption, decreased calcium intake and vitamin D insufficiency. The net result of such alterations is an increase in PTH secretion leading to an increased bone turnover and bone loss, particularly in cortical bone.[33,38] The responsibility of

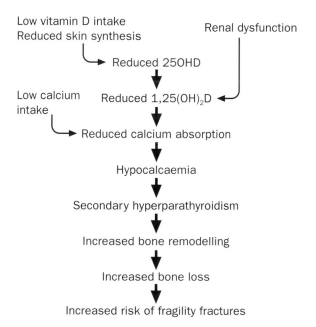

Figure 13.1 Pathophysiological mechanism of senile secondary hyperparathyroidism.

this senile secondary hyperparathyroidism for femoral fragility has been suggested by the higher PTH levels found in patients with hip fractures than in matched controls[39-41] and by histomorphometric studies of iliac crest biopsies, which have shown an increase in value of resorption parameters and a reduced cortical thickness compared with patients with vertebral fractures.[38,39] This increase in values of resorption parameters has been confirmed recently by Okano et al[42] and the non-reduction in iliac cancellous bone volume found in patients with recent hip fractures, compared with age-matched controls,[38,39] has been confirmed by Duarte et al.[43] All these data suggest that senile secondary hyperparathyroidism may play a role in the increased fragility of bone in elderly people.

The decline with age in the kidney's glomerular filtration rate does not appear to be the main determinant of the rise in PTH concentrations,[44] the main causes being low calcium intake associated with decreased intestinal calcium absorption and vitamin D insufficiency.

Calcium

The skeleton provides the calcium reserve, and dietary insufficiency is inexorably followed by a decrease in the size of calcium reserve, i.e. a decrease in bone mass inducing a corresponding decrease in bone strength.[45] Intestinal calcium absorption declines with age and, at the same time, the caloric intake itself also generally declines. Calcium requirement is the main factor controlling calcium balance; it is defined as the amount of dietary calcium required to cover obligatory losses and match the mineral required for bone accretion. The Consensus Development Conference on optimal calcium intake has recommended a daily intake of 1500 mg/day for subjects aged 65 years or over,[46] but the calcium intake in older subjects is generally lower, in the range of 500–600 mg/day in Europe and the USA.[47,48] A significant independent inverse association of dietary calcium with subsequent risk of hip fracture has been demonstrated in several studies.

The well-known Yugoslavian study of Matkowic et al[49] has shown, in two adjacent regions, that the people living in the area with high calcium content in the diet have higher values of metacarpal cortical area at all ages and there is a 50% lower incidence of hip fracture than in the other area.[49] In a Californian study, Holbrook et al[50] have found a rate of hip fracture 60% lower among men and women with a calcium intake of more than 765 mg/day than among those with an intake below 470 mg/day. In a retrospective study, Kanis et al[51] also found that the relative risk of hip fracture was 0.82 in women taking calcium, and the longer the duration of treatment the lower the associated risk. Another piece of indirect evidence in favour of calcium was given by studies showing that thiazide diuretics, which decrease urinary calcium excretion, lower the risk of hip fracture.[52,53]

Another argument for the intervention of a calcium deficit as a determinant of secondary hyperparathyroidism is the effect of an increased calcium intake on PTH concentrations in elderly women. The recent work of McKane et al[54] showed that a large calcium intake (2413 mg/day) was able to lower PTH levels by 40% to the young–normal range and normalized the increased PTH concentrations of elderly women. The same results were observed by the authors' group after supplementation of institutionalized women with calcium (1.2 g/day) and vitamin D (800 IU/day). This supplementation was able not only to normalize PTH secretion but also to reduce the hip fracture number by 23%.[55]

Vitamin D

The vitamin D status cannot be isolated from intestinal calcium absorption, particularly when calcium intake is low. Hypovitaminosis D is very frequent in elderly people even if not related to the ageing process itself. The vitamin D status is, in part, derived from dietary intake and mainly from cutaneous synthesis initiated by solar irradiation of the skin. A reduction of one or both sources leads unavoidably to vitamin D insufficiency. Many healthy older subjects going outdoors take protective action to avoid sunlight, either by use of clothing and sunscreens, or simply by just avoiding the direct path of sunlight. Old institutionalized people are often unable to go outdoors because many of them are infirm or sick. There is, in addition, as a result of the decrease in skin thickness with age, a decline in the skin's capacity to produce vitamin D_3. As a consequence, in elderly people, vitamin D status depends almost exclusively on vitamin D intake from food. There are few natural sources of vitamin D and vitamin D intake is low in countries where dairy products are not fortified.

In the review of McKenna,[56] the mean vitamin D intake was found to be 2.5 ± 1.3 µg/day in Europe, 6.2 ± 2.4 in North America and 5.2 ± 2.0 in Scandinavia (Figure 13.2). The primacy of oral intake over sunlight exposure in maintaining vitamin D stores over the winter, especially in elderly people living in western Europe and, to a lesser degree, in North America has been demonstrated. In the healthy elderly population living in North America and Scandinavia, almost 25% had low values of 25-hydroxyvitamin D (25OHD) in winter and less than 5% have low levels throughout the year.[57–59] In Europe, the prevalence of vitamin D insufficiency in winter ranges from 8% to 60%.[60] The Euronut Seneca study has evaluated the 25OHD concentrations in free living elderly people in 11 European countries during winter; overall 36% of men and 47% of women have values below 30 nmol/1, the lowest concentrations surprisingly being found in southern European towns of France, Spain and Italy.[60] Recently, in free living healthy elderly women, the authors[61] have found 39% of hypovitaminosis D (25OHD <30 nmol/l) associated with biological signs of secondary hyperparathyroidism and increased bone turnover markers (Table 13.3). The vitamin D insufficiency will lead to a small decrease of 1,25-dihydroxyvitamin D (1,25(OH)$_2$D) because the synthesis of the active metabolite is substrate dependent and will be added to the age-related decline in renal 1α-hydroxylase.[62] The lowest value of 25OHD inducing a normal synthesis of 1.25(OH)$_2$D is still not known. In clinical studies it varies from 30 nmol/l measured by Lips,[63] to

50 nmol/l measured by Peacock.[64] This mild decrease, in 1,25(OH)$_2$D leads to a decreased serum calcium which induces an increase in PTH secretion; this itself stimulates the 1α-hydroxlyation and increases 1,25(OH)$_2$D. As a consequence, the 1,25(OH)$_2$D concentration is not a reliable indicator of vitamin D insufficiency in elderly people. In addition, the cut-off must be reappraised as the basis of definition of vitamin D insufficiency.

According to several authors, it appears that there is a threshold of serum 25OHD concentration below which PTH secretion increases. This threshold varies from author to author, but appears to be higher than the classic lower limit of the normal range for 25OHD values.[65] Currently, vitamin D insufficiency is defined by a 25OHD level equal to or lower than 30 nmol/l (12 ng/ml), a value usually found in sunlight-deprived subjects, although an elevation of serum PTH level may frequently be observed with 25OHD levels above 30 nmol/l. So, the

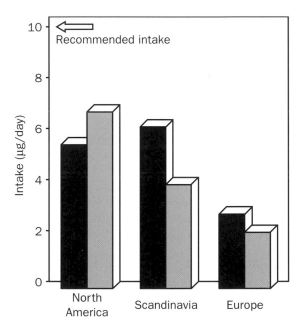

Figure 13.2 Mean of the average oral vitamin D intake in young adults ■ and elderly people ☐ from studies collated according to geographical region. (Reproduced, with permission, from McKenna.[56])

Table 13.3 Comparison of biochemical markers of bone remodeling in elderly and young women during the winter

	Elderly women living at home (EPIDOS Study) $n = 405$	Young women (OFELY Study) $n = 54$
Bone ALP (μg/ml)	15.2 ± 6.2[a]	8.5 ± 2.6
Osteocalcin (ng/ml)	24.9 ± 9.6[a]	14.9 ± 4.4
Urinary calcium (mmol/mmol Cr)	0.36 ± 0.22[b]	0.26 ± 0.15
Urinary hydroxyproline (μmol/mmol Cr)	29 ± 12[a]	19 ± 7
Cross-laps (μg/mmol Cr)	311 ± 168[a]	186 ± 108

Data are expressed as the mean ± s.d.
[a] Significantly different from young women; $p = 0.0001$.
[b] Significantly different from young women; $p = 0.001$.
ALP, alkaline phosphatase; Cr, creatinine.
EPIDOS, multicentre prospective study on risk factors for hip fractures; OFELY, prospective study of the bone loss determinants in women.
Data from Chapuy et al.[61]

lower limit of the normal range for 25OHD should reach 50 nmol/l in the study by Peacock[64] and 78 nmol/l in the study by the authors' group based on a recent survey in a large urban French adult population.[65]

Severe and prolonged 'deficiency' in vitamin D is associated with osteomalacia, characterized by defective bone, osteoid accumulation and reduced bone mineralization strength. Frank osteomalacia is very rare and has been found in less than 1% of patients with hip fractures.[38,41] In contrast, vitamin D 'insufficiency' is not capable of causing frank osteomalacia, but induces a histological picture of hyperparathyroid bone disease.[66] An interrelationship of vitamin D insufficiency, secondary hyperparathyroidism and femoral bone density has been found in elderly women[67–69] but also in middle-aged women.[70,71] For Martinez et al,[72] there was an association between low femoral BMD and low 25OHD levels in women older than 65 years. Ooms et al[67] found similar results; the best fit was obtained with a threshold at 30 nmol/l for 25OHD values and a femoral BMD of 5% higher for every 10 nmol/l 25OHD above the threshold. According to

Cummings et al[4] and Ooms et al,[67] a 25OHD level of 10 nmol/l results in a relative risk of hip fracture of 1.8. This increase in bone turnover related to secondary hyperparathyroidism was also demonstrated using the biochemical markers of bone formation and resorption.[61,72–75]

Hypovitaminosis D may play another indirect role in the incidence of hip fracture. With or without osteomalacia, it has been associated with muscle weakness, limb pain and impaired muscle function. Pain and weakness can lead to functional disability which may prevent a person from going outdoors; this, in turn, exacerbates a poor vitamin D status by suppressing exposure to sunlight. Nevertheless, no systematic studies of pain and muscle strength have been performed in an older population before and after treatment of vitamin D insufficiency. Most studies on the prevention of senile osteoporosis and fractures with vitamin D supplements failed to mention the effect on incidence of falls.[48,55,76]

In addition to falls and bone fragility, there are many other risk factors for hip fracture such as a history of maternal hip fracture, height at age 25, weight, no weight-bearing exercise, under-nutrition, current smoking and use of caffeine, etc. The hip fracture risk analysis is additive: the presence of two or less risk factors increases hip fracture risk by 1% and the presence of five or more risk factors increases hip fracture risk by 10%.[77] The addition of a low BMD to the risk factors increases hip fracture even more: the continuation of a low BMD and five risk factors has a risk of hip fracture that is 27 times greater than in a patient with normal bone mass and no risk factors.[78] The evaluation of the risk is important for the selection of intervention therapy; it may also aid in the development of strategies to change or reduce certain risk factors in order to try to reduce fracture incidence.

PREVENTION OF FALLS

The percentage of elderly people who fall increases more steeply with age after 75 years and over 90% of hip fractures in elderly people occur as a result of a fall. Measures to reduce the risk of falls seem to be the first prevention tool for hip fractures.

Until now there has been little direct evidence that specific measures prevent falls, but a series of intervention strategies are now in progress at eight American sites[9,78] called the FICSIT trials (Frailty and Injuries: Cooperative Studies of Intervention Techniques). Definitive results on fall rates are not yet available from all of the FICSIT trials, but the results published to date have shown that targeted interventions are effective in reducing them. In the study of Tinetti et al (Yale FICSIT),[79] the intervention resulted in a 12% reduction in the number of falls compared with controls. In addition, the proportion of people who had a targeted risk factor for falling was reduced with intervention group: polymedication reduced by 23% ($p = 0.009$) and balance impairment reduced by 24% ($p = 0.001$). No single and predominant risk factor has been identified so far and, because of the multifactorial aetiology of falls, unidimensional interventions are likely to be ineffective. Although it is impossible to prevent

---

Table 13.4 Fall prevention checklist

- Check that spectacles are of correct prescription and worn correctly
- Check for evidence of factors that impair walking and balance (peripheral neuropathy, arthropathy)
- Check for evidence of postural hypotension, arrhythmias
- Check for excessive use of tranquillizers, sedatives, hypnotics, antidepressants
- Pay attention to the home environment: non-slip floor surfaces; fairly high illumination throughout the house, particularly on the stairs; hand rails in the bathroom; main routes around the home free of obstacles; beds and seating easy to get into and out of

---

all falls, it is important to identify those individuals who are at greatest risk of falling. Table 13.4 presents a checklist that may be of help in identifying the main risk factors for falls, and includes individual risks and home environmental risks.

Individual risks

Exercise

In elderly people, exercise is supposed to reduce the risk of falling and to have a positive influence on BMD with, as a consequence, reduction in the risk of hip fracture.[9-14] Reduction in usual physical activity is likely to be the major reason for the doubling of age-adjusted rates of hip fracture over the past 30 years, because with increased mechanization our lives have become less physically demanding.[80] The absence of any exercise can result in an increased risk of falls and bone loss. Immobilization should be avoided as much as possible; a reduction in muscle strength resulting from a sedentary lifestyle may contribute to development of postural changes, reduced flexibility, deconditioning of the lower extremities and increased incidence of falls.[81] Exercise such as walking and climbing stairs improves muscle strength, flexibility and gait. In addition, immobilization leads directly to a reduction in bone density, particularly in weight-bearing bones such as the femur; the decline in muscle mass consequent on immobilization reduces bone density further.[80] Nevertheless, there is actually little evidence, particularly in older people, of a positive effect of exercise alone on the bone mass. Presumably physical exercise could have a positive influence on fracture outcome independent of the effect on BMD.

Vision

Elderly people depend on their visual field input to help maintain balance. Visual impairment has been found to be a risk factor for hip fracture and falls in case-control[15] and prospective studies.[16,77,82] Impaired visual acuity leads to inaccurate awareness of environmental obstacles or configuration, and consequently increases the risk of slipping or tripping accidentally. Visual deficit also increases the risk of falling by decreasing postural stability, mobility and physical function.[16] So, it is necessary to check that spectacles are of the correct prescription and worn correctly.

Medications

Medications should be reviewed with the risk of falls in mind; reducing multiple medications may be of particular interest in preventing falls. Use of psychotropic drugs was associated with an increased risk of falling in several studies[15,83] but not in that of Dargent-Molina et al[16] for which, nevertheless, anxiolytic drugs were significantly associated with the risk of hip fracture.

Hypnotics and sedative antidepressants should be avoided or their use minimized, particularly in those who already have a history of falls.

Home environment

Falls can be prevented by attention to factors in the home environment such as: floor surfaces should be non-slip; lighting should be adequate; and stairs and furniture should be easy to negotiate. Safety through prevention of falls in elderly people should be a priority in private and public spaces.

External hip protectors

It has been suggested that the main determinant of hip fractures is energy absorption rather than bone strength, and experimental studies have shown that soft tissue covering the hip may influence energy absorption during a fall; this partly explains the reduced risk of hip fractures in women who are overweight.[18] The use of energy-absorbing external hip protectors has been shown to reduce the risk of hip fracture by more than 50% in a randomized clinical study of elderly nursing home residents at high risk of falling.[84] The main problem with this hip protector is its acceptance (primary acceptance 59% and 18% after 3 months) and compliance, because only 24% of residents given the hip protector wore them regularly.[85]

PREVENTION OF BONE FRAGILITY

In the last few years, the concept of whole life prevention of bone loss has emerged.

The primary prevention of hip fracture

This may be achieved by increasing bone mass at maturity and subsequently at the onset of menopause. Theoretical calculations indicate that a relatively small increase in average bone mass would be associated with a sizeable reduction in fracture risk. As peak bone mass is influenced by environmental as well as genetic factors, the bone mass at skeletal maturing might be improved by exercise, adequate calcium intake particularly in the prepubertal

Table 13.5 Prevention of bone fragility
Attainment of a high peak bone mass during childhood and adolescence
Adequate calcium intake
Exercise
Reduction of postmenopausal bone loss
Adequate calcium and vitamin D intake
Adequate sun exposure
Hormone replacement therapy or alternatives
Exercise
Reduction of senile bone loss
Adequate calcium and vitamin D intake
Adequate sun exposure
Exercise

period, avoidance of smoking and alcohol, and attention to oestrogen deficiency status. Although the precise role of these factors is conjectural, it is important to recognize that non-hormonal (i.e. non-oestrogen-dependent) factors account for the fracture risk because they affect both men and women. Until now no drug intervention has ever been proposed for prevention of postmenopausal osteoporosis or, more logically, for prevention of hip fracture.

The secondary prevention of hip fracture

This must take place at the time of menopause when it may reduce the accelerated bone loss characteristic of this period and, later in life, prevention is still possible with drug-blocking resorption either directly with drugs such as bisphosphonates or indirectly through suppression or reduction of the increased secretion of PTH by vitamin D and calcium supplements.

Hormone replacement therapy
A great deal of evidence from prospective studies indicates that the use of hormone replace-

ment therapy (HRT) will prevent bone loss at the time of the menopause and thereafter. There are many case-control and cohort studies showing that HRT reduces the risk of femoral fractures by a mean of 50%.[86,90] This protection is, however, substantially lost within a few years of stopping HRT, a period of rapid bone loss reappearing after withdrawal of HRT that is similar in magnitude to the rapid postmenopausal bone loss of the controls who did not take oestrogen.[91] On the contrary, HRT continued for at least 10 years results in a significant decrease in hip fracture incidence.[92] Thus, HRT taken for 10 years after the menopause would defer the risk of fractures with age by 10 years. The study on 'osteoporotic fractures', a large prospective cohort study, showed a decreased risk of hip fracture (RR = 0.29) for current oestrogen users who started oestrogen within 5 years of the menopause.[37,93]

The role of oestrogens in preventing bone loss is not completely understood, but it appears to be multifactorial. It affects primarily bone resorption, with a secondary increase in bone formation as a result of the coupling of bone resorption and formation. In addition to the prevention of postmenopausal bone loss and risk of fracture, systematic review of the literature reveals consistent evidence that HRT reduces the risk of coronary heart disease by 30–50%.[92,94,95] The effects of combined oestrogen–progestogen therapy on endometrial cancer risk have not shown an increased risk compared with non-users.[92,96] The major risk of HRT seems to be the possible increase in breast cancer incidence in long-term users for whom the RR is 1.4,[97] but these data have not been confirmed by other studies.[98] A family history of breast cancer is, however, a strong argument against long-term HRT. The major new clinical finding is that oestrogen appears to be especially effective in treating older women (>65 years).[99,100] Bone turnover is reduced as much in these older women as in younger women.[92,100] A strong argument for treating women aged over 65 is that oestrogen should be continued, perhaps indefinitely, to achieve a permanent reduction in the risk of hip fracture.[92,93] The objection in older women is the resumption of menstrual cycles, but this can be overcome by using a continuous oestrogen–progestogen regimen[102] or alternatives such as tibolone.[103]

Calcium supplementation

Calcium, through its suppressive effect on PTH secretion, reduces bone turnover and may increase the BMD. It represents an important non-HRT intervention that can be used in the late postmenopausal period, particularly when calcium intake is low. Several publications indicate that calcium supplements of 0.5–2.0 g/day can reduce the postmenopausal bone loss, at least in cortical bone.[104] Only two studies have measured the effect of calcium on the femoral neck BMD,[105,106] but the only one with a high calcium supplement (1700 vs 500 mg/day), associated with vitamin D (400 IU/day), resulted in an increase in the femoral BMD.[106] As mentioned previously, calcium is probably more effective when the dietary calcium intake is low,[49,51,105] and this effect is not only on the femoral BMD but also on the risk of hip fracture. In the study of Reid et al,[107] run in late postmenopausal women, there was an increase in the hip BMD (2–4%) after 4 years of supplementation. In the studies of Chapuy et al[48] and Chevalley et al,[108] the association of calcium and vitamin D was able to reduce the femoral bone loss. The study of Chevalley et al in particular emphasized the role of calcium supplement by giving vitamin D to both controls and treated subjects, but calcium only to the treated group. In these two studies the total calcium intake was about 1700 mg/day[48] and 1400 mg/day,[108] a value that is in the range of the National Institutes of Health recommendation (1500 mg/day) and of that found by Heaney[45] to be the mean requirement for healthy postmenopausal women. The retrospective MEDOS (Mediterranean Osteoporosis) study[51] in 2086 women with a hip fracture and 3552 age-matched controls showed a reduced risk of proximal femur fracture (RR = 0.75; $p < 0.01$) in women who had received calcium supplements at some time during their lives; the duration of supplementation was universally related to the risk of fracture. In fact, in this study, women who received calcium supplements had also received drugs with recognized bone-promoting effects (i.e. oestrogens and calcitonins) and, although a calcium effect could still be detected after correction for the influence of oestrogen and/or calcitonin, it was no longer significant. The effect of calcium supplements on secondary hyperparathyroidism and bone turnover was recently confirmed by the study of McKane et al[109] who found that a mean calcium intake of 2400 mg/day was able to lower PTH levels by 40% and normalized PTH secretion in elderly women, even though it may not increase BMD or decrease fracture rate. These results are very close to those obtained by Chapuy, who used a lower dose of calcium (1200 mg vs 2400 mg) but added a supplement of 800 IU vitamin D_3 and has shown, in addition, an increase in femoral BMD and a decrease in the rate of hip fracture.[47,48]

Vitamin D supplementation

Supplementation with vitamin D in elderly people, and whether or not it is associated with calcium supplements, is based on the fact that vitamin D insufficiency is very common in elderly people and may contribute to the increased secretion of PTH and bone turnover.

A small supplement of only 220 IU daily has been shown to be capable of preventing an increase of PTH level during the winter and one of 467 IU/day lowers PTH all the year round in normal healthy postmenopausal women.[59] Doses of 400–800 IU/day lead to adequate improvement of vitamin D status and parathyroid function. Using 400 IU/day vitamin D_3, Ooms et al[67] restored normal 25OHD levels and decreased the mean PTH level by about 6–15% in elderly Dutch people. Using vitamin D_2 800 IU/day and calcium 1 g/day given to elderly people living in institutions who had vitamin D insufficiency, the authors were able to reduce PTH concentrations by 34% with normalization of 25OHD concentrations. Vitamin D supplementation also has an impact on bone density; by increasing vitamin D intake from 100 to 500 IU daily, Dawson-Hughes et al[111] were able to make a significant reduction in bone loss in the late winter and to improve the net bone density of the spine.

In a more recent study in older women (mean age 64 years), the same authors[112] have shown that a supplement of only 100 IU daily over 2 years was of marginal value in preventing femoral bone loss, with 700 IU daily giving better results. In the Decalyos study,[48] the old women treated daily, over 18 months, with 800 IU vitamin D_3 and 1.2 g calcium showed an increase of 2.7% in the BMD of the proximal femur, whereas during the same period the women in the placebo group showed a decrease in the femoral BMD of 4.6%. In the Dutch study of Ooms et al[67] daily treatment of old women (mean calcium intake = 859 mg/day) with 400 IU/day vitamin D_3 for 2 years was associated with an increase in the femoral neck BMD of 2.3% compared with the placebo group. The effects of vitamin D supplements on bone loss suggest that the correction of vitamin D insufficiency in elderly people through low doses of vitamin D may have beneficial effects on the fracture incidence. This was the aim of several recent studies.

In the Decalyos study,[48] 3270 healthy ambulatory women (mean age 84 ± 6 years), living in nursing homes, received daily either 800 IU vitamin D_3 and 1.2 g elemental calcium or a double placebo. After 18 months of follow-up, the results of the active treatment analysis showed that there was a 43% reduction in hip fractures ($p < 0.05$) and a 32% reduction in all non-vertebral fractures ($p = 0.015$) in the treated group. The results of the intention-to-treat analysis were also similar: 80 hip fractures in the vitamin D_3–calcium group and 110 in the placebo group (27% reduction; $p < 0.01$). At the same time, serum PTH decreased by 46% ($p < 0.001$) and the serum 25OHD level, low at baseline, was normalized and increased by 160% ($p < 0.001$) without change in the $1,25(OH)_2D$ levels. After a further 18 months of treatment of 1404 women, the beneficial effects of the treatment on non-vertebral fractures were confirmed. At the end of 36 months of follow-up in the intention-to-treat analysis, there were 17.2% non-vertebral fractures (255 vs 308; $p < 0.02$) and 23% fewer hip fractures (137 vs 178; $p < 0.02$) in the vitamin D_3–calcium group (Figure 13.3). The probability of hip fractures

was decreased (odds ratio or OR, 0.73; CI, 0.62–0.84) as was that of all non-vertebral fractures (OR, 0.72; CI, 0.60–0.84) (Figure 13.4). This study has pointed out the importance of vitamin D insufficiency as a determinant of senile secondary hyperparathyroidism and bone loss. Nevertheless, it was not possible to characterize the relative roles of calcium and vitamin D, although this is probably not essential because the benefit of the two nutrients are interdependent. In the Decalyos study, the potential effects of vitamin D supplements on the incidence of falls were not studied.

In addition, in a study by Heikinheimo et al,[113] 799 elderly men and women living either in residential care or in their own homes were followed for 2–5 years. In those treated with an annual injection of 150 000–300 000 IU vitamin D_2, there was a significant reduction in the number of upper limb and rib fractures, but no significant reduction in hip fractures. The reduction in hip fracture incidence reaches 22% (9.4% in the control group and 7.3% in the intervention group) which is similar to the reduction found in the Decalyos study (23%). The reason for the lack of significance was possibly the smaller sample size which might suggest that the results of supplementation with cholecalciferol and calcium were primarily the result of vitamin D rather than calcium.[113,114] In a recent, prospective, double-blind trial of 2578 men and women (mean age 80 ± 6 years) living either at home or in an institution, Lips et al[115] studied the effect of a daily supplement with 400 IU vitamin D_3. After one year of vitamin D supplementation in a subgroup of 348 women,[67] the PTH concentration was slightly but significantly reduced by 6% and the mean BMD of the femoral neck had increased by 2.3% in the vitamin D group compared with the placebo group after 2 years of treatment. Nevertheless, vitamin D supplementation did not decrease the incidence of hip fracture after a maximum treatment period of 3.5 years.

The difference observed in the results of the French and the Dutch studies may be explained by the lower dietary calcium intake in France (about 500 mg/day) than in the Netherlands (1000 mg/day) with the use of a 1200 mg cal-

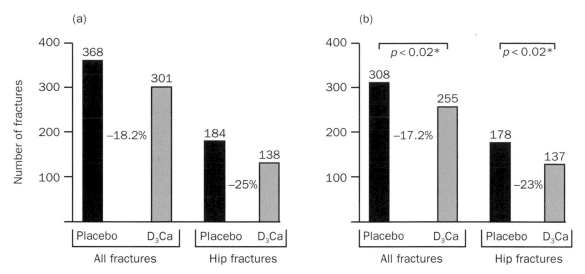

Figure 13.3 Effects of vitamin D_3 and calcium supplementation over 3 years on the number of fractures in elderly women (the Decalyos study). (a) Total number of fractures; (b) subjects with at least one fracture. *Log rank. D_3Ca, vitamin D_3–calcium supplementation.

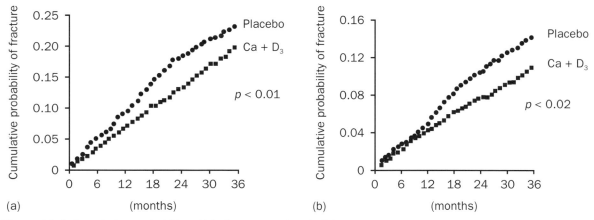

Figure 13.4 Cumulative probability of hip fractures (a) and all fractures (b) in the placebo and vitamin D_3–calcium groups (the Decalyos study). (Reproduced, with permission, from Meunier et al.[68])

cium supplement in the French study. Hip fracture incidence was lower in the Dutch study (29 per 1000 vs 40 per 1000), so its power may have been insufficient to demonstrate significant differences in the fracture rates. Nevertheless, the smaller increase in 25OHD levels and the lower reduction in PTH secretion in the Dutch study compared with the French one raised the possibility that the daily dose of 400 IU vitamin D_3 was suboptimal. These results indicate that a larger treatment effect occurred in the French study.[55]

In addition to these three prospective studies on the preventive effect of vitamin D on the hip fracture incidence, Kanis,[51] in his first retrospective report from the MEDOS study, did not find that the use of vitamin D was associated with a significant decrease in the risk fracture as was the use of calcium, oestrogen or calcitonin. When the data were reanalysed, not including all the hip fractures but only the low-energy fractures, the use of vitamin D supplement was associated with a 26% (although non-significant) decrease in the risk of hip fracture. For women aged 80 years or older, the reduction in hip fracture risk for vitamin D users was 37% ($p = 0.04$) and for those women with a body mass index (BMI) of less than $20 \, kg/m^2$ the use of vitamin D was associated with a marked and significant reduction in hip fracture risk of 55% ($p = 0.01$). In this retrospective study, vitamin D was taken for a time ranging from 1 to 20 years and the doses used were not known.

Supplementation with $1,25(OH)_2D_3$, which is the active metabolite of vitamin D, was shown, in a study of Tilyard[76] to prevent the increased incidence of vertebral fractures noted in the control group, but the effect on the incidence of hip fracture has not been studied. It must be taken into account that the active metabolite of vitamin D may cause hypercalcaemia and hypercalciuria in subjects with high calcium intake.

Bisphosphonates

Interest in bisphosphonates for the treatment of osteoporosis has been increasing in recent years.[116] All bisphosphonates are capable of strongly inhibiting bone turnover, but with the more recent compounds the relative potency has shifted in favour of inhibition of resorption by direct action on osteoclasts.[117,118] Several studies have recently shown positive effects of alendronate treatment which, after 2 or 3 years, was able to increase spine and femur BMD by 5–10%,[119,120] associated with a 50% reduction in vertebral fracture rate. There was a decrease in hip fracture rate which did not attain significance because of the low number of events; however, because there is a 3–6% increase in femur BMD with alendronate, similar to that obtained with oestrogen or vitamin D, it may be presumed that alendronate could cause a substantial reduction of hip fracture. This was recently confirmed by the preliminary results from the Fracture Intervention Trial which has shown a 50% reduction in hip fracture risk in women with low femoral neck BMD treated over 3 years with alendronate, compared with the placebo group.[121] As bisphosphonates are retained in bone, they would probably have a longer term-effect compared with that of oestrogen, which loses its effect on bone loss after withdrawal. Besides alendronate, other bisphosphonates, such as pamidronate, clodronate, tiludronate and risedronate, are undergoing extensive research for the prevention of bone loss and fractures. Even if the newer bisphosphonates appear to be very safe, long-term safety data are not yet available.[93]

CONCLUSIONS

Hip fracture is an important cause of morbidity and mortality and represents an important socioeconomic problem. Given the magnitude of the problem, in the future attention must be focused on prevention, and such a strategy should include prevention of falls and prevention of bone loss and bone fragility.

This prevention starts during childhood and adolescence with an adequate calcium intake, because it has been shown that a high calcium intake before puberty has a positive effect on peak bone mass. During adult life regular exercise and no smoking would reduce the risk of hip fracture. Both these policies can be adopted by both sexes and continued into old age. Later in life, postmenopausal oestrogen replacement therapy has been demonstrated to have a major preventive effect on the risk of hip fracture, and the consensus for the available data suggests that oestrogens prescribed early in the menopause for a minimum of 5 years result in an approximate reduction of 50% in hip fracture incidence.[86,90] Loss of this protection within a few years of stopping should, however, encourage additional prevention strategies among elderly women.

Senile secondary hyperparathyroidism appears to play an important role in decreasing femoral bone mass and increasing bone fragility. It is reversible or preventable by vitamin D and calcium supplements and these should represent a late but efficient method of preventing hip fractures. It is evident that the best solution is to increase the natural supplies – skin synthesis for vitamin D and increased consumption of dairy products for calcium – but a daily supplement with vitamin D and calcium salts can also be recommended on the basis of its absence of side effects and the frequency of hypovitaminosis D, not only in institutionalized people, but also in free living older people. In older people, prevention of bone fragility must be accompanied by prevention of falls.

The prevention of hip fracture starts early in life. At 50 years – the start of increased bone loss – subjects at risk need to be screened. Early detection of the risk of osteoporosis is necessary for prevention because the presence of oestoporosis at the hip (BMD $\geqslant$ 2.5 s.d. below the young healthy population average) is expected to increase the relative risk of hip fracture, at least in the 50-year-old woman. After 75 years, most people are at risk and screening is less important, but the prevention of hip fractures should include prevention of falls by reduction of environmental risk factors, age-related changes and iatrogenic factors, and prevention of bone fragility by calcium and vitamin D supplements. The increased incidence of hip fractures is now a socioeconomic problem that needs urgent preventive strategies for the elderly population.

REFERENCES

1. Cummings SR, Black DM, Rubin SM. Lifetime risk of hip, colle's or vertebral fracture and coronary heart disease among white postmenopausal women. *Arch Intern Med* 1989; **149:** 2445–8.
2. Obrant KS, Bengner V, Johnell O et al. Increasing age-adjusted risk of fragility fractures: a sign of increasing osteoporosis in successive generations? *Calcif Tissue Int* 1980; **44:** 157–67.
3. Cummings SR, Rubin SM, Black D. The future of hip fracture in the United States. *Clin Orthop* 1990; **252:** 163–76.
4. Cummings SR, Black DM, Nevitt MC et al. Bone density at various sites for prediction of hip fractures. *Lancet* 1993; **341:** 72–5.
5. Schott AM, Cormier C, Hans D et al. Total body and femoral neck BMD predict hip fracture in 7598 population based very elderly women. *J Bone Miner Res* 1995; **10**(suppl 1): S146.
6. Hans D, Dargent P, Schott AM et al. Ultrasound measurements predict hip fracture in elderly women independently of hip bone density. The EPIDOS study. *Lancet* 1996; **348:** 511–14.
7. Garnero P, Haussherr E, Chapuy MC et al. Markers of bone resorption predict hip fractures in elderly women. The EPIDOS prospective study. *J Bone Miner Res* 1996; **11:** 1531–8.
8. Cooper C, Melton LJ. Magnitude and impact of

osteoporosis and fractures. In: *Osteoporosis* (Marcus R, Feldman D, Kelsey J, eds). London: Academic Press, 1996: 419–34.
9. Grisso JA, Capezutti E, Schwartz A. Falls as risk factors for fractures. In: *Osteoporosis* (Marcus R, Feldman D, Kelsey J, eds). London: Academic Press, 1996: 599–611.
10. Tinetti ME, Speechley M, Ginter SF. Risk factors for falls among elderly persons living in the community. *N Engl J Med* 1988; **319:** 1701–7.
11. Hayes WC, Myers ER, Morris JN et al. Impact near the hip dominates fracture risk in elderly nursing home residents who fall. *Calcif Tiss Int* 1993; **52:** 192–8.
12. Cummings SR, Nevitt MC. A hypothesis: the cause of hip fractures. *J Gerontol* 1989; **44:** M107–11.
13. Tinetti ME. Factors associated with serious injury during falls by ambulatory nursing home residents. *J Am Geriatr Soc* 1987; **35:** 644–8.
14. Nevitt MC, Cummings SR. Type of fall and risk of hip and wrist fractures. The study of osteoporotic fractures. *J Am Geriatr Soc* 1993; **41:** 1226–34.
15. Grisso JA, Kelsey JL, Strom BL et al. Risk factors for falls as a cause of hip fracture in women. *N Engl J Med* 1991; **324:** 1326–1331.
16. Dargent Molina P, Favier F, Grandjean H et al. Fall related factors and risk of hip fractures: the

EPIDOS prospective study. *Lancet* 1996; **348:** 145–9.

17. Boland R. Role of vitamin D in skeletal muscle function. *Endocrinol Rev* 1986; **7:** 434–8.

18. Lauritzen JB, Askegaard V. Protection against hip fracture by energy absorption. *Dan Med Bull* 1992; **39:** 91–3.

19. Grisso JA, Chiu GY, Maislin G et al. Risk factors for hip fractures in men: a preliminary study. *J Bone Miner Res* 1991; **6:** 865–6.

20. Cummings SR, Kelsey JL, Nevitt MC et al. Epidemiology of osteoporosis and osteoporotic fractures. *Epidemiol Rev* 1985; **7:** 178–208.

21. Lotz JC, Hayes WC. The use of quantitative computed tomography to estimate risk of fracture of the hip from falls. *J Bone Joint Surg [Am]* 1990; **72:** 689–700.

22. Isaacs B. Clinical and laboratory studies of falls in old people prospects for prevention. *Clin Geriatr Med* 1985; **1:** 513–24.

23. Dalen N, Hellstrom LG, Jacobsen B. Bone mineral content and mechanical strength of the femoral neck. *Acta Orthop Scand* 1976; **47:** 503–8.

24. Meunier PJ. Prevention of hip fracture. *Am J Med* 1993; **95**(suppl 5A): 755.

25. Chevalley T, Rizzoli R, Nydegger V et al. Preferential low bone mineral density of the femoral neck in patients with a recent fracture of the proximal femur. *Osteoporosis Int* 1991; **1:** 147–54.

26. Duboeuf F, Braillon P, Chapuy MC et al. Bone mineral density of the hip measured with dual energy X-ray absorptiometry in normal elderly women and in patients with hip fracture. *Osteoporosis Int* 1991; **1:** 242–9.

27. Melton LJ, Atkinson EJ, O'Fallon WM et al. Long-term fracture prediction by bone mineral assessment at different skeletal sites. *J Bone Miner Res* 1993; **8:** 1227–33.

28. Marshall D, Johnell O, Wedel H. Meta analysis of how well measures of bone mineral density predict occurrence of osteoporotic fractures. *BMJ* 1996; **312:** 1254–9.

29. Van Daele PLA, Burger H, De Laet CEDH et al. Ultrasound measurement of bone. *Clin Endocrinol* 1996; **44:** 363–9.

30. Kaufman JJ, Einhorn TA. Ultrasound assessment of bone. *J Bone Miner Res* 1993; **8:** 517–25.

31. Lips P, Obrant KJ. The pathogenesis and treatment of hip fractures. *Osteoporosis Int* 1991; **1:** 218–31.

32. Uitewaal PJM, Lips P, Netelendos JC. An analysis of bone structure in patients with hip fracture. *Bone Miner* 1987; **3:** 63–73.

33. Riggs BL, Melton LJ. Evidence for two distinct syndromes of involutional osteoporosis. *Am J Med* 1983; **75:** 899–901.

34. Kassem M, Melton LJ, Riggs BL. The type I/type II model for involutional osteoporosis. In: *Osteoporosis* (Marcus R, Feldman D, Kelsey J, eds). London: Academic Press, 1996: 691–702.

35. Prestwood KM, Pilbeam CC, Berluson JA et al. The short-term effects of conjugated estrogen on bone turnover in older women. *J Clin Endocrinol Metab* 1994; **79:** 366–71.

36. Kiel DP, Felson DT, Anderson JJ et al. Hip fracture and the use of estrogens in postmenopausal women. The Framington Study. *N Engl J Med* 1987; **317:** 1169–74.

37. Cauley JA, Seeley DG, Ensrud et al. Estrogen replacement therapy and fractures in older women study of Osteoporotic Fractures Research Group. *Ann Intern Med* 1995; **122:** 9–16.

38. Lips P, Netelendos C, Jongen MJM et al. Histomorphometric profile and vitamin D status in patients with femoral neck fracture. *Metab Bone Dis Res* 1982; **4:** 85–93.

39. Johnston CC, Norton J, Khairi MRA et al. Heterogeneity of fracture syndromes in postmenopausal women. *J Clin Endocrinol Metab* 1985; **61:** 551–6.

40. Compston JE, Silver AC, Croucher PI et al. Elevated serum intact parathyroid hormone levels in elderly patients with hip fracture. *Clin Endocrinol* 1989; **31:** 667–72.

41. Benhamou CL, Chappard D, Gauvain JB. Hyperparathyroidism in proximal femur fractures: biological and histomorphometric study in 21 patients over 75 years old. *Clin Rheumatol* 1991; **10:** 144–60.

42. Okano T, Yamamoto K, Hagino et al. Iliac bone histomorphometry in Japanese women with hip fracture. In: *Bone Morphometry*, Sixth International Congress, Lexington 4–9 October 1992, 99 (abst).

43. Duarte MEL, Lauria R, Gameiro US. Structural changes in trabecular bone in patients in the hip fracture. *Bone Miner* 1992; **17**(suppl 1): 254 (abst).

44. Sherman SS, Hollis BW, Tobin JD. Vitamin D status and related parameters in a healthy population, the effects of age, sex and season. *J Clin Endocrinol Metab* 1990; **71:** 405–13.

45. Heaney RP. Nutrition and risk of osteoporosis.

In: *Osteoporosis* (Marcus R, Feldman D, Kelsey J, eds). London: Academic Press, 1996: 483–509.

46. NIH Consensus Conference. Optimal calcium intake. *JAMA* 1994; **272:** 1942–8.

47. Euronut Seneea Investigators: Cruz AA, Moreiras Valera D, Van Straveren WA et al. Intake of vitamins and minerals. *Eur J Clin Nutr* 1990; **45**(suppl 3): 121–38.

48. Chapuy MC, Arlot ME, Duboeuf F et al. Vitamin D3 and calcium to prevent hip fractures in elderly women. *N Engl J Med* 1992; **237:** 1637–42.

49. Matkowic V, Kostial K, Simonivic I et al. Bone status and fracture rates in two regions of Yugoslavia. *Am J Clin Nutr* 1979; **32:** 540–9.

50. Holbrook TL, Barrett-Connor E, Wingard D. Dietary calcium and risk of hip fracture. *Lancet* 1988; **ii:** 1046–9.

51. Kanis JA, Johnell O, Guilberg B et al. Evidence for efficacy of drugs affecting bone metabolism in preventing hip fracture. *BMJ* 1992; **305:** 1124–8.

52. Ray WA, Griffin MR, Downey W et al. Long-term use of thiazide diuretics and risk of hip fracture. *Lancet* 1989; **i:** 687–90.

53. Lacroix AZ, Wienpahl J, White LR et al. Thiazide diuretic agents and the incidence of hip fracture. *N Engl J Med* 1990; **322:** 286–90.

54. McKane WR, Khosla S, O'Fallon WM et al. A high calcium intake reverses the secondary hyperparathyroidism and decreased bone resorption in elderly women. *J Bone Miner Res* 1995; **10:** S451.

55. Chapuy MC, Arlot ME, Delmas PD et al. Effect of calcium and cholecalciferol treatment for three years on hip fractures in elderly women. *BJM* 1994; **308:** 1081–2.

56. McKenna J. Differences in vitamin D status between countries in young adults and in elderly. *Am J Med* 1992; **93:** 69–77.

57. Clemens TL, Zhou X, Myles M et al. Serum vitamin D_2 and vitamin D_3 metabolite concentrations and absorption of vitamin D_2 in elderly subjects. *J Clin Endocrinol Metab* 1986; **63:** 656–60.

58. Delvin EE, Imbach A, Copti M. Vitamin D nutritional status and related biochemical indices in an autonomous elderly population. *Am J Clin Nutr* 1988; **48:** 373–8.

59. Krall EA, Sahyoun N, Tannebaum S et al. Effect of vitamin D intake on seasonal variations in parathyroid hormone secretion in post-menopausal women. *N Engl J Med* 1989; **321:** 1777–83.

60. Van Der Wielen RP, Lowik MRH, Van der Berg H, et al. Serum 25 OHD concentrations among elderly people in Europe. *Lancet* 1995; **346:** 207–10.

61. Chapuy MC, Schott AM, Garnero P et al. Healthy elderly french women living at home have secondary hyperparathyroidism and high bone turnover in winter. *J Clin Endocrinol Metab* 1996; **81:** 1129–33.

62. Halloran BP, Portale A, Lonergan ET et al. Production and metabolic clearance of 1.25 dihydroxyvitamin D in men. Effect of advancing age. *J Clin Endocrinol Metab* 1990; **70:** 318–23.

63. Lips P, Wierzinga A, Van Ginkel FC et al. The effect of vitamin D supplementation on vitamin D status and parathyroid function in elderly subjects. *J Clin Endocrinol Metab* 1988; **67:** 644–50.

64. Peacock M, Selby PL, Francis RM et al. Vitamin D deficiency, insufficiency, sufficiency and intoxication. What do they mean? In: *Sixth Workshop on Vitamin D* (Norman A et al, eds). Berlin: Walter de Gruyter, 1985: 569–70.

65. Chapuy MC, Preziosi P, Maamer M et al. Prevalence of hypovitaminosis D in the general adult french population. *Osteoporosis Int* 1996; **6**(suppl 1): 121.

66. Rao DS, Villanueva A, Mathews SM. Histologic evaluation of vitamin D depletion in patients with intestinal malabsorption or dietary deficiency. In: *Clinical Disorders of Bone and Mineral Metabolism* (Frame B, Potts J Jr, eds). Amsterdam: Excerpta Medica, 1983: 224–6.

67. Ooms ME, Roos JC, Bezemer PD et al. Prevention of bone loss by vitamin D supplementation in elderly women: a randomized double blind trial. *J Clin Endocrinol Metab* 1995; **80:** 1052–8.

68. Meunier PJ, Chapuy MC, Arlot ME et al. Can we stop bone loss and prevent hip fractures in the elderly? *Osteoporosis Int* 1994; **4**(suppl 1): S71–6.

69. Rosen CJ, Morrison A, Zhou H et al. Elderly women in northern New England exhibit seasonal changes in bone mineral density and calciotropic hormones. *Bone Miner* 1994; **2:** 83–92.

70. Khaw KT, Sheyd MJ, Compston J. Bone density, parathyroid hormone and 25 hydroxyvitamin D concentrations in middle-aged women. *BMJ* 1992; **305:** 273–7.

71. Lukert B, Higgins J, Stoskopt M. Menopausal bone loss is partially regulated by dietary intake of vitamin D. *Calcif Tissue Int* 1992; **51:** 173–9.

72. Martinez ME, Delcampo MJ, Sanchez-Cabezudo MJ et al. Relations between calcidiol serum levels and bone mineral density in postmenopausal women with low bone density. *Calcif Tissue Int* 1994; **55**: 253–6.

73. Brazier M, Kamel S, Maamer M et al. Markers of bone remodeling in the elderly subjects: effects of vitamin D insufficiency and its correction. *J Bone Miner Res* 1995; **10**: 1753–61.

74. Szulc P, Chapuy MC, Meunier PJ et al. Serum undercarboxylated osteocalcin is a marker of the risk of hip fracture: a three year follow up study. *Bone* 1996; **18**: 487–8.

75. Van Daele PLA, Seibel MJ, Burger E et al. Case control analysis of bone resorption markers, disability and hip fracture risk: the Rotterdam study. *BMJ* 1996; **312**: 482–3.

76. Tilyard MW, Spears GFS, Thomson J et al. Treatment of postmenopausal osteoporosis with calcitriol or calcium. *N Engl J Med* 1992; **326**: 357–62.

77. Cummings SR, Nevitt MC, Browner WR et al. Risk factors for hip fracture in white women. *N Engl J Med* 1995; **332**: 767–73.

78. Miller PD. Diagnostic prediction of increased risk of hip fracture: a clinician's perspective. In: *Osteoporotic Fractures in the Elderly: Clinical Management and Prevention* (Ringe JD, Meunier PJ, eds). Stuttgart: Georg Thième Verlag, 1996: 17–24.

79. Tinetti ME, Baker DI, McAvay G et al. A multifactorial intervention to reduce the risk of falling among elderly people living with community. *N Engl J Med* 1994; **331**: 821–7.

80. Law MR, Wald NJ, Meade TJ. Strategies for prevention of osteoporosis and hip fractures. *BMJ* 1991; **303**: 453–9.

81. Sinaki M. Prevention of hip fracture: physical activity. In: *Osteoporotic Fractures in the Elderly: Clinical Management and Prevention* (Ringe JD, Meunier PJ, eds). Stuttgart: Georg Thième Verlag, 1996: 99–115.

82. Felson DT, Anderson JJ, Hannan MT et al. Impaired vision and hip fracture: The Framington study. *J Am Geriatr Soc* 1989; **37**: 495–500.

83. Ray WA, Giffin WR, Schaffner W et al. Psychotropic drug use and the risk of hip fracture. *N Engl J Med* 1987; **316**: 363–9.

84. Lauritzen JB, Pettersen MM, Lund B. Effect of external hip protectors on hip fractures. *Lancet* 1993; **341**: 11–13.

85. Hindjo K, Lauritzen JB. Influence of hip protector after 3 months. *Osteoporosis Int* 1996; **6**(suppl 1): 247.

86. Johnson RE, Specht EE. The risk of hip fracture in postmenopausal females with or without estrogen drug exposure. *Am J Publ Health* 1981; **71**: 138–44.

87. Paganini Hill A, Ross RK, Gerkins VR et al. Menopausal oestrogen therapy and hip fractures. *Ann Intern Med* 1981; **95**: 28–31.

88. Hutchinson TA, Polansky SM, Feinstein AR. Postmenopausal oestrogens protect against fractures of hip and distal radius. *Lancet* 1979; **ii**: 705–9.

89. Kiel DP, Felson DT, Anderson JJ et al. Hip fracture and the use of oestrogens in postmenopausal women. *N Engl J Med* 1987; **317**: 1169–74.

90. Grady A, Rubin SM, Petitti DB et al. Hormone replacement therapy to prevent disease and prolong life in postmenopausal women. *Ann Intern Med* 1992; **117**: 1016–37.

91. Christiansen C, Christensen MS, Transbol I. Bone mass in postmenopausal women after withdrawal of oestrogen–gestagen replacement therapy. *Lancet* 1981; **i**: 459–61.

92. Felson DT, Zhang Y, Hannon MT et al. The effect of postmenopausal oestrogen therapy on bone density in elderly women. *N Engl J Med* 1993; **329**: 1141–6.

93. Lips P. Prevention of hip fractures: drug therapy. *Bone* 1996; **18**: 159S–63S.

94. Belchetz PE. Hormonal treatment of postmenopausal women. *N Engl J Med* 1994; **330**: 1062–71.

95. Stampfer MJ, Colditz GA, Willett WC et al. Postmenopausal estrogen therapy and cardiovascular disease, the year follow up from the Nurse's health study. *N Engl J Med* 1991; **325**: 756–62.

96. Peerson I, Adam HO, Bergkvist L et al. Risk of endometrial cancer after treatment with oestrogens alone or in adjunction with progestrogens: results of a prospective study. *BMJ* 1989; **28**: 147–51.

97. Colditz GA, Hankinson SE, Hunter DJ et al. The use of estrogens and progestins and the risk of breast cancer in postmenopausal women. *N Engl J Med* 1995; **332**: 1589–93.

98. Stanford JL, Weiss NS, Voigt LF et al. Combined estrogen and progestin hormone replacement therapy in relation to risk of breast cancer in middle aged women. *JAMA* 1995; **274**: 137–42.

99. Christiansen C, Riis BJ. 17-Estradiol and continuous norethister-one: a unique treatment for established osteoporosis in elderly women. *J Clin Endocrinol Metab* 1990; **71**: 836–41.

100. Hasling C, Charles P, Jensen FT et al. A comparison of the effects of oestrogen/progestogen, high dose oral calcium, intermittent cyclic etidronate and an ADFR regime on calcium kinetics and bone mass in postmenopausal women with spinal osteoporosis. *Osteoporosis Int* 1994; **4**: 191–203.

101. Prestwood KM, Pilbeam CC, Burleson JA et al. The short-term effects of conjugated estrogen on bone turnover in older women. *J Clin Endocrinol Metab* 1994; **79**: 366–71.

102. Woodruff JD, Pickar JH. Incidence of endometrial hyperplasia in postmenopausal women taking conjugated estrogens (Premarin) with medroxyprogesterone acetate or conjugated estrogens alone. *Am J Obstet Gynecol* 1994; **170**: 1216–23.

103. Rymer J, Fogelman I, Chapman MG. The incidence of vaginal bleeding with tibolone treatment. *Br J Obstet* 1994; **101**: 53–6.

104. Dawson-Hughes B. The role of calcium in the treatment of osteoporosis. In: *Osteoporosis* (Marcus R, Feldman D, Kelsey J, eds). London: Academic Press, 1996: 1159–68.

105. Dawson-Hughes B, Dallal GE, Krall EA et al. A placebo controlled trial of calcium supplementation in postmenopausal women. *N Engl J Med* 1990; **323**: 873–83.

106. Aloia JF, Vaswani A, Yeh JK et al. Calcium supplementation with and without hormone replacement therapy to prevent postmenopausal bone loss. *Ann Intern Med* 1994; **120**: 97–103.

107. Reid IR, Ames RW, Evans MC et al. Effects of calcium supplementation on bone loss in postmenopausal women. *N Engl J Med* 1993; **328**: 460–4.

108. Chevalley T, Rizzoli R, Nydegger V et al. Effects of calcium supplements on femoral bone mineral density and vertebral fracture rate in vitamin D replete elderly patients. *Osteoporosis Int* 1994; **4**: 245–52.

109. McKane WR, Khosla S, Egan KS et al. Role of calcium intake in modulating age-related increases in parathyroid function and bone resorption. *J Clin Endocrinol Metab* 1996; **81**: 1699–703.

110. Chapuy MC, Chapuy P, Meunier PJ. Effect of calcium and vitamin D supplements on calcium metabolism in the elderly. *Am J Clin Nutr* 1987; **46**: 324–8.

111. Dawson-Hughes B, Dallal GE, Krall EA et al. Effect of vitamin D supplementation on overall bone loss in healthy postmenopausal women. *Ann Intern Med* 1991; **115**: 505–12.

112. Dawson-Hughes B, Harris SS, Krall EA et al. Rates of bone loss in postmenopausal women randomly assigned to one or two dosages of vitamin D. *Am J Clin Nutr* 1995; **61**: 1140–5.

113. Heikinheimo RJ, Inkovaara JA, Harjv EJ et al. Annual injections of vitamin D and fractures on aged bone. *Calcif Tissue Int* 1992; **51**: 105–10.

114. Torgeson D, Campbell M. Vitamin D alone may be helpful (letter). *BMJ* 1994; **309**: 193.

115. Lips P, Graafmans WC, Ooms ME et al. Vitamin D supplementation and fracture incidence in elderly persons. *Ann Intern Med* 1996; **124**: 400–6.

116. Compston JE. The therapeutic use of bisphosphonate. *BMJ* 1994; **309**: 711–15.

117. Rosen CL, Kessenich CR. Comparative clinical pharmacology and therapeutic use of bisphosphonate in metabolic diseases. *Drugs* 1996; **51**: 537–51.

118. Parfitt AM, Mundy GR, Roodman GD et al. A new model for the regulation of bone resorption with particular reference to the effect of bisphosphonates. *J Bone Miner Res* 1996; **11**: 150–9.

119. Liberman UA, Weiss SR, Brou J et al. Effect of oral alendraonate on bone mineral density and incidence of fractures in postmenopausal osteoporosis. *N Engl J Med* 1995; **333**: 1437–43.

120. Devogelaer JP, Brou H, Correa-Rotter R et al. Oral alendronate induces progressive increases in bone mass of the spine, hip, and total body over 3 years in postmenopausal women with osteoporosis. *Bone* 1996; **18**: 141–50.

121. Black DM, Cummings SR, Karpf DB et al. Randomized trial of effect of alendronate on risk of fracture in women with existing vertebral fractures. *Lancet* 1996; **348**: 1535–41.

14

Advances in the study of osteoporosis in men

E Seeman

EPIDEMIOLOGY

Fractures of the proximal femur

Hip fractures in men are a public health problem, accounting for 30% of the 1.7 million hip fractures world wide in 1990.[1,2] The predicted total number of hip fractures will be 1.2 million in men by the year 2025 (similar to the 1.1 million hip fractures in women this decade) plus the 2.8 million predicted in women (Figure 14.1). The numbers of hip fractures are increasing because the proportion of elderly people in the population is increasing. In some countries, there is also a secular increase in the age-specific incidence of hip fractures, for example, between 1970 and 1993, the age-adjusted annual incidence in Finland of hip fractures (per 100 000 people) increased from 108 to 214 in men and from 275 to 420 in women.[3] Similar secular increases have been reported in other countries, but this pattern is not global. Melton et al[4] have shown that the incidence of hip fractures has remained stable over the last 60 years in Rochester, Minnesota, and has decreased in the past few decades in men and women (Figure 14.2). In the Mediterranean Osteoporosis (MEDOS) study of hip fractures in 12 regions from France, Greece, Italy, Portugal, Spain and Turkey, the incidence of hip fractures was also more variable between countries than between sexes in one country (Figure 14.3).[5] The female : male ratio varied from 3.8 in Seville to 0.4 in rural Turkey.

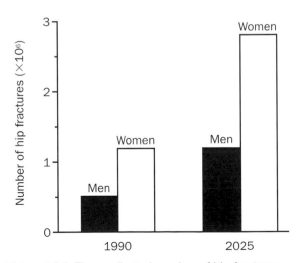

Figure 14.1 The predicated number of hip fractures by the year 2025 is 1.2 million in men (similar to the 1.1 million hip fractures in women seen in this decade) plus the 2.8 million in women. (Adapted from Cooper et al.[1])

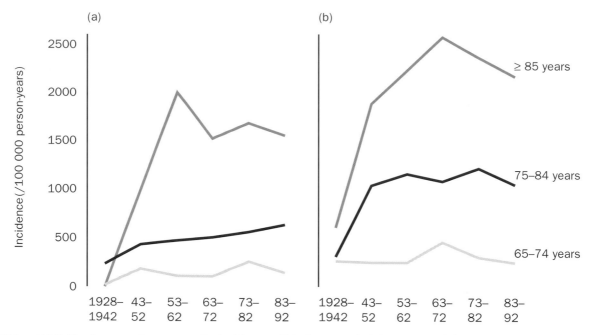

Figure 14.2 The increase in age-specific incidence of hip fractures in (a) woman and (b) men is seen in the 1950s, but there is stability or a reduction subsequently. (Adapted from Melton et al.[4])

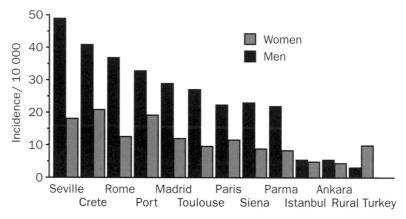

Figure 14.3 The age-specific incidence of hip fractures in men and women in southern European countries varies severalfold. (Adapted from Elffors et al.[5])

Whether ascertainment errors are responsible for this heterogeneous epidemiology across decades, between sexes in a country and in the same sex across countries is unknown but cannot be discounted.[6] Meticulous documentation of the types of fractures and greater attention to the problem of osteoporosis in men may have resulted in identification of a problem that has been present for some time, rather than reflecting an increase in its incidence. 'Incidence' is based on calculations derived from discharge records rather than being derived prospectively by surveillance of all hospitals in an area. Failure to identify all cases within a geographical region may result when there are several health providers or when hospitalization does not occur. Readmission for illnesses, hospital transfers or the occurrence of a second hip fracture may inflate the figures. Small sample sizes, particularly in groups of people aged 80+ may result in an unstable numerator whereas the population size in the age group studied, forming the denominator in the incidence calculation, is often derived from census data obtained some years previously. Groupings into 80+, 85+ are often made, as this is the age at which most hip fractures occur. Errors in the numerator and denominator may markedly alter the incidence estimates. Thus, the rising incidence across time may be an artefact of better surveillance. Retrospective analyses may result in an under-estimated incidence. The lower rates and varying sex ratios in southern Europe may result partly from more reliable case ascertainment in northern Europe.

If ascertainment errors explain only a small proportion of the heterogeneity in fracture rates, and the differing incidence figures are largely correct, then the rising and falling incidence of hip fractures across time from country to country must be caused by the rising and falling incidence of falls and trauma, or by a rise or fall in bone fragility. Likewise, the higher incidence of hip fractures in men than in women in some countries results either from men sustaining more frequent or more severe falls than women, or from men having *more* fragile bones than women in these countries.

The morbidity and mortality of hip fractures are higher in men than in women. Poór et al[7] report the mortality after hip fracture in Rochester, Minnesota; the respective case fatality in men versus women with first hip fracture was 20.7% versus 7.5% among those over 75 years of age. Of 131 men sustaining a first hip fracture as a result of moderate trauma between 1978 and 1989, 91% were over 65 years of age. Hospital mortality was 11.5% and 30-day case fatality 16%. Of the survivors, 41% recovered previous levels of functioning and almost 60% limped or required a cane. Among survivors at one year, 79% lived in a nursing home.

Lu-Yao et al[8] reported that, of the 13 167

femoral neck fractures, mortality at 12 months was higher in the men (odds ratio, OR = 1.7), in nursing home residents (odds ratio, OR = 1.5), in those with co-morbid conditions (OR = 1.7), in older people (OR = 1.1 per one year increase), and in those with pertrochanteric fractures (OR = 1.1). Mortality after 3 months was greater among black individuals (OR = 1.21).

Vertebral, forearm and other fractures

The *prevalence* of vertebral fractures in men appears to be greater than previously appreciated. Davies et al[9] suggest that there is a rise of about 30% with age in the prevalence of fractures in men and 300% in women (Figure 14.4). The prevalence in Dubbo, a community of about 30 000 people near Sydney, ranges from 10% to 25% depending on the criteria used to define fracture.[10] O'Neill et al[11] report the results of vertebral fracture prevalence among 15 570 men and women aged 50–79 years recruited from 36 centres in 19 European countries.[11] Prevalence of vertebral deformity was 20% in each sex by the Eastell method of defining a vertebral fracture, and 12% in each sex by the McClosky method. Prevalence of deformity varied by centre, with up to a threefold difference for both techniques. The prevalence of

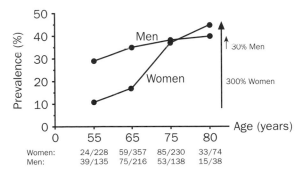

Figure 14.4 The increasing prevalence of vertebral fractures with advancing age seen in men and women aged over 50 years (899 women and 529 men). (Adapted from Davies et al.[9])

deformity appeared to be greatest for both sexes in Scandinavian centres, increased with age, and the gradient of the increase in prevalence was steeper in women than in men. This high prevalence of vertebral fractures in men is contrary to clinical experience, although clinical experience is hypothesis generating, not hypothesis testing. If the prevalence of fractures in men is similar to that in women then the fundamental view that vertebral fractures are the result of fragility caused by accelerated trabecular bone loss after menopause must be reviewed.

The *incidence* of vertebral fractures (per 1000 people per year) is about half that reported in women: 0.73 in men and 1.45 in women in Rochester, Minnesota, not one-tenth that usually reported.[12] The age-specific incidence of vertebral fractures is about 1.5/100 per year in both men and women aged around 80 years, but drops sharply in men in groups aged under 75 years (Figure 14.5). Thus, increased surveillance and awareness of the possibility that fractures are common in men may reveal the presence of a previously 'silent' or unnoticed public health problem just as has occurred in women.

The incidence of forearm fractures is low in men. The rates (per 10 000 per year) were 9 in men and 42 in women in the Trent region in the UK.[2] In Malmö, Sweden, 84 of 934 forearm fractures occurred in men.[13] The fractures are rarely fatal, and do not require hospital admission. Fractures at other sites such as the ribs, humerus, tibia and pelvis make a substantial contribution to the burden of fractures and reflect underlying bone fragility in need of prevention and treatment.

PATHOGENESIS OF BONE FRAGILITY

The risk of fracture is a function of the breaking strength of bone and the severity of the trauma. The incidence of fractures in men and women increases with advancing age as a result of the age-related increase in bone fragility and an increase in the frequency and severity of falls. Fractures occur less commonly in men than in women, less commonly in black than in white men, and less commonly in black than in white women because bone fragility is less, or trauma is less severe, in the first of each pair.

The mechanisms that may contribute to the lower bone fragility in men than in women include:[14–16]

- a higher peak bone mass and size (cross-sectional area)
- less bone loss as a percentage of the (higher) peak bone mass in men
- trabecular bone loss by thinning as a result of reduced bone formation, rather than trabecular plate perforation and loss of connectivity as occurs in women
- less cortical bone thinning as a result of less endocortical resorption and greater periosteal bone formation
- less intracortical porosity in men than in women.

The mechanisms that may account for the lower incidence of fractures in men of some ethnic groups compared with others have received limited attention. Greater bone strength in black than in white men, or in men of differing ethnic groups, may be similar to the male versus female comparisons above and include:

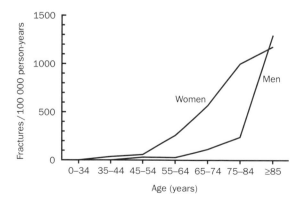

Figure 14.5 The increasing incidence of vertebral fractures in women and men. (Reproduced, with permission, from Cooper et al.[12])

- higher peak bone mass and size
- greater peak cortical thickness
- greater trabecular number, thickness or both
- lower bone turnover
- less trabecular bone loss
- trabecular bone loss by thinning rather than perforation
- less cortical bone loss by reduced endocortical resorption, less cortical porosity, more periosteal bone formation.

Whether these factors are actually responsible for the differences in fracture rates between sexes or ethnic groups is uncertain. The test of the hypothesis is to show that the difference in fracture rates between men and women, or between black and white men, diminishes when differences in bone size, shape, mass, architecture or turnover are taken into account in a multiple regression model. Alternatively, by study design, it should be possible to show that men and women with the same bone size and mass have similar fracture rates.

To understand the pathogenesis of bone fragility and the risk of fracture in old age, the following need to be done:

- Study of the growth of the structural components during the first 20 years of life – the modelling of skeletal size, shape, trabecular thickness, number, connectivity, orientation, cortical thickness to its structural peak at maturity.
- Study of the changes that take place on and within these structures during ageing – the study of bone remodelling, the means by which the skeleton replaces old with new bone, perhaps, in part, to maintain its strength and modify its architecture in accordance with its changing biomechanical requirements.

PEAK BONE MASS, SIZE AND ARCHITECTURE

Total bone mass

Bone size (cross-sectional area) is an independent determinant of bone strength.[17] The reasons why

males have bigger bones than females are uncertain. Although some studies suggest there are no size differences until puberty, the evidence is not entirely consistent. Gilsanz et al,[18] using quantitative computed tomography (QCT) in a study of 196 healthy children aged 4–20 years showed that cross-sectional areas of vertebral bodies were greater in boys (by 17% at Tanner stage I) throughout childhood and adolescence, after adjusting for age, height and weight. Vertebral height did not differ between sexes.[18] Rupich et al[19] suggest that sex and ethnic differences in total body bone mass and areal density are present in infants aged 1–18 months. The 2 years or longer of prepubertal (or non-pubertal growth) also contributes to these size differences as well as the longer and more rapid pubertal growth spurt.[20] However, only 3 cm of the 13 cm difference in height between men and women is the result of pubertal growth, 10 cm resulting from non-pubertal (prepubertal) growth.[21]

As a result of the longer non-pubertal growth in men, the non-pubertal : pubertal contribution to bone mass is 80 : 20 in males and 50 : 50 in females.[22] Thus, a smaller proportion of total bone mass at maturity may be sex hormone-dependent in men than in women. If so, then hypogonadism should result in less bone loss (as a percentage of peak) in men than in women. This assumes then there is a finite amount of sex hormone-dependent bone present, and that this amount is established at puberty (and partly during adrenarche perhaps). Likewise, delayed puberty should have a less deleterious effect in males than in females (assuming that any deficit incurred in bone mass, size or density is irreversible even when puberty finally occurs).

Of the 450 g higher bone mass in old age a greater proportion, in men than in women, is the result of the greater net amount of bone gained during growth than lost during ageing. Men gain 300 g more bone calcium during growth than women (1200 − 900 g). Net loss in men is only about 100 g during ageing and about 250 g in women. Thus, of the 450 g (1100 − 650 g) difference in total bone calcium in elderly men than in women, 300 g is the result of the greater net gain whereas only 150 g

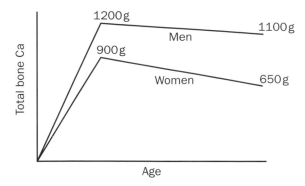

Figure 14.6 Men gain 300 g more bone calcium than women and lose less bone. Of the 450 g difference in bone mass at the end of life, 300 g results from the greater net gain whereas only 150 g results from the lesser amount lost. (Adapted from Seeman et al.[16])

is the result of the lesser net amount of bone lost (Figure 14.6).

Similar observations apply to comparisons of ethnic groups.[23] However, differences in total bone mass in old age – when fractures occur – are constituted by different combinations of bone gain and loss. For example, comparing the total bone mass of the proximal femur in old age in white, black and Mexican Americans, first for men versus women, then in black people, the higher bone mass in old age in men is the result of greater gain in men, which is partly offset by the greater net *loss in men* than women. In white and Mexican Americans, men have a higher bone mass than women in old age because they gain more and lose less. Second, for men versus men, black men have higher bone mass than white men in old age because they gain more and lose similar amounts. Black American men have higher bone mass than Mexican American men because they gain more but lose more, attenuating the difference in peak bone mass. White men gain more than Mexican American men but *lose* more, so Mexican American men have *higher bone mass* than white men in old age. Third, for women versus women, black women had higher bone mass in old age than white or

Mexican American women because they gain more and lose less. White women had the same bone mass as Mexican American women in old age because they gain more but lose more. The differing contributions of the earlier gain and later loss to bone mass in old age within and between sexes and ethnic groups are apparent. The gains and losses are net changes: the relative contributions of the endosteal and periosteal surface modelling and remodelling to *both* peak bone mass and net bone loss are unknown.

Volumetric density

The greater amount of bone gained during growth in men than in women of the same ethnic group, or in men or women of differing ethnic groups, may allow building of a bigger skeleton but not necessarily a denser skeleton. For volumetric density (the amount of bone contained within the bone) to increase during growth, increase in bone mass must be greater than the increase in bone size. For cortical bone, the volumetric bone density will increase if cortical thickness increases more greatly than the increase in external volume of the long bone containing it. For volumetric trabecular bone density of the vertebral body to increase, the increase in trabecular number or thickness must be greater than the increase in the vertebral body volume. The answers:

- Does the volumetric density of a region increase during growth?
- If so, does volumetric density increase more in men than in women, so resulting in a higher volumetric density in men?
- Does volumetric density increase more in men of one ethnic group than another?
- Does volumetric density increase more in women of one ethnic group than another?

Cortical thickness – periosteal growth and endosteal growth

Areal bone density increases during growth because size increases. Volumetric bone density is independent of age, at least in cortical bone, such as the midfemur, i.e. the proportion of bone contained within the bone is constant – increasing in proportion to the increase in bone size. Men and women are likely to have the same cortical thickness if they have the same bone size. If the male has a bigger bone, the cortical thickness is likely to be greater commensurate with the larger size. The failure of densitometric methods to account for size has led to the erroneous view that cortical bone density increases during growth. This view is prevalent because of the conventional graphic display of areal bone density increasing with age as shown in Figure 14.7.[24] When size is

taken into account, the amount of bone in the enlarging long bone is constant – volumetric bone density is independent of age because the increase in bone mineral mass and the increase in bone size are proportional. If this is true, then the factors that determine whether an individual has a higher or lower volumetric density must do so early in development, perhaps before birth.

Cortical thickness is established by the growth of cortical bone size with expansion of the periosteal surface and endosteal surface. In boys, periosteal diameter increases with advancing age and accelerates at puberty. In girls, the increase in periosteal diameter

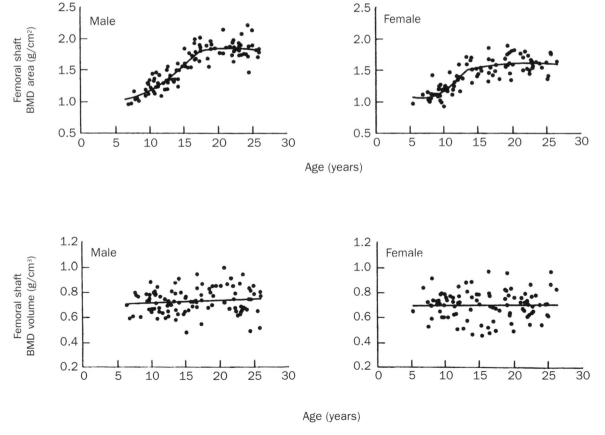

Figure 14.7 Areal and volumetric femoral shaft bone mineral density (BMD) plotted against age for males and females. (Reproduced, with permission, from Lu et al.[24])

ceases at puberty as the epiphyses close, but endocortical (or medullary) diameter decreases as endosteal bone formation occurs. In this way, periosteal growth accounts for about 80% of cortical width in men and endosteal growth contributes 20%. In girls, cortical thickness results from periosteal growth (65%) and endocortical bone formation (35%) – an oestrogen-dependent process.[25] Similar proportional contributions were found in children from Central and North America.[26] The proportional contributions in black and Asian individuals has not been studied. These two components of cortical thickness are likely to be regulated differently in females and males.[27] Medullary contraction in girls may explain the observation, by Odita,[28] in a study of 695 Nigerian boys and 583 girls, who found higher cortical thickness in girls than in boys until the age of 15 years. The temporal sequence of growth may differ from one ethnic group to another. A slower incremental rise in peak cortical area was reported in the cross-sectional study by Solomon in South African blacks.[29]

The different ways in which cortical thickness develops have implications in the pathogenesis of disease. Do some men gain more cortical bone than others at puberty by greater periosteal apposition compared with individuals with the same starting cortical mass and size? Do black men have bigger bone size because their periosteal growth is greater? If so, what regulates this growth? Are the interactions between the growth hormone–insulin-like growth factor I (IGF-I) axis and sex steroids different in black and white men (and women)? Individuals who gain a greater proportion of their peak bone mass at puberty may then lose more bone should hypogonadism result.

Delayed puberty in males may result in reduced bone size (width) because periosteal growth is testosterone dependent. Whether delayed puberty results in reduced volumetric bone density – the amount of bone in bone – remains uncertain. If so, this must be the result of reduced cortical thickness in cortical bone, and reduced trabecular numbers and/or thickness in trabecular bone. The only study examining volumetric density in adult men with a history of delayed puberty suggests that volumetric density was normal.[30] This contrasts with studies by Finkelstein et al[31,32] suggesting that men with constitutionally delayed puberty may have a low peak areal bone density in adulthood. There were two control groups: 21 men 2 years younger and 39 men 2 years older than the cases. Lumbar spine areal bone density in the cases was 1.03–0.10 g/cm² less than the younger controls, and 0.05 g/cm² less than the 60 controls combined. Results for the 39 older controls were not provided but must have been lower than for the younger controls to bring the mean from 1.13 g/cm², in the younger controls, to 1.08 g/cm² for all 60 controls; lumbar spine areal bone density should be about 1.03 g/cm² in the older controls, no different to the cases. In a follow-up study 2 years later in 18 men, radial and spinal areal bone density were reduced as reported earlier. Femoral neck areal bone density, measured for the first time, was lower than in controls: 0.88 ± 0.11 versus 0.98 ± 0.14 g/cm² ($p < 0.02$). The subjects exercised 48 ± 104 miles/week. Thirty-five per cent of the subjects ran more than 15 miles per week and 57% were regular weight lifters. The patients may have had hypogonadotrophic hypogonadism, not constitutionally delayed puberty.

The failure of densitometric methods to account for size may result in confusion. If an illness or delayed puberty reduces bone size in men and the control group has large stature, the areal bone density will be reduced because of the smaller size. If bone size is increased (e.g. failed epiphyseal closure), bone mass or mineral content may be normal or high compared with controls of smaller stature whereas volumetric density may be reduced. For example, Luisetto et al[33] reported that 42 patients with Klinefelter's syndrome had normal areal bone density (Z-scores: lumbar spine, -0.5 s.d.; femoral neck, 0.002 s.d., total femur, -0.2 s.d.).[33] Failure to account for size may have resulted in finding no deficit at the proximal femur (probably a larger bone than in controls). Thus, studies during growth must assess bone size, bone mass and volumetric density separately to avoid confusion.

Ethnic differences in peak cortical thickness In men

It seems to have been established that black individuals have greater cortical thickness than white ones, and stature varies from one ethnic group to another. These size considerations complicate the comparison across ethnic groups of areal density of predominantly cortical structures. If black men have higher areal bone density than white men (with long bones of the same external diameter), black men must have thicker cortices and/or cortices with fewer or smaller haversian canals. Trotter et al[34] reported 10–14% higher volumetric densities in black than in white people based on their study of skeletons from 40 white and 40 black people. Garn et al[25] studied 4379 white and 1589 black people. Black men had 7% higher subperiosteal, 30% higher medullary and 3% higher resultant cortical areas than white men; whether differences of this magnitude account for the ethnic and sex differences in fracture rates is unknown. By contrast, in a study of 950 South African black and 782 white individuals, Solomon[29] found that the former had *lower* cortical area (and have a lower fracture incidence) than the latter.

There is also evidence that Blacks may have more advanced skeletal age than Whites of comparable chronological age. Garn et al,[35] in a study of 1942 Blacks and 3046 Whites, showed that skeletal age was more advanced in black than in white people by about 0.6 s.d. in the women and about 0.4 s.d. in the men. Height was more advanced in Blacks of either sex by about 0.25 s.d. Thus, comparisons of black and white children, males and females, must take skeletal maturation into consideration, as well as chronological age and pubertal staging.

Comparisons of bone density in Blacks and Whites should also consider upper and lower body segment lengths.[36–39] Blacks have longer legs and shorter trunks than Whites; higher femoral neck areal density in black people may be the result of failure to adjust for the larger size. The finding of a shorter hip axis length in Blacks may be a conservative error; hip axis length may be even shorter had adjustment been made by leg length rather than by total height. Asians have similar trunk length but shorter leg length than white people. The lower bone density and shorter hip axis length reported in Japanese after adjustment for total height compared with Whites may not be observed after adjustment for leg length.

There are secular trends in upper and lower body segment lengths in Whites, Blacks and Asians.[40–45] Secular increases have been reported in upper and lower body segments in females and males. However, in some studies, secular trends were confined to one sex or one body segment. Within a community, secular trends were found in the lower, but not the higher, socioeconomic groups. Secular increases in hip axis length may parallel the changes in segment lengths. There is a secular decrease in age at puberty. Later age at puberty does not appear to result in a difference in final height, but it may contribute to changes in upper and lower body proportions. Later epiphyseal fusion may result in longer leg length; earlier epiphyseal fusion may result in shorter leg length and longer trunk length. Girls with precocious puberty have reduced height, particularly leg length and perhaps increased areal bone density as a result of the earlier maturation of the skeleton. Whether they have increased volumetric density is unknown.

The incidence of hip fractures varies markedly across Europe and across different continents.[5] These patterns may vary more between countries than between sexes. There are secular increases and decreases in hip fracture incidence during the past 50 years which vary from country to country.[4] We know little about the factors responsible for this perplexing epidemiological heterogeneity. Secular changes in the patterns of falls, the magnitude of bone loss during ageing, factors regulating peak bone mass, size, shape, volumetric density, body proportions or age at menarche 'explain' the purported shifts in fracture incidence across time, between sexes or between ethnic groups is unknown.

Trabecular structure

In contrast to cortical bone volumetric density, which appears to be independent of age, trabecular volumetric density increases during growth. Either trabecular number and/or thickness must therefore increase out of proportion to the increase in size of the vertebral body. This increase is similar in white boys and girls; they have the same trabecular number and thickness – the same volumetric trabecular bone density.[46] Quantitative computed tomography (QCT) of vertebrae L1–L3 in 25 women (aged 25–45 years) and in 18 men (aged 25–46 years) revealed no differences in cancellous or cortical bone density. Vertebral bodies in women had a lower cross-sectional area (8.22 ± 1.09 vs 10.98 ± 1.25 cm^2, $p < 0.001$) and volume (22.42 ± 2.4 vs 30.86 ± 2.6 cm^3, $p < 0.001$) than in men; these differences persisted on matching men and women for age, weight and vertebral dimensions. As a consequence, mechanical stresses within vertebral bodies are calculated to be 30–40% greater in women than in men.

Trabecular volumetric density is the same in black and white girls until puberty, when trabecular thickness increases much more in black girls, not trabecular numbers; it is trabecular thickness that is greater in black than in white women in adulthood.[47] Trabecular numbers are similar in black and white women.[48] Likewise, neither trabecular number nor thickness differs in South African black men and women, or in Japanese men and women.[29,49] Comparable data in males are lacking but some statements can be made. Black men and women have the same trabecular number and thickness. Thus, if trabecular volumetric density is greater in black than in white men this may also be the result of differences in thickness achieved at puberty. Fuggi et al,[49] using QCT, showed that Japanese men and women have similar trabecular volumetric density but lower trabecular bone density than their white counterparts.[49] These authors suggest that the differences were greater than can be explained by differences in the methods of measurement. Whether Japanese people have thinner or fewer trabeculae than white people is unknown – the lower trabecular bone density is probably in trabecular thickness rather than numbers.

Thus, bone size differs between sexes and ethnic groups – this alone may account for differences in fracture rates but the hypothesis has never been addressed. The mechanisms regulating peak bone size are unknown. The differences in size are present early – by the age of 2–4 years, if not before birth. Trabecular number and thickness are similar between sexes. Differences in trabecular volumetric density do occur in the same sex between ethnic groups and this is probably a function of differences in trabecular thickness rather than numbers.

CHANGES IN BONE MASS, SIZE AND DENSITY DURING AGEING IN MEN

Bone remodelling, replacing old with new bone, occurs on trabecular surfaces and endocortical surfaces, within cortices of bone and on periosteal surfaces. Presumably, the purpose of bone remodelling is to maintain the bone strength commensurate with biomechanical needs. However, remodelling imbalance, the failure to replace the old bone removed with the same amount of new bone, is the morphological basis of bone loss which results in trabecular fragility by trabecular thinning, perforation and loss of connectivity, and cortical fragility by endocortical resorption, increased cortical porosity and cortical thinning, which is partly offset by periosteal appositional growth.

Trabecular bone loss

The amount of trabecular bone lost in women and men at the spine is similar. Cross-sectional and longitudinal studies suggest that trabecular bone loss begins soon after attainment of peak volumetric trabecular bone density. This (seemingly surprising) observation has been made by many independent investigators using techniques such as histomorphometry, ashing and QCT.[50–55] However, trabecular bone loss in men occurs through thinning. Loss of connectivity occurs in men, but this may be less than in women. In women, bone turnover increases with advancing age and after the menopause because activation frequency (the measure of remodelling intensity) increases. As loss of trabeculae proceeds, there is less trabecular surface available for remodelling and trabecular bone loss slows.

Men have the same number of trabeculae of the same thickness as women, but they do not undergo a comparably abrupt loss of gonadal function in midlife. Thus, activation frequency may be less. If so, the amount of bone lost should also be less. However, continued remodelling may proceed by reduced bone formation and without loss of trabecular surface, so that there may be an increase in the surface available for remodelling as trabecular thinning occurs. This may result in trabecular bone loss in men that continues longer than in women. Longitudinal rates of trabecular bone loss in large numbers of elderly men and women have not received sufficient attention.

Bone loss occurs because there is a net negative remodelling balance at the basic multicellular unit (BMU) because bone formation cannot replace the amount resorbed. Whether this is a defect in the recruitment work of osteoblasts is uncertain. Jilka et al,[56] using a murine model of accelerated senescence, suggest that reduced osteoblastogenesis may contribute to the reduced bone formation. Bergman et al[57] showed that cultured marrow stromal mesenchymal stem cells from male mice aged 24 months yielded 41% fewer osteogenic progenitor cell colonies than cells from 4-month-old mice. The age-related decrease in osteoblast number and function may be the result of a reduction in the number and proliferative potential of stem cells. Whether the depth of resorption increases is uncertain. Failure of osteoclast apoptosis may occur and may be responsible for deeper resorption cavities on the endocortical surface of bone.[58]

Cortical bone loss

The term bone 'loss' is often used loosely, particularly in referring to cross-sectional derived sets of data, and in longitudinal data when there has been a fall in areal bone density. The 150 g less total bone 'loss' in men than in women is the net result of less endocortical bone resorption, greater periosteal appositional growth and less intracortical porosity in men than in women. The greater periosteal appositional growth results in a larger cross-sectional area of bone, which confers greater bending strength independent of its mass.[17] From the data by Ruff and Hayes,[17] there was little change in bending strength in men, suggesting that this was an important means of maintaining bone strength in the face of continued bone loss. If so, its regulators need to be understood and drugs aimed at increasing periosteal bone growth may result in a restoration of strength or maintenance of strength even with small gains in bone mass.

The finding that periosteal apposition at the vertebral body and midfemur occurs in men but not in women, or less so in women, suggests that this process may be androgen dependent, or partly so.[17,52] The data are difficult to interpret because periosteal apposition has been reported in women at the metacarpals.[27] Biomechanical factors may be important determinant of periosteal growth and result in site specificity. Secular trends may obscure a true increase; if height and bone width have increased in the past 70 years and there is an increase in bone width in all generations, then the increase in bone width in the 80 year old may result in increasing the bone width to that of a 20 year old. In a cross-sectional study there will be no change in bone width across age. Thus, in elderly people, bone size may be greater in men than in women because of the effects of growth before puberty, as well as the periosteal expansion that occurs during ageing.

Advanced age is associated with acceleration in bone loss. The view that bone loss decelerates in advancing age is based on cross-sectional data. Prospective studies suggest that rates of bone loss at the proximal femur accelerate with age in men and women.[59] The increased rate of bone loss is likely to be the result of continued intracortical and endocortical bone resorption. As this proceeds, cortical bone 'trabecularizes': the cortical surface available for resorption increases. More rapid rates of bone loss may not be found at the lumbar spine, perhaps because of coexistent osteoarthritis. Alternatively, trabecular surfaces available for bone resorption may decrease as trabeculae are lost. Thus, bone loss accelerates and is cortical, rather than trabecular, in origin, predisposing to hip fractures.

Cortical porosity

Reduced cortical areal bone density is also the result of increased porosity. Laval-Jeantet et al[14] showed that cortical porosity of the humerus increased from about 4% in white men and women aged 40 years to about 10% in those aged over 80 years. The fall in apparent density with age correlated with porosity. True mineral density (ash weight per volume unit of bone free of vascular channels) was unchanged.

MEN WITH VERSUS MEN WITHOUT FRACTURES

Areal bone density is reduced at the spine and proximal femur in men with spine fractures relative to age-matched and sex-matched controls. Areal bone density in men with hip fractures is reduced at the proximal femur, but not at the lumbar spine relative to age- and sex-matched controls. The lack of a deficit in areal bone density at the lumbar spine may be the result of the confounding effect of exostoses and endplate sclerosis commonly seen in elderly people.

Just as bone size is less in women than in men, reduced bone size is commonly found in men with fractures relative to age- and sex-matched controls. Vega et al[60] found reduced bone density at the lumbar spine and proximal femur in men with vertebral fractures. Vertebral area was 30% less, whereas vertebral width was 10% less, than controls. Similar observations have been made in women with vertebral fractures relative to age-matched controls with the same volumetric bone density.[61] Femoral neck width is lower in men with hip fractures.[62]

The smaller bone size may be the result of reduced peak bone size, or failure of periosteal appositional growth during advancing age. Femoral neck width increased with age ($r = 0.6$, $p < 0.0001$) and is 15% higher in men aged around 70 years than men aged 30 years (Duan Y, Seeman E, unpublished data). The lower areal bone density results partly from the confounding effect of size, as well as a reduction in the amount of bone in bone, i.e. volumetric density. The lower volumetric bone density may be the result of the attainment of a lower peak volumetric density, excessive bone loss or both. Research efforts will be needed to define the structural heterogeneity of low volumetric density in men (and in women).

BIOCHEMICAL, HISTOMORPHOMETRIC AND HORMONAL CHANGES

In women, bone loss accelerates after menopause because oestrogen deficiency results in increased bone turnover; more remodelling sites on the surface of trabecular bone, with reduced bone formation in each, result in a negative bone balance and bone loss. Bone loss in men is likely to be caused by reduced bone formation. Osteocalcin and C-terminal propeptide of type I collagen decrease with advancing age, as do doubly labelled surfaces from iliac crest bone biopsies.[62]

Markers of resorption increase or show little change.[62,63] Need et al[63] reported a fall in biochemical measurements of bone formation and a minimal rise in bone resorption with age in 147 men. Sone et al[64] measured urinary cross-linked N-telopeptide (NTX) excretion in 238 men and 214 women aged 20–79 years from a healthy Japanese population (Figure 14.8). In men, urinary NTX levels were almost stable throughout life. In women, the lowest levels were observed in the third and fourth decades, then increased by 110% with menopause.[64]

Resch et al[65] studied 27 men with spine fracture (mean age 65 years). Compared with 19 healthy men, the patients had higher alkaline phosphatase, urinary hydroxyproline and uri-

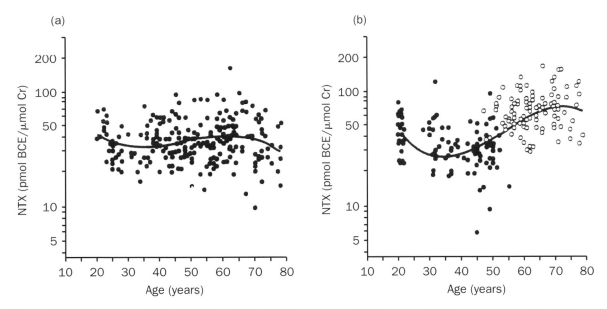

Figure 14.8 Urinary cross-linked N-telopeptides (NTX) versus age in (a) men and (b) premenopausal (solid circles) and postmenopausal women (open circles). Men, $n = 238$; women, $n = 214$. BCE, bone collagen unit; Cr, creatinine. (Reproduced, with permission, from Sone et al.[64])

nary calcium suggestive of increased bone turnover. Sharp et al[66] reported that serum procollagen I peptide, a marker of bone formation, was reduced (125.9 ± 44.6 vs 192 ± 85 ng/ml; $p < 0.002$) whereas serum collagen I telopeptide, a marker of bone resorption, was elevated in 21 men with osteoporosis compared with 44 controls (3.9 ± 1.9 vs 2.7 ± 0.7 ng/ml; $p < 0.004$). Alkaline phospatase and osteocalcin were no different to controls.

Marie et al[67] showed that reduced osteoblastic proliferative activity may be responsible for reduced bone formation in men with osteoporosis. Thymidine incorporation into DNA was normal in cells of normal people and patients with normal bone formation, and reduced in cells isolated from patients with osteoporosis who had parameters of reduced bone formation (doubly labelled surfaces, mean wall thickness, osteoblast surface and mineral apposition rate). Synthetic activity, assessed by osteocalcin responsiveness to vitamin D, was normal. Patients with osteoporosis and normal

bone formation had increased osteoclast numbers, suggesting that increased bone resorption was responsible for the reduced total bone volume in these patients.

Androgens

Testosterone or its deficiency may be one unifying factor contributing to bone size, bone turnover and volumetric bone density during growth and ageing. Testosterone may play a central role in determining the larger peak bone size in men than in women, periosteal appositional growth in men but not women, the lower bone density and bone size in men with spine or hip fractures than controls, and reduced bone formation in men.

The mechanism of action of the sex steroids is not well understood. Nakano et al[68] report that the androgen receptor, a 110-kDa protein, is located mainly in the nucleus of the osteoblastic MC3T3-E1 cell. Dihydrotestosterone and testosterone possessed similar binding affinities to the androgen receptor and both have similar potency on cell proliferation. These authors suggest that testosterone is capable of acting directly on osteoblasts, without conversion to dihydrotestosterone. Mizuno et al[69] report androgen receptor immunoreactivity localized mainly in and around the nuclei of osteoclast-like cells obtained by co-culturing mouse osteoblasts and bone marrow cells. If correct, the data suggest that androgens modulate bone resorption directly.

The sex hormone response is sex specific. Somjen et al[70] show that cell proliferation in the rat diaphysis is sex hormone specific and is stimulated by oestrogens in females only and by androgens in males only, unless gonadectomy has been carried out. Diaphyseal bone will then respond to both 17β-oestradiol and dihydrotestosterone. Administration of the appropriate hormone to gonadectomized rats restored the sex-specific response. Epiphyses showed no sex-specific responses before or after gonadectomy; however, replenishment with sex steroids resulted in acquisition of a sex-specific response in both sexes. The authors conclude that the diaphysis acquires a sex steroid specificity during development, which requires, for its maintenance, the presence of the gonadal steroid specific for each sex.

Schwartz et al[71] show that testosterone dose decreased, in a dependent fashion, the number and proliferation of male, but not female, growth zone and resting zone rat chondrocytes in vitro. Testosterone also increased collagen production in cultures of male chondrocytes only. Alkaline phosphatase-specific activity was stimulated in male growth zone cells, but not in male resting zone cells or in any female chondrocytes. The authors conclude that the effects of testosterone, at physiological concentrations, on chondrocyte differentiation in culture are dependent on the animal's sex and the maturation stage of the cell.

Testosterone is growth promoting. Orchiectomy is associated with reduced growth in size and reduced periosteal bone formation.[72] Testosterone or dihydrotestosterone restore growth and periosteal bone formation.[73]

Oestrogen is growth limiting. Oophorectomy increased longitudinal growth, periosteal bone formation and endosteal bone resorption. In trabecular bone of the proximal tibia or vertebrae, testosterone deficiency increases bone turnover and bone loss. Whether this results partly from oestrogen deficiency associated with the reduced substrate (testosterone) for aromatization is uncertain. Oestrogen and dihydrotestosterone prevent the increased bone turnover associated with orchiectomy.

Growth of genetically male rats with testicular feminization caused by androgen receptor abnormalities is reduced despite normal testosterone.[74] Trabecular bone of the proximal metaphysis is not reduced as occurs with orchiectomy. High levels of androstenedione in these animals may result in aromatization to oestrogen which prevents the increased turnover that is reported after orchiectomy. Vanderschueren et al[75] showed that vorozole, a non-steroidal aromatase inhibitor, reduced bone density at the femur and lumbar vertebrae in eugonadal male rats to a similar degree as induced by orchiectomy. Bone resorption increased by 30% in intact animals receiving vorozole and two- to threefold by orchiectomy. Inhibition of aromatization of androgens into oestrogens increases bone resorption and bone loss to a level similar to that observed with complete removal of androgens. Thus androgens may determine bone size. Oestrogens may be growth limiting and reduce bone turnover.

Haji et al[76] show that serum total testosterone remained constant until the age of 80 years and then fell in 116 healthy Japanese men aged 24–92 years. Serum-free testosterone and inhibin both declined with age, and serum luteinizing hormone (LH) and follicle-stimulating hormone (FSH) were elevated in men over 60 and 40 years old, respectively. Luteinizing hormone was inversely correlated with total and free testosterone in men over 60 years, but was positively correlated with these in younger men. Leydig cell and Sertoli cell function both decline with age. Likewise, Vermeulen et al[77] investigated 250 healthy men aged 25–100 years who show decreases in serum testosterone, dehydroepiandrosterone (DHEA) and DHEA sulphate with increases in sex hormone-binding globulin. Total testosterone levels were stable until age 55–60 years, then declined rapidly. Free testosterone started to decline earlier, accompanied by an early increase in SHBG. Plasma free testosterone, DHEA and DHEA sulphate showed a log linear decrease with age, whereas oestradiol levels were unchanged. Serum testosterone falls with age as a result of a decreased Leydig cell number, changes in hypothalamic–pituitary function and illness. Urban et al[78] showed that elderly men have an attenuated bioactive LH reserve in response to LH-releasing hormone administration.

The level of serum testosterone that may be regarded as hypogonadal in the context of skeletal health is unknown, and may be defined as the level below which bone balance becomes negative. Research is needed to determine the level of serum testosterone below which age-specific biochemical, histomorphometric and radiokinetic measures of bone formation decline, resorption increases, rates of bone loss become detectable and fracture rates increase.

An association between bone mass and testosterone has been reported in a few studies. If there is an association, this may be difficult to identify because of problems in controlling factors that influence bone density and serum testosterone and in the precision of the method of measuring serum testosterone. The variance in bone density is largely genetically determined. A single measurement of serum testosterone has a precision error of about 10–15%, and is influenced by sampling time, the presence of illness, age, body weight and other factors. There may be a threshold effect, so that the association is present below but not above a critical level of 'sufficiency'.

Total body bone mineral content (TB BMC) and bone mineral density (BMD) measured at nine sites were 4–20% higher in 49 independent, community living men aged 58–85 years than in 49 age-matched men living in extended care facilities.[79] BMD was higher in the independent group at the proximal femur, but not at the lumbar vertebrae, midshaft radius or ultradistal radius. Among the independent men, testosterone was the strongest predictor

for BMD and TB BMC, followed by body weight for TB BMC; age was the only predictor for lean body mass (LBM)/height ratio. Among the institutionalized men, testosterone correlated with femoral neck BMD only; age, low body weight and immobility were each significant predictors of BMD or body composition. Low testosterone was found in 59% of patients with hip fractures compared with 18% of controls.[80] It may be more prevalent in men with vertebral fractures.[81]

Growth hormone and insulin-like growth factor I

Growth hormone (GH) and insulin-like growth factor I (IGF-I) decrease with advancing age and may have a role in the reduced bone formation found during ageing (for more details, see Seeman[15] and Seeman[16]). IGF-I and IGF binding protein 3 (IGFBP-3) are positively associated with areal bone density. IGF-I may be reduced in men with fractures. Androgens, oestrogens and the GH–IGF-I may interact so that the effects of testosterone may in part be mediated by oestrogens and the GH–IGF-I pathway. Ageing is associated with a decline in serum DHEA sulphate. DHEA administration increases IGF-I and decreases the IGFBP-3 so that the IGF-I : BP-3 ratio is increased by 50%, increasing the bioavailability of IGF-I. Testosterone also increases IGF-I. Oestrogens induce IGF-I mRNA in rat calvaria and UMR-106 cells. Tamoxifen, an oestrogen receptor antagonist, resulted in a decrease in GH pulse amplitude, IGF-I concentration and 24-hour mean serum GH levels in eugonadal men. When hypogonadal men were given testosterone, the GH pulse amplitude, IGF-I and 24-hour mean GH levels increased and then decreased with administration of tamoxifen. Total GH secretion was reduced in older men compared with younger men and correlated with free oestradiol, not free testosterone. GH pulse amplitude also correlated with oestradiol, not testosterone. IGF-I and dihydrotestosterone increase 5α-reductase activity in human scrotal skin fibroblasts. The effect of IGF-I was 100-fold greater than the effect of dihydrotestosterone, which was reduced by addition of a monoclonal antibody against IGF-I, suggesting that its effect was mediated by local IGF-I production. Thus, androgen effects may be mediated partly by paracrine/autocrine production of growth factors.

TREATMENT

There have been no randomized controlled trials using spine or hip fracture rates as endpoints in men. Decisions must be based on the results of studies in women despite the differences in the pathogenesis of bone loss. Surrogate endpoints such as bone density, histomorphometry, markers of bone turnover and observations in animal models of osteoporosis may have to be accepted. Hypogonadism should be treated with testosterone replacement. Calcium supplements are safe and may slow bone loss. Vitamin D deficiency should be suspected, identified and treated after excluding malabsorption. Bisphosphonates may increase bone density and should be considered.

Multicentre studies will be required given the large sample sizes needed to ensure that a type 2 error is not made. Fracture rates in men aged 80+ are about 1–2 per 100 per year in the community. If this is correct, then 1260 men per group are needed to detect a 50% risk reduction produced by a drug for a 3-year study at a probability of type 1 error of 0.05 and type 2 error of 0.80 (C Cooper, personal communication). It is difficult to recruit men aged 80+ years or to conduct successful clinical trials in this age group. If trials are envisaged in men aged around 65 or 75 years, fracture rates in the placebo arm may be about 0.5 persons having fractures per 100 persons per year so that about 3740 per group will be required for 3 years. These figures are based on incidence rates in the population. Fracture rates in men selected by having bone density 2–2.5 s.d. below the young normal mean may be higher, allowing sample sizes to be more reasonable.

Theoretically, bone loss should be more amenable to treatment in men than in women because trabecular connectivity is better maintained in men. Reduced bone formation on the periosteal surface may result in greater cortical bone fragility than a comparable amount of bone loss by increased endocortical resorption, because of the biomechanical consequences of failure to add bone radially with ageing. As the biomechanical consequences of restoring bone on the periosteum may be more cost-effective than elsewhere, treatment aimed at restoring bone mass at this site may be advantageous.

Several small, open and uncontrolled studies using antiresorptive agents, such as the bisphosphonates, have been conducted in men with osteoporosis and suggest that bone density may increase at the spine. Detail and references for the work summarized below is available in reference 16. Testosterone replacement should be considered in men with hypogonadism. Anderson et al[82] studied 21 eugonadal men aged 34–73 years with vertebral crush fractures who received intramuscular injections of testosterone as Sustanon 250 fortnightly for 6 months. Lumbar spinal BMD increased by 5% ($p < 0.001$) whereas hip BMD was unchanged. There is evidence that testosterone treatment may increase bone density in eugonadal men but the trials are short term. The risk of prostatic cancer needs to be considered in any cost–benefit analysis of this approach.

Bhasin et al[83] studied 43 normal men aged 19–40 years who participated in a 10-week trial of: standardized weight-lifting three times/week plus intramuscular testosterone 600 mg each week; exercise alone; testosterone alone; or neither. In the no-exercise group, testosterone increased triceps and quadriceps size, with greater increases in strength at the bench-press and squatting. Exercise did not increase muscle size but did increase strength. Men receiving testosterone and exercise had greater increases in fat-free mass, muscle size and muscle strength than those assigned to either no-exercise group. Supraphysiological doses of testosterone, when combined with strength training, increase fat-free mass and muscle size in men, but the results do not justify use of anabolic steroids in sport because of the adverse effects.

Vitamin D supplementation may reduce the risk of hip fracture in men in nursing homes and should be considered if assessment reveals vitamin D deficiency. Screening for vitamin D deficiency is recommended as patients are often vitamin D deficient on admission to nursing homes. No benefits were reported in ambulant men receiving 1000 mg/day of calcium and 25 µg/day of cholecalciferol in a double-blind, placebo-controlled, 3-year trial.[84] 1,25-Dihydroxyvitamin D has not been studied in men. Calcitonin has been shown to reduce bone turnover in castrated men and to increase bone density in women with high turnover osteoporosis. Antifracture efficacy using calcitonin has been reported in women.[85]

Of the anabolic agents, fluoride therapy is the most efficacious in increasing bone mass. However, bone strength has not been shown to increase in the manner anticipated. The use of fluoride is inadvisable until clinical trials are designed to address the toxic–therapeutic dose spectrum of this agent. The anabolic effects of intermittent parathyroid hormone are well documented. Bone density at the lumbar spine can be increased in men with osteoporosis. Although antifracture efficacy has not been demonstrated in clinical trials there is good evidence for increased bone strength in animal studies, increased periosteal and endosteal bone formation, increased connectivity and trabecular thickness. This anabolic agent thus holds real promise in the treatment of osteoporosis in men.

The anabolic actions of GH have been addressed in several studies in women with little success. However, animal studies using IGF-I and IGFBP-3 in an oophorectomized rat model to avoid the dose-dependent hypoglycaemic effects of IGF-I administration alone, showed increases in cortical width, trabecular width, trabecular connectivity, endocortical connectivity as well as in periosteal, endocortical and trabecular bone formation rates. The use of IGF-I and pamidronate in oophorectomized rats has been shown to increase external diameter of bone, to reduce medullary width and to increase cortical thickness. Similar studies in orchiectomized animals would be of interest.

Johansson et al[86] studied 12 men aged 32–57 years with idiopathic osteoporosis. By cross-over design, subcutaneous GH (2 IU/m^2) or IGF-I (80 µg/kg) was administered for 7 days. Serum collagen propeptide of type 1 collagen (PICP) increased 29% with GH ($p < 0.001$) and 43% with IGF-I ($p < 0.001$). Osteocalcin was increased 20% by both treatments ($p < 0.001$). Urinary deoxypyridine increased 44% with GH ($p < 0.001$) and 29% with IGF-I ($p < 0.001$). Bone formation and bone resorption were both increased by GH and IGF-I, the slight differences possibly being attributable to dose.

SUMMARY

Advances have taken place in our understanding of the epidemiology and pathogenesis of osteoporosis in men, but not in its treatment. The bone fragility in old age that predisposes to fractures is a function of bone mass, size and architecture attained during growth, and the changes in these traits during ageing. Hip fractures have a higher morbidity and mortality in men than in women and are a public health problem because one-third of all hip fractures occur in men. The prevalence of spine fractures in elderly men and women is similar, and whether trauma rather than bone fragility is responsible for this observation is uncertain. The incidence of fractures may be less in men than in women because men have higher peak bone size, higher bone mass, trabecular bone loss by thinning rather than perforation, less cortical thinning because of less endocortical resorption and greater periosteal apposition, and less cortical porosity. Experimental evidence showing that these differences actually account for the sex differences in fracture rates is unavailable.

The lower areal bone density found in men with spine fractures relative to controls results from reduced bone size as well as reduced bone mass. Reduced femoral neck width may be found in men with hip fractures. The reduced bone size may be caused by attainment of a reduced peak bone size and/or failure of periosteal expansion during ageing. Testosterone deficiency may have a central role in the pathogenesis of bone fragility and may act directly, and require aromatization to oestrogen, or conversion to dihydrotestosterone. Hypogonadism during growth may contribute to a lower mineral accrual but larger bone size (failure of epiphyseal closure). The decline in testosterone with age may contribute to reduced bone formation, bone loss and decreased periosteal appositional growth during ageing. Hypogonadism is present in about 20% of elderly men in the community and in about 50% of men with spine or hip fractures. The testosterone level below which reduced bone formation occurs is unknown. Oestrogen deficiency (secondary to testosterone deficiency) may increase the percentage of bone surfaces undergoing resorption and may be partly responsible for trabecular bone loss in men. Deficiency in growth hormone and insulin-like growth factor I may contribute to reduced bone formation. Secondary hyperparathyroidism may increase bone turnover in later years of life and contribute to cortical bone loss. Many men with fractures have underlying remediable causes of bone loss, particularly hypogonadism, which should be sought with a high index of suspicion. Treatment of osteoporosis in men is uncertain because no antifracture efficacy studies have been done. Testosterone is indicated in proven hypogonadism. Bisphosphonates may prevent bone loss.

QUESTIONS

1. Is the incidence of fractures increasing in men? If so, is this the result of a secular increase in bone fragility? If so, is the cause of the increased fragility reduced peak bone mass or size, increased bone loss with age or both?
2. Is the secular increase in hip fracture incidence an artefact of better surveillance?
3. Is the incidence of falls increasing in men?
4. Is the differing incidence of fractures in men and women explained by the differences in bone size, bone density, both or neither?
5. Is the incidence and prevalence of vertebral fractures similar in women and men?
6. Is this a reflection of trauma or is the perception of osteoporosis as a problem in women rather than men incorrect?
7. As longevity in men increases, will hypogonadism assume a similar relevance as in women?
8. What is the definition of hypogonadism in the context of skeletal health?
9. What is the role of testosterone, dihydrotestosterone, oestrogen and the GH axis in bone remodelling and bone loss?
10. What is the mechanism responsible for bone remodelling on the endocortical, periosteal and intracortical surfaces of the axial and appendicular skeleton?
11. What is the role of oestrogen deficiency in bone loss in men?
12. What is the pathogenesis of bone loss on bone surfaces?
13. What are the surface-specific treatment options for osteoporosis?
14. Is the reduced bone formation in both sexes as a result to GH and IGF-I deficiency?
15. Does GH and IGF-I deficiency result partly from oestrogen deficiency in women, and testosterone deficiency (with reduced local bone marrow conversion of testosterone to oestrogen) in men?
16. Is periosteal bone formation greater in men than women because bone turnover at this surface is androgen dependent?
17. Is the failure of bone formation to 'keep up' with resorption at menopause in women, and with resorption associated with secondary hyperparathyroidism in both sexes, partly the result of GH and IGF-I deficiency?

A greater understanding of bone fragility in men and women may be achieved by considering:

- bone size, mass and volumetric density
- growth of the periosteal and endosteal surfaces of cortical bone, growth of trabecular number and thickness in men compared with women, and men of different ethnic groups, rather than integral methods of densitometry

- greater emphasis on the cellular mechanisms of reduced bone formation, as well as increased bone resorption
- the participation of cortical bone as well as trabecular bone

- the individual and interacting role of oestrogen and testosterone in the earlier gain and later loss of bone size and mass in men and women.

REFERENCES

1. Cooper C, Campion G, Melton LJ. Hip fractures in the elderly: A world-wide projection. *Osteoporosis Int* 1992; **2**: 285–9.
2. Kanis JA, Pitt FA. Epidemiology of osteoporosis. *Bone* 1992; **13**: S7–15.
3. Kannus P, Parkkari J, Sievanen H et al. Epidemiology of hip fractures. *Bone* 1996; **18**: 57S–61S.
4. Melton LJ III, Atkinson EJ, Madhok R. Downturn in hip fracture incidence. *Public Health Rep* 1996; **111**: 146–50.
5. Elffors I, Allander E, Kanis JA et al. The variable incidence of hip fracture in Southern Europe: the MEDOS Study. *Osteoporosis Int* 1994; **4**: 253–63.
6. Looker AC, Wahner HW, Dunn WL et al. Proximal femur bone mineral levels of US adults. *Osteoporosis Int* 1995; **5**: 389–409.
7. Poór G, Atkinson EJ, Lewallen DG et al. Age-related hip fractures in men: clinical spectrum and short-term outcomes. *Osteoporosis Int* 1995; **5**: 419–26.
8. Lu-Yao GL, Baron JA, Barrett JA et al. Treatment and survival among elderly Americans with hip fractures: a population-based study. *Am J Public Health* 1994; **84**: 1287–91.
9. Davies KM, Stegman MR, Heaney RP et al. Prevalence and severity of vertebral fracture: The Saunders County Bone Quality Study. *Osteoporosis Int* 1996; **2**: 160–5.
10. Jones G, Nguyen T, Sambrook PN et al. Symptomatic fracture incidence in elderly men and women: the Dubbo Osteoporosis Epidemiology Study (DOES). *Osteoporosis Int* 1994; **4**: 277–82.
11. O'Neill TW, Felsenberg D, Varlow J et al. The prevalence of vertebral deformity in European men and women: the European Vertebral Osteoporosis Study. *J Bone Miner Res* 1996; **11**: 1010–18.
12. Cooper C, Atkinson EJ, O'Fallon WM et al. Incidence of clinically diagnosed vertebral fractures: A population-based study in Rochester, Minnesota, 1985–1989. *J Bone Miner Res* 1992; **7**: 221–7.

13. Alffram, P-A, Bauer GCH. Epidemiology of fractures of the forearm. *J Bone Joint Surg [Am]* 1962; **44**: 105–14.
14. Laval-Jeantet A-M, Bergot C, Carroll R et al. Cortical bone senescence and mineral bone density of the humerus. *Calcif Tissue Int* 1983; **35**: 268–72.
15. Seeman E. Osteoporosis in men. *Am J Med* 1994; **95**: 22–8.
16. Seeman E. The dilemma of osteoporosis in men. *Am J Med* 1995; **98**(suppl 1A): 75S–87S.
17. Ruff CB, Hayes WC. Sex differences in age-related remodeling of the femur and tibia. *J Orthop Res* 1988; **6**: 886–96.
18. Gilsanz V, Boechat MI, Roe TF et al. Gender differences in vertebral body sizes in children and adolescents. *Radiology* 1994; **190**: 673–77.
19. Rupich RC, Specker BL, Lieuw-A-Fa M et al. Gender and race differences in bone mass during infancy. *Calcif Tissue Int* 1996; **58**: 395–7.
20. Preece MA. The development of skeletal sex differences at adolescence. In: *Human Adaptation* (Russo P, Gass G, eds). Sydney: Department of Biological Sciences, Cumberland College of Health Sciences, 1982: 1–13.
21. Preece MA, Pan H, Ratcliffe SG. Auxological aspects of male and female puberty. *Acta Paediatr* 1992; **383**: 11–13.
22. Gordon CL, Halton JM, Atkinson SA et al. The contributions of growth and puberty to peak bone mass. *Growth, Development Aging* 1991; **55**: 257–62.
23. Looker AC, Wahner HW, Dunn WL et al. Proximal femur bone mineral levels of US adults. *Osteoporosis Int* 1995; **5**: 389–409.
24. Lu PW, Cowell CT, Lloyd-Jones SA et al. Volumetric bone mineral density in normal subjects aged 5–27 years. *J Clin Endocrinol Metab* 1996; **81**: 1586–90.
25. Garn SM, Nagy JM, Sandusky ST. Differential sexual dimorphism in bone diameters of subjects of European and African ancestry. *Am J Phys Anthrop* 1972; **37**: 127–30.

26. Frisancho AR, Garn SM, Ascoli W. Subperiosteal and endosteal bone apposition during adolescence. *Human Biol* 1970; **42:** 639–64.

27. Garn SM. In: *The Earlier Gain and Later Loss of Cortical Bone.* Springfield, IL: CC Thomas, 1970.

28. Odita JC. Cortical bone mass in Nigerian children: an anthropometric study. *Skeletal Radiol* 1994; **23:** 49–52.

29. Solomon L. Bone density in ageing caucasian and African populations. *Lancet* 1979; **ii:** 1327–9.

30. Moore B, Briody J, Cowell CT et al. Does maturational delay affect bone mineral density? European Society of Paediatric Endocrinology, 5th Joint Meeting, Stockholm 1997, June.

31. Finkelstein JS, Neer RM, Biller BMK et al. Osteopenia in men with a history of delayed puberty. *N Engl J Med* 1992; **326:** 600–4.

32. Finkelstein JS, Klibanski A, Neer RM. A longitudinal evaluation of bone mineral density in adult men with histories of delayed puberty. *J Clin Endocrinol Metab* 1996; **81:** 1152–5.

33. Luisetto G, Mastrogiacomo I, Bonanni G et al. Bone mass and mineral metabolism in Klinefelter's syndrome. *Osteoporosis Int* 1995; **5:** 455–61.

34. Trotter M, Broman GE, Peterson RR. Densities of bones of white and Negro skeletons. *J Bone Joint Surgery [Am]* 1960; **42A:** 50–8.

35. Garn SM, Sandusky ST, Nagy JM et al. Advanced skeletal development in low-income negro children. *J Pediatr* 1972; **80:** 965–9.

36. Hamill PVV, Johnston FE, Lemeshow S. *Body Weight, Stature and Sitting Height: White and Negro Youths 12–17 years.* DHEW Publications No. (HRA) 74–1608. *Vital and Health Statistics Series 11*, No. 126, 1973 (Rockville, MA: US Dept Health, Education and Welfare).

37. Cummings SR, Cauley JA, Palermo L et al. Racial differences in hip axis lengths might explain racial differences in rates of hip fracture. *Osteoporosis Int* 1994; **4:** 226–9.

38. Mikhail MB, Vaswani AN, Aloia JF. Racial differences in femoral dimensions and their relationship to hip fractures. *Osteoporosis Int* 1996; **6:** 22–4.

39. Nakamura T, Turner CH, Yoshikawa T et al. Do variations in hip geometry explain differences in hip fracture risk between Japanese and white Americans? *J Bone Miner Res* 1994; **9:** 1071–6.

40. Meredith HV. Secular change in sitting height and lower limb height of children, youths, and young adults of Afro-black, European, and Japanese ancestry. *Growth* 1978; **42:** 37–41.

41. Malina RM, Brown KH. Relative lower extremity length in Mexican American and in American black and white youth. *Am J Phys Anthropol* 1987; **72:** 89–94.

42. Cameron N, Tanner JM, Whitehouse RH. A longitudinal analysis of the growth of limb segments in adolescence. *Ann Human Biol* 1982; **9:** 211–20.

43. Tanner JM, Hayashi T, Preece MA et al. Increase in length of leg relative to trunk in Japanese children and adults from 1957 to 1977: comparison with British and with Japanese Americans. *Ann Human Biol* 1982; **9:** 411–23.

44. Bakwin H. Secular increase in height: Is the end in sight? *Lancet* 1964: **ii:** 1195–6.

45. Reid IR, Chin K, Evans MC et al. Longer femoral necks in the young: a predictor of further increases in hip fracture incidence? *N Z Med J* 1996; **108:** 234–5.

46. Gilsanz V, Gibbens DT, Roe TF et al. Vertebral bone density in children: effect of puberty. *Radiology* 1988; **166:** 847–50.

47. Gilsanz V, Roe TF, Stefano M et al. Changes in vertebral bone density in black girls and white girls during childhood and puberty. *N Engl J Med* 1991; **325:** 1597–600.

48. Han Z-H, Palnitkar S, Rao DS et al. Effect of ethnicity and age or menopause on the structure and geometry of iliac bone. *J Bone Miner Res* 1996; **11:** 1967–75.

49. Fujii Y, Tsutsumi M, Tsunenari T et al. Quantitative computed tomography of lumbar vertebrae in Japanese patients with osteoporosis. *Bone Miner* 1989; **6:** 87–94.

50. Meunier PJ, Sellami S, Briancon D, et al. Histological heterogeneity of apparently idiopathic osteoporosis. In: *Osteoporosis. Recent Advances in Pathogenesis and Treatment* (Deluca HF, Frost HM, Jee WSS, Johnston CC, Parfitt AM, eds). Baltimore: UPP, 1990: 293–301.

51. Kalender WA, Felsenberg D, Louis O et al. Reference values for trabecular and cortical vertebral bone density in single and dual-energy quantitative computed tomography. *Eur J Radiol* 1989; **9:** 75–80.

52. Mosekilde L, Mosekilde L. Sex differences in age-related changes in vertebral body size, density and biochemical competence in normal individuals. *Bone* 1990; **11:** 67–73.

53. Genant HK, Ettinger B, Harris ST et al. Quantitative computed tomography in assessment of osteoporosis. In: *Osteoporosis: Aetiology, Diagnosis and Management* (Riggs BL, Melton LJ III, eds). New York: Raven Press, 1988: 221–50.

54. Parfitt AM, Mathews CHE, Villanueva AR et al. Relationships between surface, volume, and thickness of iliac trabecular bone in aging and in osteoporosis. *J Clin Invest* 1983; **72:** 1396–409.

55. Aaron JE, Makins NB, Sagreiy K. The microanatomy of trabecular bone loss in normal aging men and women. *Clin Orth RR* 1987; **215:** 260–71.

56. Jilka RL, Weinstein RS, Takahashi K et al. Linkage of decreased bone mass with impaired osteoblastogenesis in a murine model of accelerated senescence. *J Clin Invest* 1996; **97:** 1732–40.

57. Bergman RJ, Gazit D, Kahn AJ et al. Age-related changes in osteogenic stem cells in mice. *J Bone Miner Res* 1996; **11:** 568–77.

58. Hughes DE, Wiltschke K, Mundy GR et al. Estrogen promotes osteoclast apoptosis in vitro and in vivo. *Bone* 1995; **16**(suppl 1): 93S.

59. Ensrud KE, Palermo L, Black DM et al. Hip and calcaneal bone loss increase with advancing age: longitudinal results from the study of osteoporotic fractures. *J Bone Miner Res* 1995; **10:**1778–87.

60. Vega E, Ghiringhelli G, Mautalen C. Bone mineral density in osteoporotic men with vertebral fractures. *J Bone Miner Res* 1994; **9**(suppl 1): S383.

61. Gilsanz V, Boechat MI, Gilsanz R et al. Gender differences in vertebral size in adults: biomechanical implications. *Radiology* 1994; **190:** 678–94.

62. Clarke BL, Ebeling PR, Jones JD et al. Changes in quantitative bone histomorphometry in aging healthy men. *J Clin Endocrinol Metab* 1996; **81:** 2264–70.

63. Need AG, Morris HA, Wishart J et al. Why do men lose bone? *J Bone Miner Res* 1994; **9**(suppl 1): S320.

64. Sone T, Miyake M, Takeda N et al. Urinary excretion of type I collagen crosslinked N-telopeptides in healthy Japanese adults: age- and sex-related changes and reference limits. *Bone* 1995; **17:** 335–9.

65. Resch H, Pietschmann, Woloszczuk W et al. Bone mass and biochemical parameters of bone metabolism in men with spinal osteoporosis. *Eur J Clin Invest* 1992; **22:** 542–5.

66. Sharp CA, Worsfold M, Rowlands PR et al. Accurate prediction of spinal osteoporosis in men using a biochemical measure of collagen balance. Bone and Tooth Society Summer Meeting July 22–23, 1993. *Bone* 1994; **15:** 243.

67. Marie PJ, de Vernejoul MC, Connes D et al. Decreased DNA synthesis by cultured osteoblastic cells in eugonadal osteoporotic men with defective bone formation. *J Clin Invest* 1991; **88:** 1167–72.

68. Nakano Y, Morimoto I, Ishida O et al. The receptor, metabolism and effects of androgen in osteoblastic MC3T3-E1 cells. *Bone Miner* 1994; **26:** 245–59.

69. Mizuno Y, Orimo H, Ouchi Y et al. Do variations in hip geometry explain differences in hip fracture risk between Japanese and white Americans? *J Bone Miner Res* 1994; **9:** 1071–6.

70. Somjen D, Mor Z, Kaye AM. Age dependence and modulation by gonadectomy of the sex-specific response of rat diaphyseal bone to gonadal steroids. *Endocrinology* 1994; **134:** 809–14.

71. Schwartz Z, Nasatzky E, Ornoy A et al. Gender-specific, maturation-dependent effects of testosterone on chondrocytes in culture. *Endocrinology* 1994; **134:** 1640–7.

72. Gunness M, Orwoll E. Early induction of alterations in cancellous and cortical bone histology after orchiectomy in mature rats. *J Bone Miner Res* 1995; **10:** 17356–64.

73. Turner RT, Hannon KS, Demers LM et al. Differential effects of gonadal function on bone histomorphometry in male and female rats. *J Bone Miner Res* 1989; **4:** 557–62.

74. Vanderschueren D, Van Herck E, Geusens P et al. Androgen resistance and deficiency have different effects on the growing skeleton of the rat. *Calcif Tissue Int* 1994; **55:** 198–203.

75. Vanderschueren D, Van Herck E, De Coster R et al. Aromatization of androgens is important for skeletal maintenance of aged male rats. *Calcif Tissue Int* 1996; **59:** 179–83.

76. Haji M, Tanaka S, Nishi Y, Yanase T et al. Sertoli cell function declines earlier than Leydig cell function in aging Japanese men. *Maturitas* 1994; **18:** 143–53.

77. Vermeulen A, Kaufman JM, Giagulli VA. Influence of some biological indexes on sex hormone-binding globulin and androgen levels in aging or obese males. *J Clin Endocrinol Metab* 1996; **81:** 1821–6.

78. Urban RJ, Veldhuis JD, Blizzard RM et al. Attenuated release of biologically active luteinizing hormone in healthy aging men. *J Clin Invest* 1988; **81:** 1020–9.

79. Rudman D, Drinka PJ, Wilson CR et al. Relations of endogenous anabolic hormones and physical activity to bone mineral density and lean body mass in elderly me. *Clin Endocrinol* 1994; **40:** 653–61.

80. Stanley HL, Schmitt BP, Poses RM et al. Does hypogonadism contribute to the occurrence of a minimal trauma hip fracture in elderly men? *JAGS* 1991; **39:** 766–71.

81. Seeman E, Melton LJ, O'Fallon WM et al. Risk factors for osteoporosis in males. *Am J Med* 1983; **75:** 977–82.

82. Anderson FH, Francis RM, Faulkner K. Androgen supplementation in eugonadal men with osteoporosis: effects of 6 months of treatment on bone mineral density and cardiovascular risk factors. *Bone* 1996; **18:** 171–7.

83. Bhasin S, Storer TW, Berman N et al. The effects of supraphysiologic doses of testosterone on muscle size and strength in normal men. *N Engl J Med* 1996; **335:** 1–7.

84. Orwell WES, Oviatt SK, McClung MR et al. The rate of bone mineral loss in normal men and the effects of calcium and cholecalciferol supplementation. *Ann Intern Med* 1990; **112:** 29–34.

85. Stepan JJ, Lachman M, Zverina J et al. Castrated men exhibit bone loss: effect of calcitonin treatment on biochemical indices of bone remodelling. *J Clin Endocrinol Metab* 1989; **69:** 523–7.

86. Johansson AG, Lindh E, Blum WF et al. Effects of growth hormone and insulin-like growth factor I in men with idiopathic osteoporosis. *J Clin Endocrinol Metab* 1996; **81:** 44–8.

15

Glucocorticoid-induced osteoporosis and other forms of secondary osteoporosis

IR Reid

CONTENTS • Pathogenesis of glucocorticoid-induced osteoporosis • Epidemiology of glucocorticoid-induced osteoporosis • Interventions for prevention or treatment • Management of steroid osteoporosis • Other forms of secondary osteoporosis

Glucocorticoid drugs have revolutionized the management of a number of diseases, particularly asthma and inflammatory conditions of the joints, gastrointestinal tract and central nervous system. Despite their life-saving properties, however, they bring a substantial burden of morbidity if used long term. One of their principal complications is the development of osteoporosis. Fractures in steroid-treated patients were reported within a few years of the introduction of these drugs to clinical medicine 50 years ago, paralleling the skeletal morbidity documented by Cushing in his original description of endogenous glucocorticoid excess. This chapter considers what is known of the mechanisms by which glucocorticoids weaken the skeleton, the epidemiology of the resulting bone loss and fractures, and the increasing number of interventions that are effective in preventing and treating this problem.

PATHOGENESIS OF GLUCOCORTICOID-INDUCED OSTEOPOROSIS

Glucocorticoids affect calcium and bone metabolism at almost every level. Thus, the challenge in determining the pathogenesis of steroid-induced osteoporosis has not been to find possible mechanisms, but to determine which of the many mechanisms demonstrated are the more important.

Osteoblasts

One of the major sites of glucocorticoid action is the osteoblast. Animal and human studies of bone histomorphometry consistently demonstrate impaired bone formation, there being both a reduced rate of formation in each bone remodelling cycle and a reduced period during which it occurs.[1]

These changes are probably largely attributable to the direct action of glucocorticoids on their receptor in osteoblastic cells. Thus, there is evidence of glucocorticoid regulation of the mRNAs for type I collagen, osteocalcin, osteopontin, fibronectin, β_1-integrin, bone sialoprotein, alkaline phosphatase, collagenase and the nuclear proto-oncogenes *c-myc*, *c-fos* and *c-jun*. These effects vary with the state of osteoblast differentiation[2] and involve both transcriptional and post-transcriptional effects.[2] In osteoblast precursor cells, gene expression is modulated to produce a more differentiated osteoblastic phenotype, whereas in the mature osteoblast, cell proliferation and matrix synthesis are reduced after long-term glucocorticoid exposure. These effects may be biphasic with respect to both time and dose, with inhibition being dominant at high hormone concentrations and long exposure periods.[3,4]

Osteoblasts produce factors which act in an autocrine manner to regulate their own activity. Insulin-like growth factors (IGF) I and II act in this way, and their local synthesis is inhibited by glucocorticoids. Their local activity is modulated by the interplay of specific binding proteins and there is now evidence for a reduction in the levels of the stimulatory binding proteins, IGFBP-3 and IGFBP-5[5–7] and for increased production of IGFBP-6, an inhibitor of IGF-II activity.[8] Transforming growth factor β (TGFβ) is a further important autocrine factor modulated by glucocorticoids.[9,10]

Further evidence for the inhibition of bone matrix synthesis during steroid treatment is provided by measurements of circulating levels of the matrix protein, osteocalcin, an index of osteoblast activity. There is a dose-related reduction in this index within the first 24 hours of glucocorticoid treatment[11] which is rapidly reversible.[12] Similar changes have been reported for another marker of osteoblast activity, the circulating carboxy-terminal propeptide of type I pro-collagen.[13]

Osteoclasts

Data are contradictory regarding the effects of glucocorticoids on osteoclast activity. Most studies of bone organ culture have demonstrated an inhibitory effect of glucocorticoids on both basal and stimulated resorption.[14] More recently, however, two groups have demonstrated stimulation of bone resorption by glucocorticoids in tissue cultured in serum-free media.[15–17] These findings are consistent with the data of Shuto et al[18] demonstrating an increase in osteoclast formation after dexamethasone treatment of mouse bone marrow cultures, associated with reduced levels of granulocyte–macrophage colony-stimulating factor.[18] In contrast, studies of the effects of glu-

cocorticoids on mature osteoclasts (in the presence of serum) have suggested a cytotoxic effect.[19] Glucocorticoids have profound effects on a number of cytokines (e.g. interleukin 1, the tumour necrosis factors) and block prostaglandin synthesis. These effects may modulate the responses of osteoclasts and many other cell types to glucocorticoid excess.

Human studies are also inconsistent. Static parameters of bone resorption have been found to be increased although biochemical indices of bone resorption are usually normal, there being no increase in excretion of hydroxyproline,[20] pyridinoline[13,20] or the N-telopeptide of type I collagen.[13]

Intestinal absorption of calcium

There is consistent evidence based on both calcium balance studies and those using radioactive calcium absorption, documenting reduced intestinal absorption of calcium in glucocorticoid-treated subjects. This is demonstrable within the first 2 weeks of initiating steroid treatment, at which time serum levels of 25-hydroxyvitamin D are unchanged and those of 1,25-dihydroxyvitamin D are elevated. This implies that glucocorticoids have a direct effect on intestinal calcium absorption which may be mediated by reduced production of the vitamin D-dependent calcium-binding protein involved in intestinal calcium transport.[21]

Urinary excretion of calcium

Although infusion of hydrocortisone does not immediately affect urinary calcium excretion, calcium loss rises dramatically with longer-term glucocorticoid exposure.[20,22] Fasting urine calcium excretion is twice control levels in patients using long-term glucocorticoids and this difference remains after adjustment for serum ionized calcium levels and glomerular filtration rate, implying that it represents a direct effect on tubular reabsorption of calcium.[23]

Vitamin D

There is little evidence to support the contention that changes in vitamin D metabolism contribute significantly to the development of steroid osteoporosis. Prospective studies of patients or normal subjects beginning steroid therapy have shown no changes in 25-hydroxyvitamin D or 24,25-dihydroxyvitamin D, but significant increases in 1,25-dihydroxyvitamin D have been observed 2–15 days after initiation of therapy.[20] There is no evidence for glucocorticoid effects on concentrations of vitamin D-binding protein.[24]

Parathyroid hormone

A number of groups have found increases in circulating concentrations of parathyroid hormone (PTH) within minutes to weeks of the initiation of steroid therapy,[20,25] although this has not been universal. In cross-sectional studies of patients receiving chronic glucocorticoid therapy, elevations of PTH levels to 50–100% above those of control subjects have been reported.[25] In vitro studies of parathyroid tissue from rats,[26] cattle[27] and humans[28] suggest that hyperparathyroidism may result directly from the action of glucocorticoids on the parathyroid cell, although it is also possible that calcium malabsorption in both the gut and the renal tubule contributes. It is interesting to note that some groups have suggested that circulating calcium levels are elevated in steroid-treated subjects,[29,30] although there are many studies that have not found this. In addition to studies of PTH concentrations, there is a substantial literature suggesting an increase in osteoblast sensitivity to PTH after glucocorticoid treatment.[31–34]

Phosphate metabolism

A recent study by Cosman et al[20] demonstrated early, transient hypophosphataemia before any detectable increase in PTH concentration occurred. This was associated with a fall in tubular reabsorption of phosphate, implying a direct effect of glucocorticoid on renal phosphate handling. There is also evidence for glucocorticoid-induced phosphate malabsorption in the gut, suggesting that the body's handling of phosphate is affected in a similar way by glucocorticoids to its handling of calcium.

Sex hormones

Sex hormones are important regulators of bone metabolism, and hypogonadism in either sex is associated with the development of osteoporosis. Glucocorticoids acutely depress plasma levels of testosterone in men[35] and their chronic use is associated with a dose-dependent reduction in free testosterone concentrations of about 50%.[36] These changes appear to result from inhibition of gonadotrophin secretion and a reduction in numbers of gonadotrophin-binding sites in the testis. High-dose steroid therapy is associated with oligomenorrhoea in women, suggesting a similar effect on the pituitary–gonadal axis.

Conclusion

Of the many possible mechanisms of action of glucocorticoids on bone, those that are of substantial magnitude and consistently demonstrated in different models are the reduction in osteoblast number and activity, the malabsorption of calcium in the gut and renal tubule, and the presence of hypogonadism in male patients. These are likely to be the principal pathways by which steroid-induced osteoporosis develops. Their potential interplay is summarized in Figure 15.1

EPIDEMIOLOGY OF GLUCOCORTICOID-INDUCED OSTEOPOROSIS

Effects on bone mass

Exposure to supraphysiological doses of glucocorticoids leads to a substantial and rapid loss of bone. What limited prospective data there

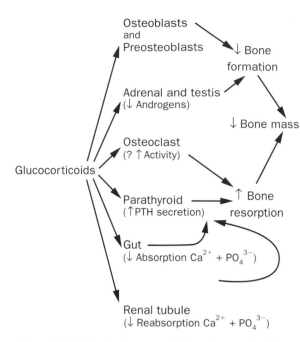

Figure 15.1 Mechanisms by which glucocorticoids produce osteopenia.

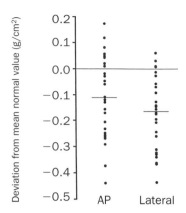

Figure 15.2 Lumbar spine bone mineral densities assessed in the anteroposterior (AP) or lateral projections of glucocorticoid-treated women. Results are shown as the absolute difference in bone density of each subject from the age-appropriate mean normal value. Note that bone densities by either technique are normally distributed about a mean that is significantly below that of the normal population ($p < 0.001$). This decrement is greater in the predominantly trabecular bone assessed in the lateral scans ($p = 0.03$). (Based on data from Reid et al.[43])

are suggest that bone loss takes place in virtually all individuals.[37,38] Bone loss is most marked in the first 12 months,[39] but continues long term, albeit at a lower rate.[40] A prospective study has shown an 8% decrement in the trabecular bone of the lumbar spine after 20 weeks of treatment with a mean dose of prednisone of 7.5 mg/day.[38] Cross-sectional studies in patients treated for periods of 5 years show that integral bone mass of the lumbar spine and proximal femur is 20% below control values.[41] Bone loss occurs more rapidly in trabecular than in cortical bone and decrements approaching 40% are seen in cross-sectional studies of the trabecular bone of the lumbar spine, whether assessed by quantitative computed tomography (QCT)[42] or by dual energy X-ray absorptiometry (DXA) in the lateral projection[43] (Figure 15.2). In cross-sectional studies, the distribution of bone density is unimodal with a standard deviation comparable to that of the normal population. This implies that there is little intersubject variability in the extent of steroid-induced bone loss. As the degree of

bone loss is usually less than the range of values in the normal population, those subjects whose pre-treatment bone densities were at the upper end of the normal range will still have 'normal' bone densities. The degree of steroid-induced bone loss is related to average steroid dose and the duration of therapy.[42,44,45]

The bone loss induced by glucocorticoids is substantially reversible after the withdrawal of these drugs. Two prospective studies have demonstrated a reaccumulation of bone density over approximately the same time span as its loss occurred.[37,38] Substantial increases in bone density have been reported after cure of Cushing's syndrome[46,47] and the author's group has demonstrated that bone density is normal in patients cured of Cushing's syndrome for a mean period of 9 years.[48] Alternate-day therapy does not, however, diminish bone loss.[49–51]

A strategy being used increasingly to limit the systemic side effects of glucocorticoids is their local administration. This still results in some systemic availability, with suppression of endogenous glucocorticoid synthesis and, often, changes in glucocorticoid-sensitive markers of bone function such as circulating osteocalcin concentrations. Several groups have reported reduced bone density in users of inhaled steroids,[52] although these studies are often confounded by previous use of oral steroids. Inhaled steroid in doses less than 1 mg/day of beclomethasone or budesonide do not affect circulating osteocalcin levels and are unlikely to have any deleterious effect on bone density in adults. Even with higher doses it seems highly probable that, for a given anti-asthmatic effect, inhaled steroids will have substantially less systemic effect than comparable doses of oral glucocorticoid. However, inhaled steroids are now being used in patients who in the past would not have received glucocorticoid therapy at all, and this may result in some subjects being exposed to a small risk of steroid osteoporosis. In this regard, the recent report from a double-blind, placebo-controlled trial of beclomethasone 200 µg twice a day in 7- to 9-year-old asthmatic children of significant growth retardation after only 6 months of treatment is a source of concern.[53]

Fractures

Studies that permit an estimate of fracture incidence in steroid users are set out in Table 15.1. Most have measured only vertebral fractures, which occur in about one-third of patients after 5–10 years of therapy. Longer periods of steroid use are associated with a greater fracture risk[61] as are other factors associated with fracture in non-users of steroids, such as age, sex and body weight.[61] Fractures at other sites are also more frequent in steroid users, the risk of hip fracture being increased 2.7-fold.[62] Patients undergoing organ transplantation may have even higher fracture risks than other steroid-treated patients, possibly because of the effects of pre-existing disease and also because of the osteopenic effects of the other immunosuppressive therapies used. Shane et al[63] have reported fracture incidences of 54% in women and 29% in men studied prospectively over a 12-month period from the time of cardiac transplantation.

INTERVENTIONS FOR PREVENTION OR TREATMENT

Calcium

As one of the main actions of glucocorticoids is to produce negative calcium balance by inhibiting absorption of this ion in both the gut and the renal tubule, providing supplemental calcium is a logical intervention to prevent this bone loss. Nilsen et al[64] compared bone loss in elderly patients with rheumatoid arthritis receiving 6 g/day microcrystalline hydroxyapatite with that in control subjects. There was a slight reduction in the rate of radial bone loss in the treated group. An uncontrolled 6-month study in children suggested improvement in bone density after supplementation with calcium and vitamin D.[65] Reid and Ibbertson[66] demonstrated a significant suppression of hydroxyproline excretion after the introduction of a 1 g/day calcium supplement in steroid-treated adults. Although this would be expected to reduce rates of bone loss, it is quite clear that a calcium supplementation alone does not completely block the development of steroid-induced osteoporosis.[67–69] This implies that steroid osteoporosis is not merely a problem of mineral balance, but is primarily related to reduced bone matrix synthesis, comparable to the wasting that occurs in soft tissues such as skin and muscle. Thus, the therapeutic task is also to reverse the catabolic effects of glucocorticoids, not merely to provide more substrate for bone synthesis.

Sex hormones

Oestrogen and testosterone are not thought specifically to interfere with the actions of glucocorticoids. Thus, their role is as a treatment for any coexisting sex hormone deficiency with a view to correcting this additional risk factor for bone loss. In premenopausal women men-

Table 15.1 Steroid use and fractures

Study	Population	Mean dose (mg/day)	Duration (years)	n	Age (years)	% Male	Fracture prevalence (%)	
							Steroid treated	Control
Ross and Lynch[54]	Cushing's syndrome	NA	NA	70	–	–	19	–
				711			36	
Adinoff and Hollister[55]	Asthmatics	–	–	128	>40	33	11 ⎫ Rib and	0
				19	44	32	42 ⎭ vertebral	0
Luengo et al[56]	Asthma	12	9	25	52	40	34 (vertebral fracture)	8 (in users of inhaled glucocorticoids)
Michel et al[57]	Rheumatoid arthritis	>5	5	46	49	0	34 (all sites)	–
		>5	5	25	55	100	8	
Laan et al[58]	Rheumatoid arthritis	7	8	12	PoM	0	42 (vertebral fracture)	19
Spector et al[59]	Rheumatoid arthritis	8	4	51	57	0	10 (vertebral fracture)	15
Lems et al[60]	Rheumatoid arthritis	6.5	4.2	52	67	13	58 (vertebral fracture)	Not available

POM, postmenopausal.
Steroid dose is mg of prednisone equivalent.

struating regularly, it does not have a place. In postmenopausal women on steroids, the increases in bone density after the institution of conventional hormone replacement therapy are at least as large as those that occur in normal postmenopausal women.[70–74]

In steroid-treated men, circulating testosterone levels are reduced by almost one-half, a factor likely to contribute to the development of osteopenia. It has recently been shown that testosterone replacement produces a 5% increase in lumbar spine bone mineral density after 12 months, as well as reversing the accumulation of body fat and loss of lean tissue which accompanies steroid therapy.[75] Androgens, in the form of anabolic steroids, have also been used for treating steroid-induced osteoporosis. They would seem to have little place in the management of men, in whom they are likely to reduce testosterone levels further. Their use in women is associated with beneficial effects on bone mass but also with virilizing side effects in almost one-half of treated patients.[76,77]

Bisphosphonates

Bisphosphonates are an attractive therapy for steroid osteoporosis because they can directly redress the imbalance between bone formation and resorption, and because they can be used in virtually all steroid-treated patients, including the young and those with no sex hormone deficiencies. They are now becoming widely used in the management of postmenopausal osteoporosis, although their efficacy was first demonstrated in the treatment of steroid osteoporosis.[67,68] In this randomized controlled trial there was a 19% increase in the density of the trabecular bone of the lumbar spine after 12 months of treatment with pamidronate, in comparison with a 9% decrease in those receiving placebo. There were smaller but statistically significant benefits in the cortical bone mass of the metacarpals. In those patients proceeding to a second year of therapy, the gains in bone density were maintained whereas there was progressive loss in the placebo group. Oral

pamidronate is not widely available but 3-monthly intravenous infusions (30 mg) of this drug also increase spinal bone density.[78]

There are now a number of studies showing that cyclic etidronate is comparably effective in steroid-treated subjects[79–82] (Figure 15.3) and this treatment has high patient acceptability because medication is only taken for 2 weeks every 3 months. The other widely available oral

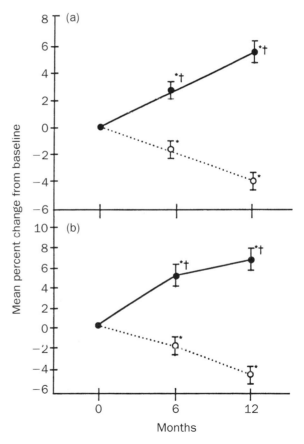

Figure 15.3 Changes in bone density in patients with established steroid-induced osteoporosis randomized to receive cyclical etidronate (filled circles) or calcium (open circles). (a) Spine (L1–L4); (b) proximal femur (total hip). Data are mean ± s.e.m. * $p < 0.02$ compared with baseline; † $p < 0.001$ compared with calcium group. (Reproduced, with permission, from Struys et al.[81])

bisphosphonate, alendronate, is now well established as an effective therapy for post-menopausal osteoporosis. Although the results of trials with this agent in steroid osteoporosis are awaited, it would seem highly likely that alendronate in a daily dose of 10 mg will produce effects comparable to those seen with etidronate or pamidronate.

Vitamin D and its metabolites

This group of compounds has been studied over a long period of time but the inconsistencies in the outcomes of the various studies mean that it is still difficult to determine their proper place in the management of steroid osteoporosis. Much of the early work in humans was carried out by Hahn and co-workers.[83] They demonstrated significant increases in forearm bone density from the use of calciferol 50 000 units three times per week plus calcium 500 mg/day.[83] In a subsequent study using 25-hydroxyvitamin D 40 µg/day, similar beneficial effects on bone density were found.[84] The group then investigated the role of calcitriol 0.4 µg/day and again found increases in forearm density, but these were no different from the increases found in the control group given calcium alone.[85] Subsequently, Braun et al[86] demonstrated a beneficial effect of alfacalcidol 2 µg/day on trabecular bone volume over a 6-month period, but Bijlsma[87] failed to show any benefit from the use of dihydrotachysterol over a 2-year study. In 1989, Di Munno et al[88] reported substantial gain in radial bone mineral content in patients starting glucocorticoids who were also given 25-hydroxyvitamin D 35 µg/day, in comparison with substantial losses in those given placebo. Sambrook et al[89] have reported a large study in which people starting glucocorticoid therapy were randomly assigned to receive calcium, calcium plus calcitriol (mean dose 0.6 µg/day) or these two agents combined with calcitonin over a 12-month period. Bone loss from the lumbar spine was −4.3%, −1.3% and −0.2% in the respective groups (Figure 15.4). There was a similar trend in distal radial bone loss which was non-signifi-

cant but no evidence whatsoever of reduced bone loss at the proximal femur (−3% in all groups). Although there was clearly benefit from the use of calcitriol, the treatment effect is less than that seen in a comparable trial in which etidronate was administered from the time of introduction of steroid therapy.[90] Furthermore several groups have documented the efficacy of etidronate in also preventing femoral bone loss[80,81] (see Figure 15.3). In contrast, one recent study of bone loss after cardiac transplantation compared the effects of alfacalcidol and etidronate.[91] Neither therapy completely prevented bone loss but the vitamin D metabolite was superior to the bisphosphonate.

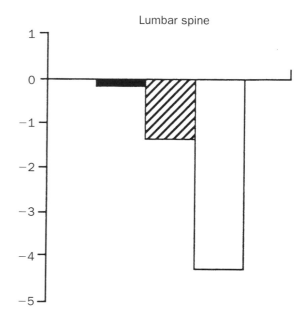

Figure 15.4 Percentage changes in bone density over one year in patients starting glucocorticoid therapy, randomized to receive also calcium, calcitonin and calcitriol (black); calcium and calcitriol (hatched); or calcium alone (open bar). There was a significant between-group difference overall, but no difference between the combined therapy group and that receiving calcitriol plus calcium. (Reproduced, with permission of the *New England Journal of Medicine*, from Sambrook et al.[69] © 1993, Massachusetts Medical Society. All rights reserved.)

It should be noted, however, that many of the patients in this study were vitamin D deficient.

Adachi et al[92] have re-examined the effect of calciferol 50 000 units/week plus calcium 1000 mg/day in a randomized controlled trial. At the end of 3 years they found no suggestion of any beneficial effect from the use of this intervention.

The relatively small number of studies and the variability of their outcomes make it difficult to determine the optimal course with respect to vitamin D and its metabolites in the prevention of steroid osteoporosis. The present author tends to use them as adjunctive therapy to either sex hormone replacement or bisphosphonates, in the patient with severe steroid osteoporosis, or as a second-line therapy in patients for whom these other agents are not acceptable.

Fluoride

The fluoride ion is a potent osteoblast mitogen capable of producing sustained gains in lumbar spine bone density with long-term therapy. This unique beneficial effect is counterbalanced by its interference with normal mineralization of bone when present in bone crystal at high concentrations. These opposing effects have made it difficult to translate fluoride's beneficial effects on bone mass into reduced fracture incidence in postmenopausal osteoporosis. Work is continuing in this condition to find the appropriate therapeutic window for its effective use. It is, in theory, an attractive agent for use in steroid osteoporosis because its greatest effects are on trabecular bone, the site of greatest bone loss in steroid-treated subjects. There is now clear evidence that it can increase spinal bone density[93,94] and increase trabecular bone volume of the iliac crest[95] in steroid-treated subjects. However, its antifracture efficacy in this context remains to be established and it should not be used as a first-line agent in steroid-induced osteoporosis. Its cautious use may have a role as an adjunctive therapy in patients with severe bone loss.

Calcitonin

Calcitonin acts via specific receptors on osteoclasts, reducing bone resorption. It has been used in some countries for the management of postmenopausal osteoporosis, although its effectiveness is thought to be less than that of hormone replacement therapy or bisphosphonates. There have now been several controlled trials in steroid-treated subjects, suggesting that it slows or prevents bone loss.[96-98] Thus, calcitonin is likely to be effective, but its side effects and costs make it less attractive than sex hormone therapy or the bisphosphonates.

Bone-sparing glucocorticoids

Deflazacort is a derivative of prednisone which has been suggested to exert less deleterious effects on calcium and bone metabolism than prednisone itself. Thus, studies have demonstrated less marked hypercalciuria,[99,100] lesser effects on intestinal calcium absorption,[99] reduced bone loss[101-104] and less growth retardation in children treated with deflazacort.[105,106] However, all these studies assumed that the potency of prednisone relative to deflazacort was 1.2. Recently, there has been a re-examination of the relative potencies of these two glucocorticoids with the finding that the relative potency is really 1.4–1.8.[107,108] Thus, much of the earlier literature may be invalid because it has compared non-equivalent doses of the two agents. A recent study of bone density changes in patients with polymyalgia rheumatica, in which doses were adjusted to produce symptom control, also suggested that the glucocorticoid potency of deflazacort has been over-estimated in the past, and demonstrated no bone-sparing effect of this agent.[109]

MANAGEMENT OF STEROID OSTEOPOROSIS

Patient assessment

In addition to determining the average dose and duration of steroid therapy, assessment of the steroid-treated patient should include other factors relevant to bone health, which form a part of the assessment of any subject at risk of osteoporosis. Thus, a full medical and drug history is necessary, including menstrual history, dietary calcium intake, smoking history, alcohol intake, use of other osteopenic drugs and measurement of body weight. Past fracture history is an important predictor of future risk. In the patient without a previous history of fractures, bone density measurement is the key step in the assessment of future risk, and thus the need for pharmacological measures to increase bone mass. Glucocorticoids primarily deplete trabecular bone, so density measurement at a site rich in trabecular bone is most appropriate. Dual energy X-ray absorptiometry assessment of the lumbar spine in the anteroposterior projection is often adequate, although exclusion of the cortical posterior processes by use of lateral scanning is preferable.[43,110] Computed tomography is also able specifically to assess trabecular bone in the spine.

It is important to assess the sex hormone status of men and premenopausal women. The occurrence of regular menses provides presumptive evidence for oestrogen sufficiency, but in the absence of this measurement of serum oestradiol is required. The reductions in serum testosterone occurring in steroid-treated men are usually asymptomatic, so measurement of testosterone levels is needed to determine whether sex hormone replacement might be indicated. There is no evidence that other biochemical assessments of calcium metabolism are helpful in predicting rates of steroid-induced bone loss.[42]

Devising a therapeutic regimen

In any patient at risk of steroid-induced osteoporosis, minimization of steroid dose and optimization of the local administration of steroids should take place. Advice regarding the correction of other risk factors for osteoporosis should be offered (e.g. increasing exercise, cessation of smoking, moderation of alcohol intake, optimization of dietary calcium intake). In patients

whose bone density is above the mean normal value for young adults, their immediate risk of fracture can be assumed to be low and further intervention may not be necessary unless they have just begun glucocorticoids. Such patients should have a further measurement of bone density after 6–24 months (depending on their steroid dose and the previous duration of therapy) to determine whether progressive bone loss is occurring and, thus, more aggressive intervention may be necessary. Patients with a bone density between the mean normal value and 1–2 standard deviations (s.d.) below it are in a transitional range over which the fracture risk increases fourfold. They may be managed conservatively, as discussed above, or with therapeutic interventions depending on other risk factors, their steroid dose and previous duration of therapy. Those on higher steroid doses can expect to have greater bone loss as can those who have only recently started taking these drugs.

Patients with bone densities lower than this level and those with a previous history of low trauma fractures would usually be offered treatment. Correction of sex hormone deficiency in women is effective and well tolerated, and carries with it other likely benefits, such as the prevention of cardiovascular disease. In men, it is well tolerated and often leads to significant improvements in the sense of well-being, but the need for parenteral administration and the possible exacerbation of prostate disease may be a relative contra-indication in some subjects. Bisphosphonates are increasingly available and are generally well tolerated. Etidronate occasionally causes exacerbation of pre-existing inflammatory bowel disease, and aminobisphosphonates such as alendronate sometimes cause oesophageal or gastric irritation. In the rare patient in whom neither sex hormone replacement nor bisphosphonates are appropriate, vitamin D metabolites are likely to be beneficial. In patients with severe disease, all of these three modalities can be combined. Rarely, bone loss may be sufficiently severe that the addition of fluoride as well might be considered.

Calcitonin and anabolic steroids both require parenteral administration and both cause significant side effects; in addition calcitonin is expensive. The use of these interventions is therefore limited. Recent studies have somewhat tempered enthusiasm for the use of deflazacort although the significant reductions in bone loss, found in earlier studies of its use, imply a steep dose–response between steroid dose and bone loss when doses are being given that are only modestly above physiological levels. This reinforces the importance of minimizing the dose of steroid used as well as the duration for which these drugs are administered.

OTHER FORMS OF SECONDARY OSTEOPOROSIS

The number of conditions known to be associated with low bone density is steadily increasing as a result of the wide availability of bone densitometers in recent years. The practising physician is likely to be daunted by the number of these conditions (see Table 15.2) but, in fact, there is only a fairly small number of underlying mechanisms that contribute to secondary bone loss. The conditions in Table 15.2 have been categorized according to these mechanisms. This categorization is to some extent arbitrary, and obviously some conditions should appear under more than one heading.

Table 15.2 Conditions associated with osteoporosis

Inflammatory disorders	**Disorders associated with immobilization**
Rheumatoid arthritis	Parkinson's disease
Inflammatory bowel disease	Poliomyelitis
Cystic fibrosis	Cerebral palsy
Bone marrow disorders	Paraplegia
Multiple myeloma	**Defective synthesis of connective tissue**
Mastocytosis	Osteogenesis imperfecta
Leukaemia	Marfan's syndrome
Disorders associated with hypogonadism	Homocystinuria
Athletic amenorrhoea	**Endocrinological disorders**
Haemochromatosis	Thyrotoxicosis
Turner's syndrome	?Hyperparathyroidism
Klinefelter's syndrome	**Miscellaneous**
Post-chemotherapy	Pregnancy/lactation
Hypopituitarism	Ankylosing spondylitis
Disorders associated with low body weight	Hypercalciuric nephrolithiasis
Anorexia nervosa	**Drugs**
Type 1 diabetes mellitus	Glucocorticoids
Disorders associated with malabsorption	Alcohol
Coeliac disease	Caffeine
Post-gastrectomy	Medroxyprogesterone acetate
Liver disease	Anticonvulsants
Total parenteral nutrition	Methotrexate
	Heparin
	Cyclosporin

Even before the era of bone densitometry, skeletal rarefraction and the occurrence of fractures were noted in chronic inflammatory conditions such as rheumatoid arthritis. The same is true of bone marrow disorders such as multiple myeloma and mastocytosis. Both these groups of conditions probably lead to bone loss through over-production of bone-resorbing factors either locally or systemically. Cytokines such as interleukin 1 (IL-1), IL-6, the tumour necrosis factors and leukaemia inhibitory factor are likely to be involved. In rheumatoid arthritis, bone loss is most marked adjacent to joints, possibly because these are the sites of maximum inflammation, but possibly as a result of disuse attributable to local pain. In multiple myeloma, diffuse osteoporosis can occur in addition to the local osteolytic lesions at the site of myeloma deposits. The bisphosphonates may be useful in preventing both of the complications of this condition.

Sex hormone deficiency in both sexes results in bone loss, and is also associated with increased levels of osteolytic cytokines in the bone microenvironment. The list of causes of hypogonadism given in Table 15.2 is simply for purposes of illustration. Any disease or medication that reduces sex hormone levels will usually lead to loss of bone mass. Hypogonadism is a very common finding in many chronic diseases.

In women, ovarian function is dependent on maintenance of a minimum body weight. Thus, in conditions such as anorexia nervosa, hypogonadism is a major contributor to bone loss. However, in both sexes and at all times of life, body weight itself influences bone mass. A number of mechanisms probably contribute, including the effects of the high insulin and amylin levels that are seen in obesity, but production of oestrone in adipocytes and the response of the skeleton to the loading provided by higher body weight may also be significant.[111] In type 1 diabetes mellitus, small and variable decreases in bone density have been reported. Insulin deficiency, low body weight, acidosis and glycosylation of matrix proteins may contribute, but fractures are not a major clinical problem in this condition. In type 2 dia-

betes, bone density tends to be increased[112] possibly because of the presence of hyperinsulinaemia. As for hypogonadism, low body weight is a frequent accompaniment of chronic illness and will contribute to the bone loss in many of the conditions listed in Table 15.2. This is particularly true of diseases of the gastrointestinal tract. These conditions result in weight loss, but also in malabsorption of specific nutrients such as calcium and vitamin D. There is recent evidence that bilirubin is toxic to osteoblasts and this may exacerbate bone loss in cholestatic conditions.[113]

Bone, like muscle, responds to use, and extreme bone loss is seen after complete immobilization following a fracture. Less marked but significant bone loss occurs in a variety of neurological conditions that interfere with the use of the limbs. In some of these, such as Parkinson's disease,[114] there is also an increased frequency of falling, which compounds the problem and leads to higher fracture frequency.

The structural integrity of bone is dependent on that of its matrix proteins. The classic forms of osteogenesis imperfecta result in fractures from the start of life, but some milder variants may not present until adulthood. In individuals with reduced bone strength as a result of inherited connective tissue disorders, the loss of bone that takes place after the menopause can result in the development of symptomatic fractures.

The importance of insulin in promoting osteoblast growth has been alluded to above. At least two other hormones have significant direct actions on bone: thyroid and parathyroid hormones. Excess of either of these hormones is associated with reduced bone mass. In hyperthyroidism, bone mass increases after cure of thyroid disease. Data are conflicting regarding bone loss in hyperparathyroidism, although many authorities believe that cortical bone mass, at least, is significantly reduced.[115,116]

Normal pregnancy is not associated with significant bone loss and there is only minor loss during normal lactation, which is corrected after weaning.[117] Very rarely, severe trabecular bone loss can occur in the last trimester of preg-

nancy or during the first few months of lactation. Available data suggest that this is associated with high bone turnover, which could be
the result of increased release of PTH-related
peptide from either the pregnant uterus and/or
the lactating breast.[118]

Several recent studies have documented
reduced bone density in ankylosing spondylitis.
In advanced cases, the presence of syndes-
mophytes artefactually elevates spinal bone
density measurements. However, this extraver-
tebral calcification does not increase vertebral
strength and the incidence of vertebral fractures
is increased in this condition.[119] There is increasing evidence for reduced bone mass in subjects
with hypercalciuric nephrolithiasis.[120] This is
consistent with data from normal individuals
showing an inverse relationship between urine
calcium loss and bone density.[121]

Alcohol is one of the most common drugs
associated with bone loss. At daily intakes of
20–40 g ethanol, a deleterious effect on bone
density has not been consistently demonstrated.
However, at higher intakes, particularly in men,
osteoporotic fractures do occur. This may be the
result of the hypogonadism and liver disease
which themselves result from alcohol abuse,
although there is also evidence of a direct toxic
effect of alcohol on osteoblasts. Caffeine
increases urinary calcium loss and some studies
have shown high caffeine intakes to be associated with reduced bone mass.[112] In some databases, this has only been found when a low
dietary calcium intake coexists with high use of
caffeine.

Medroxyprogesterone acetate is a progestational agent used in some countries as a
hormonal contraceptive. It suppresses
gonadotrophin release, resulting in anovulation
and hypo-oestrogenaemia. Its long-term use is
associated with reductions of spinal bone density by almost 10%. These reductions are
reversible when normal ovarian function is
restored.[122]

A number of anticonvulsant drugs induce
the activity of hepatic enzymes which catabo-
lize vitamin D. In the past, frank osteomalacia

was reported in some epileptic patients. This is
more likely to occur if there are other factors
contributing to the low vitamin D levels, such
as low sunlight exposure or poor diet. Some
recent studies have suggested that low vitamin
D levels and the resulting hyperparathyroidism
may be associated with modest decreases in
bone density,[123] but atraumatic fractures are
seldom seen without other risk factors being
present.

Skeletal complications from the use of
methotrexate were initially reported in children, and the same syndrome has recently been
reported in adults.[124] Patients on this drug for
more than 6 months may complain of severe
pain in the distal tibia and may develop fractures at this site. The symptoms resolve after
discontinuation of the drug. Methotrexate use
also seems to be associated with generalized
bone loss, although it is hard to know to what
extent these findings are attributable to the
underlying illness for which the methotrexate is
being administered.

Case reports of fractures associated with
long-term heparin use appeared in the 1960s.
At the present time, chronic administration of
this drug is limited to pregnant women, about
2% of whom will develop fractures.[125] The
mechanism by which heparin produces osteoporosis has not been fully elucidated although
animal studies have shown that its use is associated with hyperparathyroidism and reduced
levels of 1,25-dihydroxyvitamin D.

Cyclosporin is a widely used immunosuppressive agent, particularly in association with
organ transplantation. It was hoped that its
introduction would reduce the problems of
osteoporosis experienced by immunosup-
pressed patients, through decreasing use of glucocorticoids. Although other steroid side effects
have become less common, cyclosporin itself
seems to cause bone loss via increased bone
turnover, so some of the highest incidences of
fractures are seen in cardiac and liver transplant recipients,[63,126] although pre-existing
osteopenia may also contribute to some of this
morbidity.

REFERENCES

1. Dempster DW. Bone histomorphometry in glucocorticoid-induced osteoporosis. *J Bone Miner Res* 1989; **4:** 137–41.

2. Shalhoub V, Conlon D, Tassinari M et al. Glucocorticoids promote development of the osteoblast phenotype by selectively modulating expression of cell growth and differentiation associated genes. *J Cell Biochem* 1992; **50:** 425–40.

3. Gallagher JA, Beresford JN, MacDonald BR et al. Hormone target cell interactions in human bone. In: *Osteoporosis* (Christiansen C, ed.). Copenhagen: Osteopress, 1984: 431–9.

4. Dietrich JW, Canalis EM, Maina DM et al. Effects of glucocorticoids on fetal rat bone collagen synthesis in vitro. *Endocrinology* 1979; **104:** 715–21.

5. Chevalley T, Strong DD, Mohan S et al. Evidence for a role for insulin-like growth factor binding proteins in glucocorticoid inhibition of normal human osteoblast-like cell proliferation. *Eur J Endocrinol* 1996; **134:** 591–601.

6. Gabbitas B, Pash JM, Delany AM et al. Cortisol inhibits the synthesis of insulin-like growth factor-binding protein-5 in bone cell cultures by transcriptional mechanisms. *J Biol Chem* 1996; **271:** 9033–8.

7. Okazaki R, Riggs BL, Conover CA. Glucocorticoid regulation of insulin-like growth factor-binding protein expression in normal human osteoblast-like cells. *Endocrinology* 1994; **134:** 126–32.

8. Gabbitas B, Canalis E. Cortisol enhances the transcription of insulin-like growth factor-binding protein-6 in cultured osteoblasts. *Endocrinology* 1996; **137:** 1687–92.

9. Centrella M, McCarthy TL, Canalis E. Glucocorticoid regulation of transforming growth factor beta 1 activity and binding in osteoblast-enriched cultures from fetal rat bone. *Mol Cel Biol* 1991; **11:** 3390–6.

10. Oursler MJ, Riggs BL, Spelsberg TC. Glucocorticoid-induced activation of latent transforming growth factor-beta by normal human osteoblast-like cells. *Endocrinology* 1993; **133:** 2187–96.

11. Reid IR, Chapman GE, Fraser TRC et al. Low serum osteocalcin levels in glucocorticoid-treated asthmatics. *J Clin Endocrinol Metab* 1986; **62:** 379–83.

12. Godshalk MF, Downs RW. Effect of short-term glucocorticoids on serum osteocalcin in healthy young men. *J Bone Miner Res* 1988; **3:** 113–15.

13. Lems WF, Gerrits MI, Jacobs JWG et al. Changes in (markers of) bone metabolism during high dose corticosteroid pulse treatment in patients with rheumatoid arthritis. *Ann Rheum Dis* 1996; **55:** 288–93.

14. Caputo CB, Meadows D, Frisz LG. Failure of estrogens and androgens to inhibit bone resorption in tissue culture. *Endocrinology* 1976; **98:** 1065–8.

15. Lowe C, Gray DH, Reid IR. Serum blocks the osteolytic effect of cortisol in neonatal mouse calvaria. *Calcif Tissue Int* 1992; **50:** 189–92.

16. Gronowicz G, McCarthy MB, Raisz LG. Glucocorticoids stimulate resorption in fetal rat parietal bones in vitro. *J Bone Miner Res* 1990; **5:** 1223–30.

17. Reid IR, Katz J, Ibbertson et al. The effects of hydrocortisone, parathyroid hormone and the bisphosphonate APD on bone resorption in neonatal mouse calvaria. *Calcif Tissue Int* 1986; **38:** 38–43.

18. Shuto T, Kukita T, Hirata M et al. Dexamethasone stimulates osteoclast-like cell formation by inhibiting granulocyte-macrophage colony-stimulating factor production in mouse bone marrow cultures. *Endocrinology* 1994; **134:** 1121–6.

19. Tobias J, Chambers TJ. Glucocorticoids impaire bone resorptive activity and viability of osteoclasts disaggregated from neonatal rat long bones. *Endocrinology* 1989; **125:** 1290–5.

20. Cosman F, Nieves J, Herbert J et al. High-dose glucocorticoids in multiple sclerosis patients exert direct effects on the kidney and skeleton. *J Bone Miner Res* 1994; **9:** 1097–105.

21. Tohmon M, Fukase M, Kishihara M et al. Effect of glucocorticoid administration on intestinal, renal and cerebellar calbindin-D28K in chicks. *J Bone Miner Res* 1988; **3:** 325–31.

22. Gray RES, Doherty SM, Galloway J et al. A double-blind study of deflazacort and prednisone in patients with chronic inflammatory disorders. *Arthritis Rheum* 1991; **34:** 287–95.

23. Reid IR, Ibberston HK. Evidence for decreased tubular reabsorption of calcium in glucocorticoid-treated asthmatics. *Hormone Res* 1987; **27:** 200–4.

24. Braun JJ, Juttman JR, Visser TJ et al. Short-term effect of prednisone on serum 1,25-hydroxy-vitamin D in normal individuals and in hyper-

and hypoparathyroidism. *Clin Endocrinol* 1982; **17**: 21–8.

25. Fucik RF, Kukreja SC, Hargis GK et al. Effect of glucocorticoids on function of the parathyroid glands in man. *J Clin Endocrinol Metab* 1975; **40**: 152–85.

26. Au WYW. Cortisol stimulation of parathyroid hormone secretion by rat parathyroid glands in organ culture. *Science* 1976; **193**: 1015–17.

27. Sugimoto T, Brown AJ, Ritter C et al. Combined effects of dexamethasone and 1,25-dihydroxyvitamin D_3 on parathyroid hormone secretion in cultured bovine parathyroid cells. *Endocrinology* 1989; **125**: 638–41.

28. Butler RC, Davie MWJ, Worsfold M et al. Bone mineral content in patients with rheumatoid arthritis: relationship to low-dose steroid therapy. *Br J Rheumatol* 1991; **30**: 86–90.

29. Bikle DD, Halloran B, Fong L et al. Elevated 1,25-dihydroxyvitamin-D levels in patients with chronic obstructive pulmonary disease treated with prednisone. *J Clin Endocrinol Metab* 1993; **76**: 456–61.

30. Hattersley AT, Meeran K, Burrin J et al. The effect of long- and short-term corticosteroids on plasma calcitonin and parathyroid hormone levels. *Calcif Tissue Int* 1994; **54**: 198–202.

31. Chen TL, Feldman D. Glucocorticoid receptors and actions in subpopulations of cultured rat bone cells. *J Clin Invest* 1979; **63**: 750–8.

32. Hahn TJ, Halstead LR. Cortisol enhancement of PTH-stimulated cyclic AMP accumulation in cultured fetal rat long bone rudiments. *Calcif Tissue Int* 1979; **29**: 173–5.

33. Titus L, Rubin JE, Lorang MT et al. Glucocorticoids and 1,25-dihydroxyvitamin D_3 regulate parathyroid hormone stimulation of adenosine 3',5'-monophosphate-dependent protein kinase in rat osteosarcoma cells. *Endocrinology* 1988; **123**: 1526.

34. Zajac JD, Livesey SA, Michelangeli VP et al. Glucocorticoid treatment facilitates cyclic adenosine 3',5'-monophosphate-dependent protein kinase response in parathyroid hormone-responsive osteogenic sarcoma cells. *Endocrinology* 1986; **118**: 2059–64.

35. Doerr P, Pirke KM. Cortisol-induced suppression of plasma testosterone in normal adult males. *J Clin Endocrinol Metab* 1976; **43**: 622–9.

36. Reid IR, France JT, Pybus J et al. Low plasma testosterone levels in glucocorticoid-treated male asthmatics. *BMJ* 1985; **291**: 574.

37. Rizzato G, Montemurro L. Reversibility of exogenous corticosteroid-induced bone loss. *Eur Respir J* 1993; **6**: 116–19.

38. Laan RFJM, Vanriel PLCM, Vandeputte LBA et al. Low-dose prednisone induces rapid reversible axial bone loss in patients with rheumatoid arthritis – a randomized, controlled study. *Ann Intern Med* 1993; **119**: 963–8.

39. Lo Cascio V, Bonucci E, Imbimbo B et al. Bone loss in response to long-term glucocorticoid therapy. *Bone Miner* 1990; **8**: 39–51.

40. Saito JK, Davis JW, Wasnich RD et al. Users of low-dose glucocorticoids have increased bone loss rates: A longitudinal study. *Calcif Tissue Int* 1995; **57**: 115–19.

41. Reid IR, Evans MC, Wattie DJ et al. Bone mineral density of the proximal femur and lumbar spine in glucocorticoid-treated asthmatic patients. *Osteoporosis Int* 1992; **2**: 103–5.

42. Reid IR, Heap SW. Determinants of vertebral mineral density in patients receiving chronic glucocorticoid therapy. *Arch Intern Med* 1990; **150**: 2545–8.

43. Reid IR, Evans MC, Stapleton J. Lateral spine densitometry is a more sensitive indicator of glucocorticoid-induced bone loss. *J Bone Miner Res* 1992; **7**: 1221–5.

44. Hall GM, Spector TD, Griffin AJ et al. The effect of rheumatoid arthritis and steroid therapy on bone density in postmenopausal women. *Arthritis Rheum* 1993; **36**: 1510–16.

45. Mateo L, Nolla JM, Rozadilla A et al. Bone mineral density in patients with temporal arteritis and polymyalgia rheumatica. *J Rheumatol* 1993; **20**: 1369–73.

46. Lufkin EG, Wahner HW, Bergstralh EJ. Reversibility of steroid-induced osteoporosis. *Am J Med* 1988; **85**: 887–8.

47. Hermus AR, Huysmans DA, Smals AG et al. Remarkable improvement of osteopenia after cure of Cushing's syndrome. *Horm Metab Res* 1994; **26**: 209–10.

48. Manning PJ, Evans MC, Reid IR. Normal bone mineral density following cure of Cushing's syndrome. *Clin Endocrinol* 1992; **36**: 229–34.

49. Chesney RW, Mazess RB, Rose P et al. Effect of prednisone on growth and bone mineral content in childhood glomerular disease. *Am J Dis Child* 1978; **132**: 768–72.

50. Gluck OS, Murphy WA, Hahn TJ et al. Bone loss in adults receiving alternate day glucocorticoid therapy. *Arthritis Rheum* 1981; **24**: 892–8.

51. Ruegsegger P, Medici TC, Anliker M. Corticosteroid-induced bone loss. A longitudi-

nal study of alternate day therapy in patients with bronchial asthma using quantitative computed tomography. *Eur J Clin Pharmacol* 1983; **25:** 615–20.

52. Marystone JF, Barrett-Connor EL, Morton DJ. Inhaled and oral corticosteroids – their effects on bone mineral density in older adults. *Am J Pub Health* 1995; **85:** 1693–5.

53. Doull I, Freezer N, Holgate S. Osteocalcin, growth, and inhaled corticosteroids – a prospective study. *Arch Dis Child* 1996; **74:** 497–501.

54. Ross EJ, Linch DC. Cushing's syndrome – killing disease: discriminatory value of signs and symptoms aiding early diagnosis. *Lancet* 1982; **ii:** 646–9.

55. Adinoff AD, Hollister JR. Steroid-induced fractures and bone loss in patients with asthma. *N Engl J Med* 1983; **309:** 265–8.

56. Luengo M, Picado C, Del Rio L et al. Vertebral fractures in steroid dependent asthma and involutional osteoporosis: a comparative study. *Thorax* 1991; **46:** 803–6.

57. Michel BA, Bloch DA, Fries JF. Predictors of fractures in early rheumatoid arthritis. *J Rheumatol* 1991; **18:** 804–8.

58. Laan RFJM, van Riel PLCM, van Erning LJThO et al. Vertebral osteoporosis in rheumatoid arthritis patients: effect of low dose prednisone therapy. *Br J Rheumatol* 1992; **31:** 91–6.

59. Spector TD, Hall GM, McCloskey EV et al. Risk of vertebral fracture in women with rheumatoid arthritis. *BMJ* 1993; **306:** 558.

60. Lems WF, Jahangier ZN, Jacobs JWG et al. Vertebral fractures in patients with rheumatoid arthritis treated with corticosteroids. *Clin Exp Rheumatol* 1995; **13:** 293–7.

61. Michel BA, Bloch DA, Wolfe F et al. Fractures in rheumatoid arthritis – an evaluation of associated risk factors. *J Rheumatol* 1993; **20:** 1666–9.

62. Cooper C, Coupland C, Mitchell M. Rheumatoid arthritis, corticosteroid therapy and hip fracture. *Ann Rheum Dis* 1995; **54:** 49–52.

63. Shane E, Rivas M, Staron RB et al. Fracture after cardiac transplantation – a prospective longitudinal study. *J Clin Endocrinol Metab* 1996; **81:** 1740–6.

64. Nilsen KH, Jayson MIV, Dixon AStJ. Microcrystalline calcium hydroxyapatite compound in corticosteroid-treated rheumatoid patients: a controlled study. *BMJ* 1978; **2:** 1124.

65. Warady BD, Lindsley CB, Robinson RG et al. Effects of nutritional supplementations on bone mineral status of children with rheumatic diseases receiving corticosteroid therapy. *J Rheumatol* 1994; **21:** 530–5.

66. Reid IR, Ibbertson HK. Calcium supplements in the prevention of steroid-induced osteoporosis. *Am J Clin Nutr* 1986; **44:** 287–90.

67. Reid IR, King AR, Alexander CJ et al. Prevention of steroid-induced osteoporosis with (3-amino-1-hydroxypropylidene)-1,1-bisphosphonate (APD). *Lancet* 1988; **i:** 143–6.

68. Reid IR, Heap SW, King AR et al. Two-year follow-up of bisphosphonate (APD) treatment in steroid osteoporosis. *Lancet* 1988; **ii:** 1144.

69. Sambrook P, Birmingham J, Kelly P et al. Prevention of corticosteroid osteoporosis – a comparison of calcium, calcitriol, and calcitonin. *N Engl J Med* 1993; **328:** 1747–52.

70. Lukert BP, Johnson BE, Robinson RG. Estrogen and progesterone replacement therapy reduces glucocorticoid-induced bone loss. *J Bone Miner Res* 1992; **7:** 1063–9.

71. Grey AB, Cundy TF, Reid IR. Continuous combined oestrogen/progestin therapy is well tolerated and increases bone density at the hip and spine in post-menopausal osteoporosis. *Clin Endocrinol* 1994; **40:** 671–7.

72. Reid IR, Grey AB. Corticosteroid osteoporosis. *Baillière's Clin Rheumatol* 1993; **7:** 573–87.

73. Macdonald AG, Murphy EA, Capell HA et al. Effects of hormone replacement therapy in rheumatoid arthritis – a double blind placebo-controlled study. *Ann Rheum Dis* 1994; **53:** 54–7.

74. Studd JWW, Savvas M, Johnson M. Correction of corticosteroid-induced osteoporosis by percutaneous hormone implants. *Lancet* 1989; **i:** 339.

75. Reid IR, Wattie DJ, Evans MC et al. Testosterone therapy in glucocorticoid-treated men. *Arch Intern Med* 1996; **156:** 1173–7.

76. Need AG. Corticosteroids and osteoporosis. *Aust N Z J Med* 1987; **17:** 267–72.

77. Adami S, Fossaluzza V, Rossini M et al. The prevention of corticosteroid-induced osteoporosis with nandrolone decanoate. *Bone Miner* 1991; **15:** 72–81.

78. Gallacher SJ, Fenner JAK, Anderson K et al. Intravenous pamidronate in the treatment of osteoporosis associated with corticosteroid dependent lung disease – an open pilot study. *Thorax* 1992; **47:** 932–6.

79. Worth H, Stammen D, Keck E. Therapy of steroid-induced bone loss in adult asthmatic

with calcium, vitamin D, and a diphosphonate. *Am J Respir Crit Care Med* 1994; **150:** 394–7.

80. Diamond T, McGuigan L, Barbagallo S et al. Cyclical etidronate plus ergocalciferol prevents glucocorticoid-induced bone loss in postmenopausal women. *Am J Med* 1995; **98:** 459–63.

81. Struys A, Snelder AA, Mulder H. Cyclical etidronate reverses bone loss of the spine and proximal femur in patients with established corticosteroid-induced osteoporosis. *Am J Med* 1995; **99:** 235–42.

82. Gregoire AJP, Kumar R, Everitt B et al. Transdermal oestrogen for treatment of severe postnatal depression. *Lancet* 1996; **347:** 930–3.

83. Hahn TJ, Hahn BH. Osteopenia in patients with rheumatic diseases: principles of diagnosis and therapy. *Semin Arthritis Rheum* 1976; **6:** 165–88.

84. Hahn TJ, Halstead LR, Teitelbaum SL et al. Altered mineral metabolism in glucocorticoid-induced osteopenia. *J Clin Invest* 1979; **64:** 655–65.

85. Dykman TR, Haralson KM, Gluck OS et al. Effect of oral 1,25-dihydroxy-vitamin D and calcium on glucocorticoid-induced osteopenia in patients with rheumatic diseases. *Arthritis Rheum* 1984; **27:** 1336–43.

86. Braun JJ, Birkenhager-Frenkel DH, Rietveld Jr AH et al. Influence of 1α(OH)D3 administration on bone and bone mineral metabolism in patients on chronic glucocorticoid treatment; a double-blind controlled study. *Clin Endocrinol* 1983; **18:** 265–73.

87. Bijlsma JWJ, Raymakers JA, Mosch C et al. Effect of oral calcium and vitamin D on glucocorticoid-induced osteopenia. *Clin Exp Rheumatol* 1988; **6:** 113–19.

88. Di Munno O, Beghe F, Favini P et al. Prevention of glucocorticoid-induced osteopenia: Effect of oral 25-hydroxyvitamin D and calcium. *Clin Rheumatol* 1989; **8:** 202–7.

89. Waterhouse DM, Calzone KA, Mele C et al. Adherence to oral tamoxifen – a comparison of patient self-report, pill counts, and microelectronic monitoring. *J Clin Oncol* 1993; **11:** 1189–97.

90. Mulder H, Struys A. Intermittent cyclical etidronate in the prevention of corticosteroid-induced bone loss. *Br J Rheumatol* 1994; **33:** 348–50.

91. Van Cleemput J, Daenen W, Geusens P et al. Prevention of bone loss in cardiac transplant recipients – a comparison of biphosphonates and vitamin D. *Transplantation* 1996; **61:** 1495–9.

92. Adachi JD, Bensen WG, Bianchi F et al. Vitamin D and calcium in the prevention of corticosteroid induced osteoporosis – a 3 year followup. *J Rheumatol* 1996; **23:** 995–1000.

93. Rizzoli R, Chevalley T, Slosman DO et al. Sodium monofluorophosphate increases vertebral bone mineral density in patients with corticosteroid-induced osteoporosis. *Osteoporosis Int* 1995; **5:** 39–46.

94. Guaydier-Souquieres G, Kotzki PO, Sabatier JP et al. In corticosteroid-treated respiratory diseases, monofluorophosphate increases lumbar bone density – a double-masked randomized study. *Osteoporosis Int* 1996; **6:** 171–7.

95. Meunier PJ, Briancon D, Chavassieux P et al. Treatment with fluoride: bone histomorphometric findings. In: *Osteoporosis* (Christiansen C, Johansen JS, Riis BJ, eds). Copenhagen: Osteopress, 1987: 824–8.

96. Rizzato G, Tosi G, Schiraldi G et al. Bone protection with salmon calcitonin (sCT) in the long-term steroid therapy of chronic sarcoidosis. *Sarcoidosis* 1988; **5:** 99–103.

97. Luengo M, Picado C, Del Rio Le et al. Treatment of steroid-induced osteopenia with calcitonin in corticosteroid-dependent asthma. *Am Rev Respir Dis* 1990; **142:** 104–7.

98. Montemurro L, Schiraldi G, Fraioli P et al. Prevention of corticosteroid-induced osteoporosis with salmon calcitonin in sarcoid patients. *Calcif Tissue Int* 1991; **49:** 71–6.

99. Caniggia A, Marchetti M, Gennari C et al. Effects of a new glucocorticoid, oxazacort, on some variables connected with bone metabolism in man: a comparison with prednisone. *Int J Clin Pharmacol* 1977; **15:** 126–34.

100. Gray RES, Doherty SM, Galloway J et al. A double-blind study of deflazacort and prednisone in patients with chronic inflammatory disorders. *Arthritis Rheum* 1991; **34:** 287–95.

101. Lo Cascio V, Bonnucci E, Imbimbo B et al. Bone loss after glucocorticoid therapy. *Calcif Tissue Int* 1984; **36:** 435–8.

102. Gennari C, Imbimbo B. Effects of prednisone and deflazacort on vertebral bone mass. *Calcif Tissue Int* 1985; **37:** 592–3.

103. Loftus J, Allen R, Hesp J et al. Randomized, double-blind trial of deflazacort versus prednisone in juvenile chronic rheumatoid arthritis: a relatively bone-sparing effect of deflazacort. *Paediatrics* 1991; **88:** 428–36.

104. Olgaard K, Storm T, Wowern NV et al. Glucocorticoid induced osteoporosis in the

lumbar spine, forearm and mandible of nephrotic patients. A double-blind study on the high-dose long-term effects of prednisone versus deflazacort. *Calcif Tissue Int* 1992; **50:** 490–7.

105. Balsan S, Steru D, Bourdeau A et al. Effects of long-term maintenance therapy with a new glucocorticoid, deflazacort, on mineral metabolism and statural growth. *Calcif Tissue Int* 1987; **40:** 303–9.

106. Aicardi G, Milani S, Imbimbo B et al. Comparison of growth retarding effects induced by two different glucocorticoids in pre-pubertal sick children: an interim long-term analysis. *Calcif Tissue Int* 1991; **48:** 283–7.

107. Dimunno O, Imbimbo B, Mazzantini M et al. Deflazacort versus methylprednisolone in polymyalgia rheumatica: clinical equivalence and relative antiinflammatory potency of different treatment regimens. *J Rheumatol* 1995; **22:** 1492–8.

108. Weisman MH. Dose equivalency of deflazacort and prednisone in the treatment of steroid dependent rheumatoid arthritis. In: *Proceedings of the 4th International Symposium on Osteoporosis* (Christiansen C, Riis B, eds). 4th International Symposium on Osteoporosis, Copenhagen, 1993: 515.

109. Krogsgaard MR, Thamsborg G, Lund B. Changes in bone mass during low dose corticosteroid treatment in patients with polymyalgia rheumatica – a double blind, prospective comparison between prednisolone and deflazacort. *Ann Rheum Dis* 1996; **55:** 143–6.

110. Finkelstein JS, Cleary RL, Butler JP et al. A comparison of lateral versus anterior–posterior spine dual energy x-ray absorptiometry for the diagnosis of osteopenia. *J Clin Endocrinol Metab* 1994; **78:** 724–30.

111. Reid IR, Legge M, Stapleton JP et al. Regular exercise dissociates fat mass and bone density in premenopausal women. *J Clin Endocrinol Metab* 1995; **80:** 1764–8.

112. Bauer DC, Browner WS, Cauley JA et al. Factors associated with appendicular bone mass in older women. *Am Intern Med* 1993; **118:** 657–65.

113. Janes CH, Dickson ER, Okazaki R et al. Role of hyperbilirubinemia in the impairment of osteoblast proliferation associated with cholestatic jaundice. *J Clin Invest* 1995; **95:** 2581–6.

114. Revilla M, Delasierra G, Aguado F et al. Bone mass in parkinson's disease – a study with three methods. *Calcif Tissue Int* 1996; **58:** 311–15.

115. Silverberg SJ, Bilezikian JP. Evaluation and management of primary hyperparathyroidism. *J Clin Endocrinol Metab* 1996; **81:** 2036–40.

116. Grey AB, Stapleton JP, Evans MC et al. Accelerated bone loss in postmenopausal women with mild primary hyperparathyroidism. *Clin Endocrinol* 1996; **44:** 697–702.

117. Sowers M, Randolph J, Shapiro B et al. A prospective study of bone density and pregnancy after an extended period of lactation with bone loss. *Obstet Gynecol* 1995; **85:** 285–9.

118. Reid IR, Wattie DJ, Evans MC et al. Post-pregnancy osteoporosis associated with hypercalcaemia: a case report and literature review. *Clin Endocrinol* 1992; **37:** 298–303.

119. Cooper C, Carbone L, Michet CJ et al. Fracture risk in patients with ankylosing spondylitis: a population based study. *J Rheumatol* 1994; **21:** 1877–82.

120. Pietschmann F, Breslau NA, Pak CYC. Reduced vertebral bone density in hypercalciuric nephrolithiasis. *J Bone Miner Res* 1992; **7:** 1383–8.

121. Reid IR, Ames R, Evans MC et al. Determinants of total body and regional bone mineral density in normal postmenopausal women – a key role for fat mass. *J Clin Endocrinol Metab* 1992; **75:** 45–51.

122. Cundy T, Cornish J, Evans MC et al. Recovery of bone density in women who stop using medroxyprogesterone acetate. *BMJ* 1994; **308:** 247–8.

123. Valimaki MJ, Tiihonen M, Laitinen K et al. Bone mineral density measured by dual-energy x-ray absorptiometry and novel markers of bone formation and resorption in patients on antiepileptic drugs. *J Bone Miner Res* 1994; **9:** 631–7.

124. Zonneveld IM, Bakker WK, Dijkstra PF et al. Methotrexate osteopathy in long-term, low-dose methotrexate treatment for psoriasis and rheumatoid arthritis. *Arch Dermatol* 1996; **132:** 184–7.

125. Dahlman TC. Osteoporotic fractures and the recurrence of thromboembolism during pregnancy and the puerperium in 184 women undergoing thromboprophylaxis with heparin. *Am J Obstet Gynecol* 1993; **168:** 1265–70.

126. Sambrook PN, Kelly PJ, Fontana D et al. Mechanisms of rapid bone loss following cardiac transplantation. *Osteoporosis Int* 1994; **4:** 273–6.

16

Quality of life in osteoporosis

P Lips

CONTENTS • Consequences of osteoporosis • Quality of life assessment • Osteoporosis questionnaires • Conclusion

Osteoporosis leads to fractures which cause pain and disability. These may be moderate and temporary as in the case of distal forearm fracture or severe and chronic after several vertebral crush fractures. Hip fracture often leads to severe functional impairment, especially with walking, necessitating change of residence. Clinical studies have indicated that there is only a moderate correlation between pain and the number of vertebral fractures, whereas disability often correlates better with the number of vertebral fractures.[1,2] Functional impairment and pain lead to social dysfunction and may have psychological impact.[3] Lack of energy and depression are common findings in osteoporotic patients, and these are all components of quality of life. The effect of treatment of osteoporosis may be quantified as a decrease of fracture incidence, an increase of bone mineral density, a change in biochemical markers of bone turnover or an improvement in quality of life. The last relates more directly to the overall functioning of the patient. For this purpose, questionnaires have been developed for use in the individual patient or in clinical trials. Assessment of quality of life has been mentioned as a prerogative for the testing of new osteoporosis treatments.[4,5]

CONSEQUENCES OF OSTEOPOROSIS

Epidemiological studies have estimated that less than half of all vertebral deformities may come to clinical attention.[6,7] Of course, these deformities may have other causes such as Scheuermann's disease, osteoarthritis or trauma, which are more common in men. The occurrence of a vertebral fracture may either pass unnoticed or lead to severe pain, which abates in the months or years after fracture.[2] A new vertebral fracture may lead to a relapse of pain. Chronic pain may persist and this is more likely when several vertebral fractures have occurred. Although pain intensity does not necessarily increase with subsequent fractures, dysfunction often parallels the number of vertebral fractures. A clinical study in 70 patients with osteoporosis showed a good correlation between impairment of self-care and spine deformity index.[1]

The score of the Sickness Impact Profile, a generic (non-specific) quality of life questionnaire, was higher with multiple vertebral fractures than with a single vertebral fracture, and was even more elevated after hip fracture.[8]

Virtually all patients with hip fracture are operated on and pain usually is not a severe problem. However, most patients have functional disability with dressing, and walking upstairs and outside.[9–13] A study of 120 patients who sustained a hip fracture showed significant disability 6 months after the fracture.[9] Although 86% could dress independently before hip fracture, only 49% were able to do so 6 months after the fracture. For independent transfer the data were 90% before and 32% after the fracture. For independent walking and stair climbing the numbers were 75% and 63% before hip fracture and 15% and 8% 6 months after the fracture. There are few data on quality of life after distal forearm fracture or proximal humerus fracture.

QUALITY OF LIFE ASSESSMENT

Quality of life can be defined as the assembly of the functional, social and psychological well-being of a person.[14–16] It may be assessed by covering various aspects of well-being in an interview. In the last few decades, many instruments have been developed for the assessment of quality of life in the general population or in specific patient groups. Quality of life questionnaires may be generic, i.e. aimed at assessing general state of health and not directed at one disease, or specific, i.e. aimed at a specific population, function or disease. Generic questionnaires may be more time-consuming but, on the other hand, can be used in various populations and situations and may detect unexpected effects. They also enable comparison between different diseases. Examples of generic questionnaires are the Sickness Impact Profile,[17] Nottingham Health Profile,[18] the McMaster Health Index Questionnaire[19] and the Short Forms of the Medical Outcomes Study.[20]

Disease-specific questionnaires may be more efficient because they do not contain redundant questions. On the other hand, rare or unexpected symptoms may be missed. Examples of specific questionnaires are the Arthritis Impact Scale, the Irritable Bowel Questionnaire and the Geriatric Depression Scale. Disease-specific questionnaires are probably more valid, i.e. agree better with grade of disease. They should

	Generic	Disease-specific
Examples	Nottingham Health Profile	Arthritis Impact Scale
	Sickness Impact Profile	Irritable Bowel Questionnaire
	MOS Short Form 36	Geriatric Depression Scale
Population selectivity	Assesses general health	Focused on specific problems
	Useful in various populations	Makes sense to the patient
	Detects unexpected effects	Misses unexpected effects
	Facilitates comparison between diseases	Not suitable for other diseases
	May detect co-morbidity	
Time	Takes more time	Efficient
		Less burden to patient
Sensitivity	Reduced for specific diseases	Sensitive for one disease

Table 16.1 Characteristics of generic and disease-specific questionnaires for quality of life

have a higher sensitivity to change, i.e. better parallel improvement or deterioration of disease. Some advantages of generic questionnaires are the possibility of comparing quality of life in different diseases and supplying normative data for the general population.[21] Patients with osteoporosis, especially those with hip fracture, may be of advanced age and show considerable co-morbidity. This might be assessed as well with a generic instrument. Some properties of generic and disease-specific questionnaires are summarized in Table 16.1.

Quality of life questionnaires are multidimensional. They contain modules for the assessment of pain, activities of daily living, mobility, social function and emotional well-being. A questionnaire should be tested on repeatability (short-term reproducibility) and validity. The last indicates how far it agrees with grade of disease, which in the case of osteoporosis is with the number of (vertebral) fractures. Some questionnaires are meant for self-administration by the patient whereas others should be administered by an interviewer. The latter may add subjective interpretation. On the one hand, self-administration enables widespread use of the questionnaire; on the other, it may lead to misunderstanding and missed values.

Questionnaires also differ in the way they show different degrees of illness; they may be meant for more healthy or more ill people. In a large population study in the UK, the Nottingham Health Profile showed a black and white picture on one end of the scale whereas the Short Form 36 yielded more grey values.[20] This depends on the answer categories for the questions where there are two in the Nottingham Health Profile and five in the Short Form 36.

OSTEOPOROSIS QUESTIONNAIRES

Over the past few years, a tendency has arisen to develop disease-specific questionnaires. Several studies in patients with vertebral osteoporosis have shown that functional limitations in activities of daily living, household activities,

social activities and mood changes, such as lack of energy and depression, are at least as specific as back pain. Quality of life questionnaires for osteoporosis may be used in epidemiological studies, health economics or clinical trials.[22]

Extensive studies have been performed by Ross et al at the Hawaii Osteoporosis Center using an 11-question disability survey.[2] The questions related to pain or discomfort with various movements, walking and activities of daily living. It was shown that new vertebral fractures occurring during the study (incident fractures) were associated with more pain and disability than prevalent vertebral fractures (Figure 16.1). The pain and disability lasted for several years after the occurrence of the vertebral fracture. A more basic approach was used by Cook and colleagues.[23] They identified items by examining generic questionnaires and interviewing rheumatologists, rheumatology nurses, physiotherapists and patients. Their initial questionnaire contained 168 items in five domains and it was to be administered by an

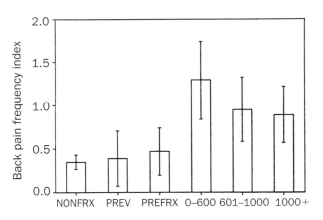

Figure 16.1 Back pain frequency index in subjects without fractures, prevalent fracture (PREV), before fracture (PREFRX) and at various times after an incident fracture (0–600, 601–1000, 1000+ days after fracture). (Reproduced, with permission, from Ross et al.[2])

interviewer. The questionnaire was evaluated in 100 women with at least one vertebral fracture.

The highest scores were related to pain, difficulty in lifting and carrying objects, and fear of falls and fractures. The results correlated fairly well with the Sickness Impact Profile but the relationship with grade of disease as assessed by radiographs or densitometry was poor. A Working Party of the European Foundation for Osteoporosis has developed a specific questionnaire for patients with established vertebral osteoporosis, i.e. with at least one vertebral fracture.[24] This questionnaire was made to be used in clinical trials. It includes 54 questions

and visual analogue scales in the seven domains: pain, activities of daily living (ADL), housekeeping, mobility, leisure and social activities, general health perception, and emotion. The questionnaire can be completed by the patient in about 20 minutes. Currently, versions in eight languages are available. Preliminary results of validation in a multicentre study showed good reproducibility and discrimination between patients with vertebral osteoporosis and control subjects (Table 16.2). Other specific questionnaires which have been developed for osteoporosis include the Osteoporosis Assessment Questionnaire (OPAQ) comprising

Table 16.2 Some questions of the questionnaire for quality of life of the European Foundation for Osteoporosis (Qualeffo)

	Question	Answer	κ	OR (95% CI)
3	How severe is your back pain at its worst?	( ) no back pain ( ) mild ( ) moderate ( ) severe ( ) unbearable	0.69	2.1 (1.6–2.7)
10	Do you have problems with dressing?	( ) no difficulty ( ) a little difficulty ( ) moderate difficulty ( ) may need some help ( ) impossible without help	0.71	2.7 (1.6–4.3)
19	Can you get up from a chair?	( ) without difficulty ( ) with a little difficulty ( ) with moderate difficulty ( ) with great difficulty ( ) only with help	0.70	2.5 (1.6–4.0)
33	How often did you visit friends or relatives during the last 3 months?	( ) once a week or more ( ) once or twice a month ( ) less than once a month ( ) never	0.62	1.3 (1.0–1.8)

The repeatability (within subject agreement: κ) was tested by repeating the questionnaire in the same subjects within 4 weeks. The discrimination between patients with osteoporosis and control subjects is presented as the odds ratio (OR) with 95% confidence interval (95% CI). (Reproduced with permission, from Lips et al.[24])

79 questions[25] and the Osteoporosis Targeted Quality of Life Questionnaire, comprising 32 items in three domains (physical difficulties, adaptations and fears) developed for cross-sectional population studies.[26,27] The last was validated and showed good internal consistency and reproducibility. It showed moderate to good correlations with the Short Form 36 and discriminated between osteoporosis and osteopenia. When choosing a specific questionnaire, cultural differences should also be taken into account.

Osteoporosis is a disease of postmenopausal women and elderly people. As stated before, it is often associated with significant co-morbidity. Other chronic diseases, e.g. cardiovascular, neurological and locomotor diseases, may also impair quality of life to a significant degree and these may determine the outcome in patients with hip fracture. For assessing co-morbidity or 'burden of disease', the use of a generic quality of life instrument may complement the use of a specific osteoporosis questionnaire. In elderly people, the scope of a questionnaire is limited. Functional tests may give a better picture of physical limitations, such as mobility impairment.[3,28]

CONCLUSION

Osteoporotic fractures lead to functional limitations which impair household activities, mobility and social life, and may lead to decreased self-esteem, anxiety and depression. These facts can be assessed by a multidimensional quality of life questionnaire. Specific instruments are now available for osteoporotic patients. These may be used in epidemiology and clinical trials. Generic quality of life questionnaires may also be used in osteoporotic patients to assess general health and co-morbidity, or to facilitate comparison with other patient groups. The data obtained with a specific questionnaire can be completed by functional testing in order to quantify the physical limitations.

REFERENCES

1. Leidig G, Minne HW, Sauer P et al. A study of complaints and their relation to vertebral destruction in patients with osteoporosis. *Bone Miner* 1990; **8:** 217–29.
2. Ross PD, Davis JW, Epstein RS et al. Pain and disability associated with new vertebral fractures and other spinal conditions. *J Clin Epidemiol* 1994; **47:** 231–9.
3. Lyles KW, Gold DT, Shipp KM et al. Association of osteoporotic vertebral compression fractures with impaired functional status. *Am J Med* 1993; **94:** 595–601.
4. Kanis JA, Geusens P, Christiansen C on behalf of the Working Party of the Foundation. Guidelines for clinical trials in osteoporosis. A position paper of the European Foundation for Osteoporosis and Bone Disease. *Osteoporosis Int* 1991; **1:** 182–8.
5. Reginster JY, Compston JE on behalf of the Group for the Respect of Ethics and Excellence in Science. Recommendations for the registration of new chemical entities used in the prevention and treatment of osteoporosis. *Calcif Tissue Int* 1995; **57:** 247–50.
6. Spector TB, McCloskey EV, Doyle DV et al. Prevalence of vertebral fracture in women and the relationship with bone density and symptoms: the Chingford study. *J Bone Miner Res* 1993; **8:** 817–22.
7. O'Neill TW, Felsenberg D, Varlow J et al. The prevalence of vertebral deformity in European men and women: the European Vertebral Osteoporosis Study. *J Bone Miner Res* 1996; **11:** 1010–18.
8. Kanis J, McCloskey EV. Epidemiology of vertebral osteoporosis. *Bone* 1992; **13:** S1–S10.
9. Marotolli RA, Berkman LF, Cooney LM. Decline in physical function following hip fracture. *J Am Geriatr Soc* 1992; **40:** 861–6.
10. Magaziner J, Simonsick EM, Kashner TM et al. Predictors of functional recovery one year following hospital discharge for hip fracture: a prospective study. *J Gerontol A Biol Sci Med Sci* 1990; **45:** 101–7.
11. Chrischilles EA, Shireman T, Wallace R. Costs and health effects of osteoporotic fractures. *Bone* 1994; **15:** 377–86.
12. Jalovarra P, Virkkunen H. Quality of life after

hemiarthroplasty for femoral neck fracture. *Acta Orthop Scand* 1991; **62:** 208–17.

13. Greendale GA, Barrett-Connor E, Ingles S et al. Late physical activity and functional effects of osteoporotic fracture in women: the Rancho Bernardo Study. *J Am Geriatr Soc* 1995; **43:** 955–61.

14. Fitzpatrick R, Fletcher A, Gore S et al. Quality of life measures in health care I. Applications and issues in assessment. *BMJ* 1992; **305:** 1074–7.

15. Fletcher A, Gore S, Jones D et al. Quality of life measures in health care II. Design, analysis and interpretation. *BMJ* 1992; **305:** 1145–8.

16. Spiegelhalter DJ, Gore SM, Fitzpatrick R et al. Quality of life measures in health care III: resource allocation. *BMJ* 1992; **305:** 1205–9.

17. Bergner M, Bobbitt RA, Carter WB et al. The sickness impact profile: development and final revision of a health status measure. *Med Care* 1981: **19:** 787–805.

18. Hunt S, McEwen J, McKenna SP. Measuring health status: a new tool for clinicians and epidemiologists. *J R Coll Gen Pract* 1985; **35:** 185–8.

19. Guyatt GH, Feeney DH, Patrick DL. Measuring health-related quality of life. *Ann Intern Med* 1993; **70:** 225–30.

20. Brazier JE, Harper R, Jones NMB et al. Validating the SF36 health survey questionnaire: new outcome measures for primary care. *BMJ* 1992; **305:** 160–4.

21. Jenkinson C, Coulter A, Weight L. Short form 36 (SF 36) health survey questionnaire: normative data for adults of working age. *BMJ* 1993; **306:** 1437–40.

22. Kanis JA, Minne HW, Meunier PJ et al. Quality of life and vertebral osteoporosis. *Osteoporosis Int* 1992; **2:** 161–3.

23. Cook DJ, Guyatt GH, Adachi JD et al. Quality of life issues in women with vertebral fractures due to osteoporosis. *Arthritis Rheum* 1993; **36:** 750–6.

24. Lips P, Cooper C, Agnusdei D et al. Quality of life as outcome in the treatment of osteoporosis: the development of a questionnaire for quality of life by the European Foundation for Osteoporosis. *Osteoporosis Int* 1997; **7:** 36–8.

25. Silverman SL, Go K, Tou K. What is the quality of life of patients with osteoporosis? *J Bone Miner Res* 1996; **11:** S357 (abst).

26. Lydick E, Ross PD, Dwyer J et al. Development of an osteoporosis targeted quality of life questionnaire. *Osteoporosis Int* 1996; **6:** (abst).

27. Chandler JM, Lydick E, Martin AR et al. Measurement characteristics of an osteoporosis targeted quality of life survey. *J Bone Miner Res* 1996; **11:** S357 (abst).

28. Graafmans WC, Ooms ME, Hofstee HMA et al. Falls in the elderly: a prospective study of risk factors and risk profiles. *Am J Epidemiol* 1996; **143:** 1129–36.

Preclinical evaluation of new therapeutic agents for osteoporosis

P Ammann, R Rizzoli and J-P Bonjour

CONTENTS • **Importance of preclinical studies in the development of antiosteoporotic drugs** • **Animal models of osteoporosis** • **Conclusions**

Animal models are of major importance for understanding the pathophysiology of various human diseases at the cellular and molecular levels. In the late 1960s most experimental research conditions in the bone field shifted from animal investigation settings to in vitro systems, with the widespread use of tissue and particularly cell cultures. Thanks to the tremendous progress in molecular genetics, it is now possible to analyse in vivo the role of many factors affecting bone and mineral metabolism. Therefore, from the start of the current decade a reverse trend is occurring with an increasing use of animal experiments in the approach to fundamental questions about the mechanisms involved in the pathophysiology of bone diseases, including osteoporosis. Besides molecular genetics, the remarkable progress made in quantitative image analysis has provided new investigational tools applicable to animal experimentation and to patients with osteoporosis. With the aim of a better understanding of human disease, these technical advances have enabled the development of animal models of osteoporosis in several laboratories. These models are playing a crucial role in the development of new preventive and curative antiosteoporotic therapies.

IMPORTANCE OF PRECLINICAL STUDIES IN THE DEVELOPMENT OF ANTIOSTEOPOROTIC DRUGS

In the development of antiosteoporotic agents, the main objective of preclinical studies is to demonstrate the agent's efficacy in appropriate animal models of osteoporosis and to establish the relationship between the effects on bone mass and bone strength induced by drugs. Other important specific objectives are:

- to assess bone tolerance, i.e. to determine whether the quality of skeletal tissue is maintained with long-term exposure to the agent
- to understand the mechanism of action of the drug.

The results of the preclinical studies will determine whether a new agent should be tested in humans and, if so, the investigations will help to identify the subjects and endpoints required in the different phases of the clinical evaluation.

Several registration authorities have enacted guidelines for the evaluation of antiosteoporotic drugs. The most resounding text on this matter is that made available by the Division of Metabolism and Endocrine Drug Products from the Food and Drug Administration (FDA) in the USA. This text,[1] published in 1994 and entitled 'Guidelines for preclinical and clinical evaluation of agents used in the prevention or treatment of postmenopausal osteoporosis', deserves a critical consideration because its worldwide acceptance will have marked consequences on the future development of antiosteoporotic drugs. The recommendations contained in the April 1994 version of the FDA guidelines have been justifiably influenced by the results of clinical trials, suggesting that drug-induced increase in bone mass may not invariably be associated with a significant commensurate reduction in fracture rate. The possibility of such a dissociation between changes in bone mass and bone strength is certainly an important, if not the most important, aspect that must be considered in the development of new antiosteoporotic agents, particularly those that have the capability of restoring skeletal mass. Accordingly, it is fully understandable that the 1994 FDA guidelines recommended the development of programmes aimed at evaluating whether drug effects on bone mass are accompanied by commensurate effects on bone strength. In fact, quite a substantial portion of the recommendations concerns the preclinical evaluation which was not detailed in the penultimate FDA guidelines in 1985. In the 1994 version, it is stated in the paragraph introducing the preclinical evaluation that

> In addition to toxicity studies required for all new drugs, preclinical studies of bone quality should be performed for drugs to be used in the prevention and intervention of osteoporosis.

It should be noted that, in the 1994 FDA guidelines, 'bone quality is considered to be comprised of architecture, mass and strength of bone'. Further, it is recognized that there is no adequately validated clinical technique for noninvasively assessing bone strength:

> ... but animal studies provide an opportunity to directly examine bone mass, architecture and strength. Thus, the primary objective of preclinical studies is to demon-

strate that long-term treatment with a specific agent will not lead to deleterious effects on bone quality.

In other words, animal studies should permit researchers to identify whether a drug results in abnormal architecture or in the production of bone in which strength is not positively correlated with change in bone mass and architecture. The secondary objective of animal studies, according to the 1994 FDA guidelines, is to demonstrate efficacy. The following is a series of recommendations for these preclinical guidelines:

- The study design which should reflect the clinical indications.
- The animal models (two species, one of which must be the ovariectomized rat; the other will be selected from larger remodelling species at the discretion of the sponsor).
- The use of biochemical markers of bone turnover (pyridinium cross-links, bone specific alkaline phosphatase, osteocalcin).
- Bone mass/density measurement (noninvasive techniques such as dual energy X-ray absorptiometry should be associated with bone ash weight determination).
- Analysis of bone architecture and dynamics (using light microscopy and polarized light microscopy for examining bone collagen arrangement; histomorphometry).
- Biomechanical testing of bone strength (bending, torsional and compression tests).

It appears that most of these recommendations are scientifically sound and quite reasonable in terms of feasibility. However, one stipulation concerning the treatment duration (12 months in ovariectomized rats) is highly disputable, because it is based on limited data about the number of complete resorption and formation cycles per year.

However, the most controversial aspect of the 1994 FDA guidelines is the impact of the preclinical results on the clinical evaluation process. On the one hand, the guidelines specify that the preclinical studies are critical for establishing the relationship between bone mass and bone strength for the drug in question, but, on the other, the results of these preclinical studies will only influence the duration of the clinical trial and not the primary efficacy endpoint. Indeed, fracture evaluation in clinical trials will be required to demonstrate the efficacy of any new antiosteoporotic drug, with the exception of oestrogen. If further applied in the USA and accepted by registration authorities in other countries, this very strict requirement could have tremendous implications for the future development of antiosteoporotic drugs. Indeed fracture rate evaluation in clinical trials is a very difficult task requiring enormous investments from the patients, the medical investigator team and of course the sponsors. Such a difficult requirement would be understandable if (1) the diagnosis of osteoporosis was dependent on the presence of fracture and (2) there was no reliable animal model of osteoporosis.

There is now a large consensus, including the World Health Organization, that defines osteoporosis as 'a disease characterized by low bone mass and microarchitectural deterioration of bone tissue, leading to enhanced bone fragility and a consequent increase in fracture risk'.[2] Thus, the decrease in bone mass with change in microarchitecture and consecutive increased fragility represents the disease, whereas 'spontaneous' or low stress fractures represent a complication of the disease that may or may not occur. Indeed, the osteoporotic fracture is a stochastic event, depending upon several internal and external factors which are not directly related to the osteoporotic process. For instance, in the case of hip fractures, the propensity to fall, the impact near the proximal femur and the local energy absorption by soft tissues are all independent factors.

For many years, experts used to state that there was no animal model of osteoporosis. This view was based chiefly on a definition of osteoporosis that made the occurrence of 'spontaneous' fracture the hallmark or key feature of the disease mandatory to the diagnosis. However, animal models of osteoporosis consistent with the definition mentioned above definitely exist. Indeed, the effects of potential preventive and curative therapies for human osteoporosis can now be reliably evaluated in well-characterized animal models (see below). Therefore, it is now quite possible to elaborate drug development guidelines where the respective 'job specifications' of preclinical versus clinical studies are clearly defined, particularly with respect to mechanical resistance testing, on the basis of well-accepted scientific knowledge. Such a complementary preclinical and clinical programme would avoid the necessity of multicentre clinical trials involving several thousand patients testing one single antiosteoporotic compound. Obviously, the reason for this recruitment of a very large number of patients stems from selecting the fracture rate as the endpoint of antiosteoporotic clinical trials. By analogy, this would correspond to selecting cardiovascular complications as the only endpoint worth evaluating in clinical trials on essential hypertension.

One can understand the rationale for considering the complication(s) of the disease as the most valuable endpoint of a clinical trial. However, the future of antiosteoporotic drug development may well be drastically hampered if difference in fracture rate, with the huge number of patients it requires for a valid statistical assessment, becomes the main endpoint of clinical trials. There is a way to avoid this undesirable orientation. Indeed, it is scientifically sound to envisage a complementary preclinical–clinical programme to assess the efficacy of an antiosteoporotic drug. Thus, it can be conceived that preclinical studies carried out in the most reliable animal models, i.e. the most predictive with respect to human calcium and bone metabolism, and drug responsiveness, will be aimed at testing drug efficacy on bone mass/mineral density, microarchitecture and mechanical resistance in well-controlled conditions. Then, clinical trials in phase III of drug investigation will concentrate on testing efficacy on bone mass/mineral density, and possibly in a limited number of subjects on bone microarchitecture as assessed by histomorphometry, but not on fracture rate. Such a clinical programme will drastically reduce the number of patients necessary for demonstrating drug efficacy. If the results on bone mass/mineral density and possibly microarchitecture are similar to those observed in the selected animal models, and assuming that bone tolerance and overall safety are substantiated, there is good reason to think that the drug will exert the same effect on bone mechanical resistance in humans as demonstrated in animals. Post-marketing surveillance with a well-organized reporting procedure could provide information on the influence of the drug on fracture rate in the long term. Such a distribution of task assignment between preclinical and clinical programmes deserves to be given serious consideration in order to make the progress of preclinical research available to the osteoporotic patients within a reasonable period of time and at an acceptable cost.

ANIMAL MODELS OF OSTEOPOROSIS

General consideration

Animal species

So far, preclinical studies have been carried out in various mammalian species: mice, rats, rabbits, (mini)pigs, ewes, dogs, monkeys and, more recently, ferrets. The animal species are selected if their basal bone remodelling pattern is histodynamically quite comparable to that observed in humans and/or if their response to calciotropic or osteotropic agents is similar to that observed in human subjects. The criteria also include the possibility that a relatively rapid and significant bone mass loss can be induced. In addition, the animal is selected according to a series of other criteria such as: availability, biological homogeneity of individual specimen, ease of handling and experimentation on, purchase price, cost for maintenance and cultural sensitivity, which may exclude the use of a given species in some countries.

Manoeuvres

Various manoeuvres have been used to induce bone mass loss in experimental animals: ovariectomy, orchiectomy, low calcium diet in lactating animals, immobilization by using a plaster cast, hemichordectomy, sciatic denervation or skeletal

unloading, including the space flight model. Some rodent strains display spontaneous signs of osteoporosis which can be associated with accelerated ageing. Recently, the transgenic technique has been used in mice with the generation of a severe bone disease resembling human involutional osteoporosis. Similarities of the therapeutic response in these different models with humans remain to be assessed. Nevertheless, data obtained in some models can already be considered to be highly predictive of human reaction. This is the case for the adult ovariectomized rat model in which the results of several therapeutic interventions mimic observations made in postmenopausal osteoporotic women. In addition to those mentioned above, models of fracture healing could be integrated in research and development programmes on antiosteoporotic drugs. Obviously, ethical considerations are an important determinant in the choice of the osteoporosis-inducing manoeuvre.

Experimental conditions that do no mimic human osteoporosis, and thereby cannot be considered true 'models' of this disease, can, however, be very useful for selecting molecules of potential interest. This is the case for experimental settings where potency of antiosteoclastic drugs is assessed in animals treated with an enhancer of bone resorption.

Endpoints

A series of variables can be evaluated by either invasive or non-invasive techniques: histomorphometry, ex vivo culture of bone-forming or bone-resorbing organs or cells, chemistry of bone tissue, biochemistry of bone markers present in blood and urine, metabolic balance of calcium combined with radioactive calcium kinetics, radiogrammetry of bone radiographs, neutron activation analysis of whole-body calcium, single and dual photon absorptiometry, quantitative computed tomography (QCT) and, more recently, dual energy X-ray absorptiometry (DXA). Assessment of the resistance to mechanical stress is a very important endpoint which has to be included in preclinical development programmes, particularly in curative studies when an investigational drug is shown to restore bone in patients with low bone mass.

Mechanical competence can be tested at several sites of the skeleton where bone mass can be measured either in vivo or ex vivo, including vertebral body, femoral neck and long bone metaphysis.

The choice of the variables to be measured should be made according to the stage of drug development. Screening aimed at determining the antiresorptive potency of new compounds does not require the same sophistication, time- and money-consuming techniques as studies that elucidate drug influence on various aspects of remodelling. The same differential and progressive approach should be considered when dealing with a stimulator of bone formation.

Specific considerations

Animal species and manoeuvres
The adult ovariectomized rat

To evaluate drugs that could eventually be utilized for the prevention and/or treatment of postmenopausal osteoporosis, the adult ovariectomized rat represents a very convenient and reliable model.[3-7] Rats, like humans, have cancellous bone undergoing remodelling. In adult rats, ovariectomy is followed after a relatively short period by an increase in bone turnover which is associated with accelerated bone loss and permanent bone mass deficit at several skeletal sites, including vertebral bodies, the

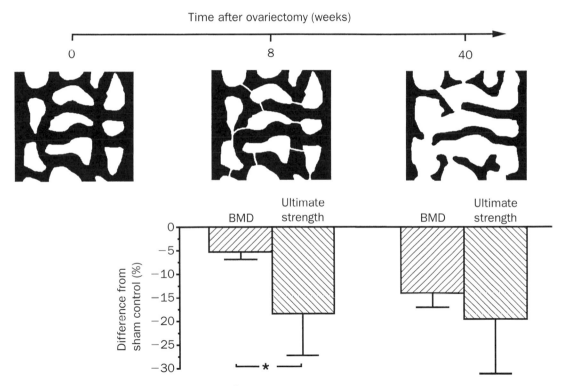

Figure 17.1 Bone mineral density (BMD, g/cm^2) and bone strength (ultimate strength, N) were evaluated 8 and 40 weeks after ovariectomy or sham operation, at the level of the lumbar spine in adult Sprague–Dawley rats. Values of ovariectomized rats are expressed as percentage difference compared with the sham. All animals were pair-fed a diet containing 1.2% Ca and 0.8% inorganic phosphate. Measurement of BMD was performed by dual energy X-ray absorptiometry (Hologic 1000) and bone strength was assessed by compression of an isolated vertebral body. A discrepancy between bone mass loss and decreased bone strength was observed 8 and 40 weeks after ovariectomy, which might reflect the early (8 weeks after ovariectomy) perforation of trabeculae (alteration of connectivity) followed by the thinning of trabeculae (40 weeks after ovariectomy). *$p < 0.05$.

proximal femur and long bone metaphysis such as distal femur or proximal tibia.[8,9] The microarchitectural alteration in the cancellous network is very similar, if not identical, to that observed in postmenopausal (and age-dependent) osteoporosis, including osteoclastic perforation and thinning of the trabecular elements.[4,10–16] This phenomenon is reflected by the observation that, in rats early after ovariectomy, a discrepancy between bone mass loss and decreased bone strength can be observed (Figure 17.1).

The characteristics of the adult rat model, the experimental conditions and the aims of the study have to be precisely defined. An adult rat model implies that, as for humans, the animals have reached a 'peak bone mass'. Some specific differences between strains might be observed and should be taken into account. Indeed, the level of skeletal maturity strongly influences the effects of ovariectomy on bone mass. Ovariectomy performed when peak bone mass is fully attained induces a decrease in bone mass. In contrast, an ovariectomy performed before the attainment of peak bone mass is associated with a slight decrease in bone mass and mostly with a marked slow-down of bone mass acquisition (Figure 17.2). A tight control of the food intake ('pair-feeding') of all experimental groups is mandatory in order to avoid introducing higher dietary intakes as a variable. Furthermore, accuracy of in vivo DXA measurement might be influenced by soft tissue modification.[8,9]

A number of antiosteoporotic drugs have been shown to exert effects on bone mass very similar to those observed in postmenopausal women.[17–21] Nevertheless, the adult ovariectomized rat model, at least in the experimental conditions

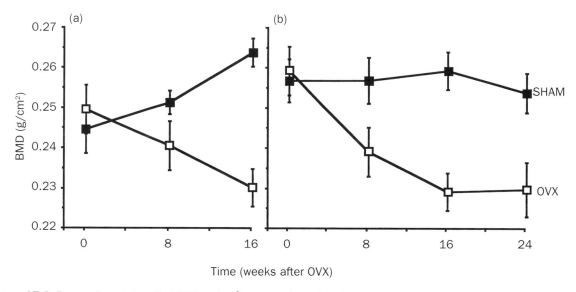

Figure 17.2 Bone mineral density (BMD, g/cm^2) was evaluated before and every 8 weeks after ovariectomy (OVX) or sham operation (SHAM) in (a) 4- or (b) 6-month-old Sprague–Dawley rats. All the animals were pair-fed a diet containing 1.2% Ca and 0.8% inorganic phosphate. Measurement of BMD was performed by dual energy X-ray absorptiometry (Hologic 1000). The results indicate that the bone loss induced by ovariectomy depends on the skeletal maturity. Thus, ovariectomy performed when peak bone mass is fully attained induces a decrease in bone mass. In contrast, ovariectomy performed before peak bone mass is reached is associated with a slight decrease in bone mass and with a marked decrease in the rate of bone mass acquisition.

used so far, has some limitations that have to be recognized. A low spontaneous cortical bone remodelling is observed in the usual dietary laboratory conditions.[3] There is an incomplete closure of some but not all epiphyseal plates in 'adult' animals. Nevertheless the thickness of the growth line is drastically reduced and partially mineralized, reducing the capacity of growth.[22] The fact that the adult rats maintain some degree of bone modelling should not be considered as a drawback because enlargement of the external envelope by periosteal apposition is also observed at several sites of the human adult skeleton.[23,24]

Other rat models

Adult or aged rats can be submitted to other manipulations that are capable of modifying bone mass and/or turnover. These include castration in males,[25–31] nutritional deficiency (particularly calcium deprivation-induced osteoporosis)[3,32,33] and immobilization.[34–38] A model of corticosteroid-induced osteoporosis has not been yet validated in rats.

Young growing rats are potential models for the study of factors that can influence bone mass accrual and thereby affect peak bone mass. Furthermore, young growing rats can provide useful information on the short-term effects of drugs on bone resorption such as in the retinoid-induced bone resorption model,[39,40] calcium kinetics and balance,[41] or calciotropic hormone levels. However, as inhibitors of bone resorption prevent bone remodelling of the primary spongiosa, a young growing rat model is not useful for measuring an osteogenic drug effect.[93]

Mice models

Adult ovariectomized mice[42,43] can also be used as a model of postmenopausal osteoporosis. As non-invasive measurement of bone mass and mechanical properties was recently adapted to mice, these animals represent a promising model.[42] Thus, the amount of agent necessary for an in vivo study could be markedly reduced in mice compared with rats (size). This advantage is especially appreciated when the availability or price of a drug represents a limiting

factor for undertaking an in vivo investigation.

Models of congenitally osteoporotic mice are also available. SAM/P6 mice (senescence accelerated mouse) are characterized by a low peak bone mass at skeletal maturity and develop fractures later on.[44–46] Transgenic mice models have been developed to examine the physiological or pathophysiological role of several molecules on bone metabolism. Models actually available consist of mice with null mutation for interleukin 6 (IL-6),[47] osteocalcin,[48] tumour necrosis factor (TNF) and IL-1 receptor,[49] and mice with over-expression of TNF-neutralizing receptor[42] or transforming growth factor β (TGFβ).[50] Transgenic mice with alterations of constitutive bone collagen are also described.[51] They will prove useful for understanding the pathophysiology of osteoporosis as well as mechanisms of action of drugs. Genetic variability in adult bone density was observed among inbred strains of mice and might represent a model for the investigation of the genetics of osteoporosis.[52]

Non-rodent species models

To complete the information gained from investigations carried out in rodent species, a non-murine model should also be used. This model should not only confirm the data obtained in murine species, but also provide information that cannot be obtained in rats or mice. In this regard, an animal model exhibiting a more extensive cortical bone remodelling than the rat should be an important selection criterion. The model has to be validated by the demonstration that osteoporosis (as defined above) can be induced at relevant skeletal sites by manoeuvres such as hypogonadism and calcium deprivation. To simulate as closely as possible the human situation, it is preferable to use non-rodent animals at peak bone mass.

Various species (primates, pigs, sheep, ferrets, dogs) have been investigated and have demonstrated advantages. The effect of ovariectomy on bone mass and the response to treatment might differ in these different models. For instance, the *ferret*[53,54] model exhibits changes in bone remodelling and bone loss after ovariectomy. Haversian bone remodelling was also observed. However, the duration of the daily light exposure could in itself influence oestrogen level and bone mass. Further investigations aimed at evaluating the responses to inhibitors of bone resorption and stimulators of bone formation still need to be carried out in order to compare the responses to those of humans. Controversial information concerning the effect of ovariectomy in *dogs*[55–63] have been reported. Nevertheless, this model has the advantage of clearly demonstrating haversian bone remodelling. The *mini-pig*[64–68] seems also to represent a good model of evolved mammalian because ovariectomy increased bone turnover and induced bone loss. As in humans, fluoride and bisphosphonate treatment of pigs induced an increase in bone mass. Histomorphometric parameters in old *sheep*[69–73] are very close to those found in humans. However, the effects of ovariectomy on bone mass still need to be precisely investigated. As cycles are dependent on light exposition, strict conditions about maintenance have to be applied. The most appropriate model is non-human *primates*[6,74–79] which exhibit menstrual cycles and reproductive hormonal patterns similar to those observed in premenopausal women and develop high bone turnover and osteoporosis, at least at the spinal level, after ovariectomy. Nevertheless, the handling of animals, their supply and ethical concerns might prevent their use.

In rabbits, dogs and, more recently, sheep, corticosteroid treatment has been found to induce changes in bone formation indices with or without alteration in bone resorption variables similar to what has been observed in human subjects.[80,81] Despite the complexity, inhomogeneity and controversial pathophysiology of human glucocorticoid-induced osteoporosis, these species can be useful in the assessment of drugs aimed at preventing or treating corticosteroid-induced osteoporosis.

Measurement of bone mass and geometry (or macroarchitecture)

Several techniques can be used, either in vivo or ex vivo, to assess bone mass, areal or volumetric bone mineral density in small and/or large animals: neutron activation analysis of whole-body calcium,[82] single or dual photon absorptiometry (SPA, DPA); single or dual X-ray absorptiometry (SXA, DXA);[8,9,83–85] and peripheral QCT (pQCT).[86,87] The selected technique should be validated in terms of both precision and accuracy for the animal species selected. As for human use, strict control of quality of the machine has to be regularly performed.

Techniques such as DXA allow the measurement of areal bone mineral density in the axial and peripheral skeleton (spine, femur including the femoral neck, and tibia). In long bones, metaphyseal (with predominantly trabecular bony tissue) and diaphyseal (essentially made of cortical bone) regions can be selectively measured and values correlated with those obtained from bone strength tests applied to the same skeletal sites. Peripheral quantitative computed tomography has the ability to analyse trabecular and cortical bone separately and also to assess cortical thickness or width. Both DXA and pQCT can be used to monitor drug or manipulation effects on bone geometry, and relate any changes in the macrostructure to the results obtained by histomorphometry and biomechanical testing (Figure 17.3).[9,88] The development of such techniques and their adaptation to small animals have resulted in major advances in the field because they allow non-invasive in vivo measurement of bone mass and geometry. Microradiography can also be used to assess semiquantitative changes in geometry and cortical and trabecular bone volume. In growing rats, the so-called Schenk's test has been widely used to assess the potency of antiresorbing agents.[89]

In the future, techniques using pQCT or magnetic resonance imaging (MRI) technology will be available to approach in vivo microarchitecture.[90,91] A recent study has also indicated that ultrasonography will become available for use in small animals.[92]

In relation to the initial site of fracture in osteoporotic human adults, special attention should be paid to assessment of the effect of treatment on epiphyseal, metaphyseal, intertrochanteric and femoral neck cortices. This pertains to the assessment of bone 'quality' by histomorphometry and biomechanics.

	Experimental conditions			
	OVX (vehicle)	OVX + APD	OVX + IGF-I	OVX + APD + IGF-I
Experimental data				
External diameter (mm)	2.81 ± 0.04	2.82 ± 0.05	2.91 ± 0.03	2.98 ± 0.06 *
Cortical thickness (mm)	0.63 ± 0.01	0.68 ± 0.02 *	0.64 ± 0.02	0.71 ± 0.01 *
Bone surface (mm^2)	4.51 ± 0.12	4.55 ± 0.16	4.61 ± 0.11	5.10 ± 0.13 *

Conceptual view

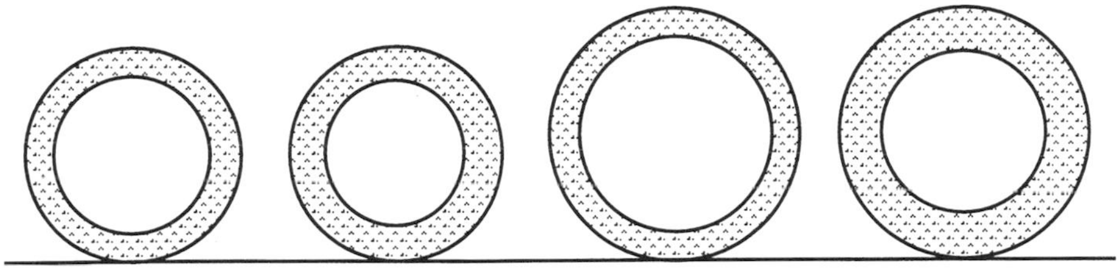

Figure 17.3 Ovariectomized osteoporotic 6-month-old Sprague–Dawley rats were treated for 6 weeks with pamidronate (APD) and/or IGF-I. The animals were pair-fed a diet containing 1.2% Ca and 0.8% inorganic phosphate. Midshaft tibia dimensions (diameters, cortical thicknesses and bone surfaces) were measured using image analysis after section performed at the level of the middle of the tibia. The results are expressed as means ± s.e.m. (mm or mm^2) and indicate that IGF-I increases the diameter of the bone and that pamidronate (inhibitor of bone resorption) treatment increases cortical thickness; these effects appear to be additive. These results underline the importance of structural analysis of bone, especially when they contribute to bone strength. *$p < 0.05$ as compared with OVX controls.

Bone histology

Bone histomorphometry is a necessary tool for understanding the mechanisms of action of new therapeutic agents on bone remodelling and for assessing some important components of bone quality in animals treated long term. Histologically, several components of bone quality can be assessed including: microarchitecture, texture of bone matrix reflected by the presence of lamellar or woven bone, and the possible appearance of mineralization defects. Defects in each of these factors can jeopardize bone strength.

Bone histomorphometry[69,70,93–95] performed on undecalcified sections is the only method that gives access to a direct and precise analysis of the effects of new drugs on trabecular and cortical bone at both cellular and tissue levels. In each compartment, whether cortical or trabecular, an assessment of the effects on bone modelling and on bone remodelling can be made. Modelling is a process in which bone formation and bone resorption are not coupled and which is responsible for the growth and shaping of bones. Bone remodelling is characterized by a spatial and temporal coupling of bone formation and resorption. In young and adult rats, both modelling and remodelling are present. In adult larger animals, such as primates, sheep, dogs, rabbits, pigs or ferrets, remodelling is present. The tetracycline double-labelling procedure or use of other fluorochromes can provide dynamic information on bone mineralization and bone formation, and permit the introduction of the dimension of time into the quantitative analysis.

Various bones can be used depending on the animal species: tibia, femur, vertebrae or iliac crest. The samples should be handled in a laboratory that has expertise in embedding, sectioning, staining and the use of digitizing image analysis systems. High quality sections are a prerequisite to any quantitative analysis.

Assessment of trabecular bone should include various static parameters of bone formation (trabecular bone volume or trabecular area; marrow cavity area; osteoid surface, volume and width; osteoblast surface), bone resorption (eroded surface, osteoclast surface, osteoclast number), microarchitecture and connectivity parameters (trabecular number, width and separation; node numbers; free end numbers; mineral apposition rate [from interlabelling width]; mineralizing surfaces [doubly labelled surfaces and half singly labelled surfaces]); bone formation rate and activation frequency. Investigation of cortical bone should investigate bone area, porosity and width, haversian mineral apposition rate and end-haversian eroded surface.[94,95]

Assessment of the mechanical properties of bone

Mechanical properties of bone represent an important aspect of the investigation of any curative or preventive treatment because improvement of bone strength corresponds to an improvement of bone fragility and possible decreased risk of fracture (the essential goal of any treatment).

Several tests can be used for the evaluation of mechanical properties of bones harvested from small and large animals. Changes in the strength of a long bone diaphysis are classically tested by applying three- or four-point bending and torsion tests. Compression or a combination of bending–compression tests can also be used to assess the mechanical resistance of vertebral bodies and the femoral neck. Indentation test can be used to evaluate purely trabecular bone.

The mechanical properties of bone can be directly determined by analysing the load–deformation relationship (respectively stress–strain curve).[96–98] This analysis provides information on:

- The *intrinsic stiffness*, a characteristic that is independent of bone size but reflects the stiffness of the bony 'material' corresponding to the slope of the load–deformation curve.
- The *failure load (breaking strength)*, corresponding to the maximal load that the bone can tolerate (for the bending test, the maximal load is also expressed as the bending moment).
- The *energy absorption*, which is a measure of bone toughness and corresponds to the area under the curve up to the maximal load.

Additional information on possible changes in the 'brittleness' of the bone can be obtained by determining the area under the curve after the *yield point* which separates the *elastic* from the *plastic* deformation region. To get reliable measures, care should be taken to preserve and test the specimens in standardized conditions. Preservation in alcohol or formaline, or immersion in another liquid, could alter the mechanical properties. Prolonged exposure to air could result in drying the tested bone and in alteration of the stiffness.[88,98]

The relative contribution of trabecular as against cortical tissue, to the overall bone strength can vary markedly according to the skeletal sites. The two types of bony tissues can be differentially influenced not only by the kind of manoeuvres inducing osteoporosis, but also by the tested drugs. Therefore, the tests should be performed at several skeletal sites so that the drug effects are not only assessed by the mechanical resistance of the vertebral bodies and the midshaft regions of long bones, but also, using available information, by the osteo-densitometric and histomorphological evaluations at the levels of epiphyseal, metaphyseal, intertrochanteric and femoral neck cortices. At the spinal level it can also be informative to assess the mechanical properties (compressive failure load and stiffness) of both the vertebral whole body and the vertebral trabecular core.[98–101] Techniques of preparation of the vertebral body that preserve its integrity are preferred to others that result in destruction of the proximal and distal ends.

Results obtained by the above-mentioned biomechanical tests should take into account changes in bone size and shape.[9,19,88,98] The combined evaluation of the geometrical and mechanical alterations allows distinction between changes in the intrinsic property of the bone laid down during the treatment period and those resulting from modifications caused by the size and shape of the skeleton. This assessment is particularly important for drugs that accumulate in bone and may alter the quality of the organic and/or crystal material. For instance, such a distinction can be made in bending tests carried out on long bone diaphyses by measuring the cross-sectional moment of inertia (a measure of the distribution of bony tissue around the central or neutral axis), whereas, at the level of the proximal femur, both the axial length and the cross-sectional moment of inertia of the femoral neck should be measured. The moment of inertia has to be measured with great precision by using either an image-analysing system or point-counting techniques. Calculation of the moment of inertia from cylindrical or oval approximation of the cross-sectional geometry of the long bones should be avoided because it can provide inaccurate results.[102]

For vertebral bodies, ultimate strength and intrinsic stiffness data obtained from craniocaudal compressive tests should also be analysed in relation to the drug effects on bone mass, geometry (three-dimensional architecture of the vertebral body) and material property of the bony tissue. The nature of the drug effects should be assessed by analysing the relationship between bone mass and bone strength.

Biochemical markers of bone turnover

The measurement of biochemical markers of bone turnover could be useful in short-term studies aimed at determining the full dose range of the drug. In long-term studies they can only be considered as secondary endpoints. Osteodensitometric, histomorphometric and biomechanical measurements represent the primary endpoints. Modification of these parameters of bone turnover have to be interpreted in the light of bone mass modification.

Preference should be given to those bone-formation or bone-resorption biochemical markers for which there is experimental evidence indicating that the plasma concentration and/or the urinary excretion varies in relation to some well-defined dynamic histomorphometric parameters.

Various markers for bone resorption could be suggested, such as pyridinium cross-links[103–105] or hydroxyproline,[106] but urinary excretion of molecules previously deposited in bone, such as tetracycline,[106] can also be used. Fasting urinary calcium excretion remains a useful variable to estimate *net* bone resorption. Bone formation could be appreciated by determination of bone-specific alkaline phosphatase and osteocalcin. Studies on the kinetics of radioactive calcium coupled with calcium balance measurements can provide useful information on the effect of the drug on calcium deposition (i.e. bone formation) and release (i.e. bone resorption) at the level of the whole skeleton.

Study design

Drug administration

Type of intervention: curative or preventive

Administration of drugs basically designed for preventive therapy should be started simultaneously with or immediately after the osteoporosis-inducing manoeuvre.

Administration of drugs designed for curative therapy should be started once the osteoporotic state is fully expressed.

Treatment administration

The treatment schedule should simulate those intended to be used in clinical trials, e.g. continuous, intermittent, combined, sequential or cyclic. The toxicity of a drug may vary markedly according to its mode of administration. This possibility should be taken into account in the design of the experiments.

Dosage

The full dose range should be determined in relatively short time studies using appropriate screening models with endpoints such as: bone mass non-invasively determined by DXA or QCT, calcium balance, bone resorption and formation biomarkers.

For long-term studies, including bone mass, bone architecture, histomorphometry microstructural analysis and bone strength as endpoints, three doses are required: a first with which a minimal response (or half-maximal response) can be expected; a second that is optimally effective; and, for safety reasons, a third that is 5–10 times the optimum effective dose.

Treatment duration

There is no firm experimental evidence that would allow the reliable setting of the duration of treatment by taking into account the estimate of the formation/resorption period for trabecular bone. Indeed, this estimate can vary greatly within a given species according to experimental conditions. The lifespan of remodelling units is shorter in small animals, such as rats, than in larger species. It is arbitrarily proposed that, in monkeys, the drug should be applied for a period half that selected for human exposure and, in rats, five times shorter.

Pharmacokinetics

As for any other new drugs, appropriate experiments should be carried out in at least two species in order to get information on bioavailability, pharmacokinetics and distribution, and excretion and metabolism.

Assessment of bone tolerance

Chronic toxicity studies should be used to assess the long-term effects of the drug on bone quality. The most critical endpoints to consider with respect to skeletal toxicity are: growth impairment, mineralization defects, reduced bone mass, increased fragility, impairment of fracture healing, and complete and irreversible blockage of bone turnover (i.e. 'frozen bone' genesis). The assessment should be made using most of the above-mentioned methods.

Drugs affecting bone metabolism may influence the repair process of bone fracture through callus formation bridging both bone ends, callus mineralization and internal remodelling at the fracture site. Therefore, it is recommended that it should be examined whether the administration of the drug impairs the fracture healing processes.

For the evaluation of the healing process it is recommended that both radiological and histological examinations are used. In addition, mechanical tests should be performed to determine the quality of the fracture union, such as bending, torsion and/or tensile tests.[107–110]

Minimal preclinical requirements before starting clinical trials

There is a large body of evidence in the field of osteoporosis that adequate preclinical evaluation in terms of pharmacodynamics and bone quality, as defined above, can predict the therapeutic success or failure of drugs when used to prevent or improve osteoporosis. Therefore, it appears to be both scientifically and ethically valid to require a reasonably well-documented preclinical evaluation before initiating a clinical programme. This evaluation should include at least pharmacodynamic and bone tolerance data obtained by osteodensitometric, histomorphometric and biomechanical methods. Some information on the mechanism of action should also be required because it could influence the design of clinical trials.

CONCLUSIONS

A preclinical/clinical complementary programme for the assessment of the efficacy of new antiosteoporotic drugs is mandatory. Preclinical studies carried out in the most reliable animal models (i.e. the most predictive with respect to human calcium and bone metabolism, and drug responsiveness) are aimed at testing drug efficacy on bone mass/mineral density, microarchitecture and mechanical resistance in well-controlled conditions. Then, clinical trials in phase III of the drug investigation concentrate on testing efficacy on bone mass/mineral density, and possibly on bone microarchitectures as assessed by histomorphometry in a limited number of subjects, but not on fracture rate. Such a clinical programme will drastically reduce the number of patients necessary to demonstrate drug efficacy. In cases where the results on bone mass/mineral density and possibly microarchitecture are similar to those observed in the selected animal models, and assuming that both bone tolerance and overall safety are warranted, it can be anticipated that the drug will exert the same effect on bone mechanical resistance in humans as demonstrated in animals. Phase IV studies (post-marketing surveillance) with well-organized reporting procedure could,

in the long term, provide information on the influence of the drug on fracture rate. Such a distribution of task assignment between preclinical and clinical programmes should make the progress of preclinical research available to the osteoporotic patients within a reasonable period of time.

ACKNOWLEDGEMENTS

Part of the notions presented in this chapter were discussed in the Training Course organized by Professor Pierre Delmas for the European Foundation for Osteoporosis (Lyon: 29–31 January 1996; 27–29 January 1997). Different aspects of the animal models were also discussed within a group brought together by the World Organization of Osteoporosis in February 1996; the foregoing text has been influenced by the valuable conceptual and technical comments made by Drs John Kanis, Pierre Meunier, Toshitaka Nakamura and John Wark. Research on animal models developed in the authors' laboratory were supported by the Swiss National Foundation (Grant 32-32411.91).

REFERENCES

1. Guidelines for preclinical and clinical evaluation of agents used in the prevention or treatment of postmenopausal osteoporosis. Division of Metabolism and Endocrine Drug Products. Food and Drug Administration. Draft April (1994).

2. Peck WA, Burckhardt P, Christiansen C et al. Consensus development conference: diagnosis, prophylaxis, and treatment of osteoporosis. *Am J Med* 1993; **94**: 646–50.

3. Frost HM, Jee WSS. On the rat model of human osteopenias and osteoporoses. *Bone Miner* 1992; **18**: 227–36.

4. Kalu DN, Liu CC, Hardin RR et al. The aged rat model of ovarian hormone deficiency bone loss. *Endocrinology* 1989; **124**: 7–16.

5. Kalu DN. The ovariectomized rat as a model of postmenopausal osteopenia. *Bone Miner* 1991; **15**: 175–91.

6. Schnitzler CM, Ripamonti U, Mesquita JM. Bone histomorphometry in baboons in captivity. *Bone* 1993; **14**: 383–7.

7. Wronski TJ, Yen CF. The ovariectomized rat as an animal model for postmenopausal bone loss. *Cells Materials* 1991; **5**(suppl 1): 69–74.

8. Ammann P, Rizzoli R, Slosman D et al. Sequential and precise in vivo measurement of bone mineral density in rats using dual energy X-ray absorptiometry. *J Bone Miner Res* 1992; **7**: 311–6.

9. Maugars Y, Ammann P, Rizzoli R et al. Accurate prediction of rat proximal femur bone strength by in vivo DXA measurement of bone mass and femoral neck geometry. *J Bone Miner Res* 1995; **10**: S358 (abst).

10. Dempster DW, Li XF, Birchman R et al. On the mechanism of cancellous bone loss in the ovariectomized rat. In: *Calcium Regulating*

Hormones and Bone Metabolism (Cohn DV, Gennari C, Tashjian Jr AJ, eds). Amsterdam: Elsevier Science, 1992: 460–4.

11. Jee WSS. The aged rat model for bone biology studies. *Cells Materials* 1991; **5**(suppl 1): 131–42.

12. Li XJ, Jee WSS, Ke HZ et al. Age-related changes of cancellous and cortical bone histomorphometry in female Sprague–Dawley rats. *Cells Materials* 1991; **5**(suppl 1): 25–35.

13. Shen V, Dempster DW, Birchman R et al. Loss of cancellous bone mass and connectivity in ovariectomized rats can be restored by combined treatment with parathyroid hormone and estradiol. *J Clin Invest* 1993; **91**: 2479–87.

14. Wronski TJ, Dann LM, Scott KS et al. Long-term effects of ovariectomy and aging on the rat skeleton. *Calcif Tissue Int* 1989; **45**: 360–6.

15. Wrosnki TJ, Dann LM, Scott KS et al. Endocrine and pharmacological suppressors of bone turnover protect against osteopenia in ovariectomized rats. *Endocrinology* 1989; **125**: 810–6.

16. Wronski TJ, Dann LM, Horner SL. Time course of vertebral osteopenia in ovariectomized rats. *Calcif Tissue Int* 1990; **46**: 101–10.

17. Ammann P, Rizzoli R, Caverzasio J et al. IGF-1 and pamidronate increase bone mineral density in ovariectomized adult rats. *Am J Physiol* 1993; **265**: 770–6.

18. Ammann P, Rizzoli R, Caverzasio J et al. Effects of bisphosphonate tiludronate on bone resorption, calcium balance, and bone mineral density. *J Bone Miner Res* 1993; **8**: 1491–8.

19. Jorgensen PH, Bak B, Andreassen TT. Mechanical properties and biochemical composition of rat cortical femur and tibia after long-term treatment with biosynthetic human growth hormone. *Bone* 1991; **12**: 353–9.

20. Mitlak BH, Burdette-Miller P, Schoenfeld D et al. Sequential effects of chronic human PTH (1–84) treatment of estrogen-deficiency osteopenia in the rat. *J Bone Miner Res* 1996; **11**: 430–9.

21. Toolan BC, Shea M, Myers ER et al. Effects of 4-amino-1-hydroxybutylidene bisphosphonate on bone biomechanics in rats. *J Bone Miner Res* 1992; **7**: 1399–406.

22. Kimmel DB. Quantitative histologic changes in the proximal tibial growth cartilage of aged female rats. *Cells Materials* 1991; **5**(suppl 1): 19–24.

23. Beck TJ, Ruff CB, Scott WW et al. Sex differences in geometry of the femoral neck with aging – a structural analysis of bone mineral data. *Calcif Tissue Int* 1992; **50**: 24–9.

24. Ringe JD. Hip fractures in men. *Osteoporosis Int* 1986; **6**(suppl 3): S48–51.

25. Danielsen CC, Mosekilde L, Andreassen TT. Long-term effect of orchidectomy on cortical bone from rat femur – bone mass and mechanical properties. *Calcif Tissue Int* 1992; **50**: 169–74.

26. Hock JM, Gera I, Fonseca J et al. Human parathyroid hormone (1–34) increases bone mass in ovariectomized and orchidectomized rats. *Endocrinology* 1988; **122**: 2899–904.

27. Saville PD. Changes in skeletal mass and fragility with castration in the rat: a model of osteoporosis. *Am Geriat Soc* 1969; **17**: 155–66.

28. Vanderschueren D, Vanherck E, Suiker AMH et al. Bone and mineral metabolism in aged male rats – short and long term effects of andogen deficiency. *Endocrinology* 1992; **130**: 2906–16.

29. Vanderschueren D, Van Herck E, Schot P et al. The aged male rat as a model for human osteoporosis: evaluation by nondestructive measurements and biomechanical testing. *Calcif Tissue Int* 1993; **53**: 342–7.

30. Vanderschueren D, Jans I, Vanherck E et al. Time-related increase of biochemical markers of bone turnover in androgen-deficient male rats. *Bone Miner* 1994; **26**: 123–31.

31. Verhas M, Schoutens A, L'Hermite-Baleriaux M et al. The effect of orchidectomy on bone metabolism in aging rats. *Calcif Tissue Int* 1986; **39**: 74–7.

32. Kalu DN, Hardin RR, Cockerham R et al. Aging and dietary modulation of the rat skeleton and parathyroid hormone. *Endocrinology* 1988; **115**: 1239–47.

33. Kalu DN, Masoro EJ, Yu BP et al. Modulation of age-related hyperparathyroidism and senile bone loss in Fischer rats by soy protein and food restriction. *Endocrinology* 1988; **122**: 1847–54.

34. Fleisch H, Russell RGG, Simpson B et al. Prevention by a diphosphonate of immobilization 'osteoporosis' in rats. *Nature* 1969; **223**: 211–12.

35. Globus RK, Bikle DD, Morey-Holton E. The temporal response of bone to unloading. *Endocrinology* 1986; **118**: 733–42.

36. Jee WSS, Wronski TJ, Morey ER et al. Effects of spaceflight on trabecular bone in rats. *Am J Physiol* 1983; **244**: R310–4.

37. Wronski TJ, Morey ER. Effect of spaceflight on periosteal bone formation in rat. *Am J Physiol* 1983; **244**: R305–9.

38. Zhang RW, Supowit SC, Klein GL et al. Rat tail suspension reduces messenger RNA level for growth factors and osteopontin and decreases the osteoblastic differentiation of bone marrow stromal cells. *J Bone Miner Res* 1995; **10**: 415–23.

39. Stutzer A, Fleisch H, Trechsel U. Short- and long-term effects of a single dose of bisphosphonates on retinoid-induced bone resorption in thyroparathyroidectomized rats. *Calcif Tissue Int* 1988; **43**: 294–9.

40. Trechsel U, Fleisch H. Effect of a retinoid on Ca and Vitamin D metabolism in thyroparathyroidectomized (TPTX) rats. In: *Vitamin D. A Chemical Biochemical and Clinical Update.* Berlin: Walter de Gruyter & Co., 1985: 51–2.

41. Ammann P, Rizzoli R, Fleisch H. Influence of the disaccharide lactitol on intestinal absorption and body retention of calcium in rats. *J Nutr* 1988; **118**: 793–5.

42. Ammann P, Rizzoli R, Bonjour JP et al. Transgenic mice expressing high levels of soluble tumor necrosis factor receptor-1 are protected against bone loss caused by estrogen deficiency. *J Clin Invest* 1997; **99**: 1699–1703.

43. Weiss A, Arbell I, Steinhagen-Thiessen E et al. Structural changes in aging bone: Osteopenia in the proximal femurs of female mice. *Bone* 1991; **12**: 165–72.

44. Kawase M, Tsuda M, Matsuo T. Accelerated bone resorption in senescence-accelerated mouse (SAM-P/6). *J Bone Miner Res* 1989; **4**: 359–64.

45. Matsushita M, Tsuboyama T, Kasai R et al. Age-related changes in bone mass in the senescence-accelerated mouse (SAM). *Am J Pathol* 1986; **125**: 276–83.

46. Tsuboyama T, Takahashi K, Yamamuro T et al. Cross-mating study on bone mass in the spontaneously osteoporotic mouse (SAM-P/6). *Bone Miner* 1993; **23**: 57–64.

47. Poli V, Balena E, Fattori E et al. Interleukin-6 deficient mice are protected from bone loss caused by estrogen depletion. *EMBO J* 1994; **13**: 1189–96.

48. Ducy P, Desbois C, Boyce B et al. Increased bone formation in osteocalcin-deficient mice. *Nature* 1996; **382**: 448–52.

49. Vargas SJ, Naprte A, Glaccum et al. Interleukin-6 expression and histomorphometry of bones from mice deficient in receptors for interleukin-1 or tumor necrosis factor. *J Bone Miner Res* 1996; **11**: 1736–43.

50. Erlebacher A, Derynck R. Increased expression of TGF-beta 2 in osteoblasts results in an osteoporosis-like phenotype. *J Cell Biol* 1996; **132**: 195–210.

51. Bonad J, Jepsen KJ, Mansoura MK et al. A murine skeletal adaptation that significantly increases cortical bone mechanical properties. *J Clin Invest* 1993; **92**: 1691–705.

52. Beamer WG, Donahue LR, Rosen CJ et al. Genetic variability in adult bone density among inbred strains of mice. *Bone* 1996; **18**: 397–403.

53. Li XJ, Stevens ML, Mackey MS et al. The ferret: skeletal responses to treatment with PTH. *J Bone Miner Res* 1994; **9**(suppl 1): S258 (abst).

54. Mackey MS, Stevens ML, Ebert DC et al. The ferret as a small animal model with BMU-based remodeling for skeletal research. *Bone* 1995; **17**: 191S–6S.

55. Dannucci GA, Martin RB, Patterson-Buckendahl P. Ovariectomy and trabecular bone remodeling in the dog. *Calcif Tissue Int* 1987; **40**: 194–9.

56. Faugere MC, Fanti P, Friedler RM et al. Bone changes occurring early after cessation of ovarian function in beagle dogs: a histomorphometric study employing sequential biopsies. *J Bone Miner Res* 1990; **5**: 263–72.

57. Karambolova KK, Snow GR, Anderson C. Differences in periosteal and corticoendosteal bone envelope activities in spayed and intact beagles: a histomorphometric study. *Calcif Tissue Int* 1985; **41**: 665–8.

58. Kimmel DB. The oophorectomized beagle as an experimental model for estrogen-depletion bone loss in the adult human. *Cells Materials* 1991; **5**(suppl 1): 75–84.

59. Malluche HH, Faugere MC, Rush M et al. Osteoblastic insufficiency is responsible for maintenance of osteopenia after loss of ovarian function in experimental beagle dogs. *Endocrinology* 1986; **119**: 2649–54.

60. Motoie H, Nakamura T, O'uchi N et al. Effects of the bisphosphonate YM175 on bone mineral density, strength, structure, and turnover in ovariectomized beagles on concomitant dietary calcium restriction. *J Bone Miner Res* 1995; **10**: 910–20.

61. Podbesek R, Edouard C, Meunier PJ et al. Effects of two treatment regimes with synthetic human parathyroid hormone fragment on bone formation and the tissue balance of trabecular bone in greyhounds. *Endocrinology* 1983; **112**: 1000–6.

62. Shen V, Dempster DW, Birchman R et al. Lack

of changes in histomorphometric, bone mass, and biochemical parameters in ovariohysterectomized dogs. *Bone* 1992; **13:** 311–6.

63. Snow GR, Anderson C. The effects of 17 b-estradiol and progestagen on trabecular bone remodeling in oophorectomized dogs. *Calcif Tissue Int* 1986; **39:** 198–205.

64. Fratzl P, Schreiber S, Roschger P et al. Effects of sodium fluoride and alendronate on the bone mineral in minipigs: a small-angle x-ray scattering and backscattered electron imaging study. *J Bone Miner Res* 1996; **11:** 248–53.

65. Lafage MH, Balena R, Battle MA et al. Comparison of alendronate and sodium fluoride effects on cancellous and cortical in minipigs. A one year study. *J Clin Invest* 1995; **95:** 2127–33.

66. Mosekilde L, Kragstrup J, Richards A. Comprehensive strength, ash weight, and volume of vertebral trabecular bone in experimental fluorosis in pigs. *Calcif Tissue Int* 1987; **40:** 318–22.

67. Mosekilde L, Weisbrode SE, Safron JA et al. Calcium-restricted ovariectomized Sinclair S-1 minipigs: an animal model of osteopenia and trabecular plate perforation. *Bone* 1993; **14:** 379–82.

68. Stevens ML, Sacco-Gibson N, Combs KS et al. Evaluation of skeletal parameters in the Sinclair S-1 minipig: histomorphometric assessment of skeletal changes at 3 months post-ovariectomy. *J Bone Miner Res* 1994; **9:** S258 (abst).

69. Chavassieux P, Pastoureau P, Boivin G et al. Dose effects on ewe bone remodeling of short-term sodium fluoride administration. A histomorphometric and biochemical study. *Bone* 1991; **12:** 421–7.

70. Chavassieux P, Pastoureau P, Boivin G et al. Fluoride-induced bone changes in lambs during and after exposure to sodium fluoride. *Osteoporosis Int* 1991; **2:** 26–33.

71. Hornby SB, Ford SL, Mase CA et al. Skeletal changes in the ovariectomized ewe and subsequent response to treatment with 17b oestradiol. *Bone* 1995; **17**(4): 389S–94S.

72. Newman E, Turner AS, Wark JD. The potential of sheep for the study of osteopenia: Current status and comparison with other animal models. *Bone* 1995; **16:** 277S–84S.

73. Turner AS, Alvis M, Myers W et al. Changes in bone mineral density and bone-specific alkaline phosphatase in ovariectomized ewes. *Bone* 1995; **17:** 395S-402S.

74. Balena R, Toolan BC, Shea M et al. The effects of 2-year treatment with the aminobisphosphonate alendronate on bone metabolism, bone histomorphometry, and bone strength in ovariectomized nonhuman primate. *J Clin Invest* 1993; **92:** 2577–86.

75. Hodgen GD, Goodman AL, O'Connor A et al. Menopause in rhesus monkeys: model for study of disorders in the human climatcteric. *Am J Obstet Gynecol* 1977; **127:** 581–4.

76. Lundon KL, Grynpas M. The longterm effect of ovariectomy on the quality and quantity of cortical bone in the young Cynomolgus monkey: comparison of density fractionation and histomorphometric techniques. *Bone* 1993; **14:** 389–95.

77. Mann DR, Gould KG, Collins DC. A potential primate model for bone loss resulting from medical oophorectomy or menopause. *J Lab Clin Med* 1990; **71:** 105–10.

78. Miller C, Weaver DS, McAlister JA et al. Effects of ovariectomy on vertebral trabecular bone in the cynomolgus monkey. *Calcif Tissue Int* 1986; **38:** 62–5.

79. Pope NS, Gould KG, Anderson DC et al. Effects of age and sex on bone density in the rhesus monkey. *Bone* 1989; **10:** 109–12.

80. Deloffre P, Hans D, Rumelhart C et al. Comparison between bone density and bone strength in glucocorticoid-treated aged ewes. *Bone* 1995; **17:** 409S–14S.

81. Quarles LD. Prednisone-induced osteopenia in beagles: variable effects mediated by differential suppression of bone formation. *Endocrinol Metab* 1992; **26:** E136–41.

82. Hefti E, Trechsel U, Bonjour JP et al. Increase of whole-body calcium and skeletal mass in normal and osteoporotic adult rats treated with parathyroid hormone. *Clin Sci* 1982; **62:** 389–96.

83. Jayo MJ, Rankin SE, Weaver DS et al. Accuracy and precision of lumbar bone mineral content by DPA in live female monkeys. *Calcif Tissue Int* 1991; **49:** 438–40.

84. Safadi M, Shapira D, Leichter I et al. Ability of different techniques of measuring bone mass to determine vertebral bone loss in aging female rats. *Calcif Tissue Int* 1988; **42:** 375–82.

85. Turner AS, Mallinckrodt CH, Alvis MR et al. Dual-energy X-ray absorptiometry in sheep: experiences with in vivo and ex vivo studies. *Bone* 1995; **17**(4): 381S–8S.

86. Ferretti JL. Perspectives of pQCT technology associated to biomechanical studies in skeletal

research employing rat models. *Bone* 1995; **17:** 353S–64S.

87. Gasser JA. Assessing bone quantity by pQCT. *Bone* 1995; **17:** 145S–54S.

88. Ammann P, Rizzoli R, Meyer J-M, Bonjour J-P. Bone density and shape as determinants of bone strength in IGF-I and/or pamidronate-treated ovariectomized rats. *Osteoporosis Int* 1996; **6:** 219–27.

89. Schenk R, Merz WA, Mülbauer R et al. Effect of e t h a n e - 1 - h y d r o x y - 1 , 1 - d i p h o s p h o n a t e (C12MDP) on the calcification and resorption of cartilage and bone in the tibial epiphysis and metaphysis of rats. *Calcif Tissue Res* 1973; **11:** 196–214.

90. Hipp JA, Jansujwicz A, Simmons CA et al. Trabecular bone morphology from micro-magnetic resonance imaging. *J Bone Miner Res* 1996; **11:** 286–92.

91. Rüegsegger P, Koller B, Müller R. A microtomographic system for the nondestructive evaluation of bone architecture. *Calcif Tissue Int* 1996; **58:** 24–9.

92. Amo C, Revilla M, Hernandez ER et al. Correlation of ultrasound bone velocity with dual-energy x-ray bone absorptiometry in rat bone specimens. *Invest Radiol* 1996; **31:** 114–7.

93. Bourrin S, Palle S, Rupier R et al. Effects of physical training on bone adaptation in three zones of the rat tibia. *J Bone Miner Res* 1995; **10:** 1745–52.

94. Parfitt AM. Bone histomorphometry: standardization of nomenclature, symbols and units. *J Bone Miner Res* 1987; **2:** 595–610.

95. Parfitt AM. Stereologic basis of bone histomorphometry: the theory of quantitative microscopy and reconstruction of the third dimension. In *Bone Histomorphometry: Techniques and Interpretation* (Recker RR, ed.). Boca Raton, FL: CRC Press, 1983: 53–89.

96. Einhorn TA. Bone Strength: the bottom line. *Calcif Tissue Int* 1992; **51:** 333–9.

97. Hayes WC, Gerhart TN. Biomechanics of bone: applications for assessment of bone strength. *Bone Miner Res* 1995; **3:** 259–94.

98. Turner CH, Burr DB. Basic biomechanical measurements of bone: a tutorial. *Bone* 1993; **14:** 595–608.

99. Granhed H, Johnson R, Hansson T. Mineral content and strength of lumbar vertebrae: a cadaver study. *Acta Orthop Scand* 1989; **60:** 105–9.

100. Lang SM, Moyle DD, Berg CEW et al. Correlation of mechanical properties of vertebral trabecular bone with equivalent mineral density as measured by computed tomography. *J Bone Joint Surg [Am]* 1988; **70:** 1531–8.

101. Mosekilde L, Danielsen CC. Biomechanical competence of vertebral trabecular bone in relation to ash density and age in normal individuals. *Bone* 1987; **8:** 79–85.

102. Kenedi RM. *Textbook of Biochemical Engineering.* Glasgow: Blackie, 1980: 39–73.

103. Egger CD, Muhlbauer RC, Felix R et al. Evaluation of urinary pyridinium crosslink excretion as a marker of bone resorption in the rat. *J Bone Miner Res* 1994; **9:** 1211–19.

104. Pecile A, Netti C, Sibilia V et al. Comparison between urinary pyridinium cross-links and hydroxylysine glycosides in monitoring the effects of ovariectomy and 17 beta-estradiol replacement in aged rats. *J Endocrinol* 1996; **150:** 383–90.

105. Torjman C, Lhumeau A, Pastoureau P et al. Evaluation and comparison of urinary pyridinium crosslinks in two rat models of bone loss – ovariectomy and adjuvant polyarthritis – using a new automated HPLC method. *Bone Miner* 1994; **26:** 155–67.

106. Claassen N, Potgieter HC, Seppa M et al. Supplemented gamma-linolenic acid and eicosapentaenoic acid influence bone status in young male rats: effects on free urinary collagen crosslinks, total urinary hydroxyproline, and bone calcium content. *Bone* 1995; **16:** 385S–92S.

107. Bonnarens F, Einhorn TA. Production of a standard closed fracture in laboratory animal bone. *J Orthop Res* 1984; **2:** 97–101.

108. Carter DR, Hayes WC. Bone compressive strength: The influence of density and strain rate. *Science* 1976; **194:** 1174–6.

109. Einhorn TA, Bonnarens F, Burstein AH. The contributions of dietary protein and mineral to the healing of experimental fractures. A biomechanical study. *J Bone Joint Surg [Am]* 1986; **68:** 1389–95.

110. Friedman RJ, Parent T, Draughn RA. Production of a standard closed fracture in the rat tibia. *J Orthop Trauma* 1994; **8:** 111–5.

Index